PRICE-POTTENGER

Price-Pottenger was originally founded in 1952 as the Santa Barbara Medical Research Foundation and became the Weston A. Price Memorial Foundation in 1965. The name was later changed to the Price-Pottenger Nutrition Foundation to include the important work of Dr. Francis M. Pottenger, Jr., MD. In 2016, we simplified our name to Price-Pottenger to reflect the wide appeal the foundation has achieved.

We are a nonprofit 501 (c)(3), tax-exempt, public education ~~~~ ~~~~ ablished to maintain the unique collection of ~~~~ ~~~~ Weston A. Price, DDS. We are dedicated to cc  ion and *Physical Degeneration*, along with his ~ to the public in perpetuity.

Membership fees and donations allow ~~~~ ssion of educating the public on health and nutrition based on scientific and anthropological evidence that can help them attain a high state of health for themselves and future generations. We accomplish this through articles, blogs, and audio/visual programs on our website, as well as through classes we offer and books we sell.

The foundation also maintains extensive archives and a library of over 10,000 books and publications, which include the works of not only Dr. Price, but also those of Dr. Francis M. Pottenger, Jr.; Dr. Royal Lee; Dr. Melvin Page; Dr. Emanuel Cheraskin; Dr. William Albrecht; and many other great nutrition pioneers.

It is our hope that the understanding and application of the principles taught by Dr. Price, and brought forth so eloquently in this book, will help humanity prevent and reverse the physical degeneration that has become so prevalent today.

—*The Board of Directors of Price-Pottenger*

Price-Pottenger
7890 Broadway • Lemon Grove, CA 91945
email: info@price-pottenger.org
website: www.price-pottenger.org

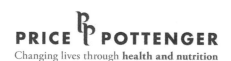

PRICE P POTTENGER
Changing lives through **health and nutrition**

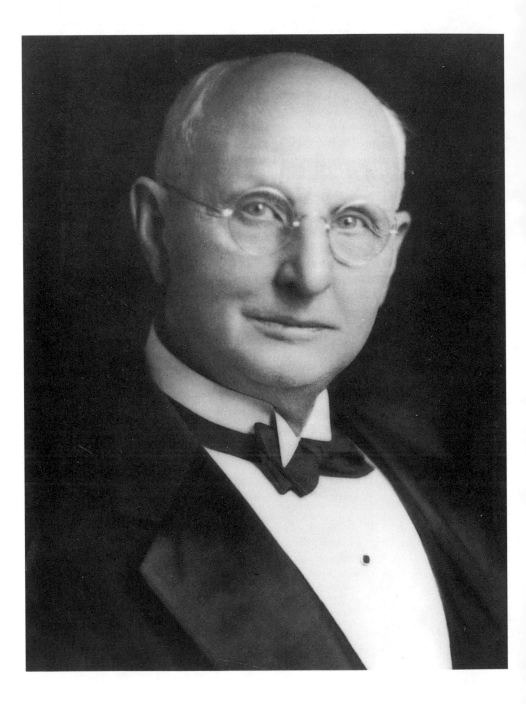

Nutrition and Physical Degeneration

8th Edition

Weston A. Price, D.D.S.

With forewords to previous editions by
Earnest A. Hooton, Professor of Anthropology,
Harvard University,

William A. Albrecht, Ph.D.

and Granville F. Knight, M.D.

PUBLISHED BY
PRICE-POTTENGER
7890 Broadway
Lemon Grove, CA 91945

Nutrition and Physical Degeneration is intended solely for information and education, and not as medical advice. Please consult a medical or health professional if you have questions about your health.

NUTRITION AND PHYSICAL DEGENERATION

Copyright © 1939, 1945 by Weston A Price; © 1970, 1989, 1997, 2003, 2004, 2006, 2008 by the Price-Pottenger Nutrition Foundation.

24th Printing, 2018

Library of Congress Cataloging-in-Publication Data

Price, Weston A. (Weston Andrew)
    Nutrition and physical degeneration / Weston A Price : with
foreworded from the original edition by Earnest Albert Hooton,
Granville Frank Knight, and Abram Hoffer-6th ed.
    p. c
    Includes bibliographical references and index.
    ISBN 13: 978-0-916764-20-3
    ISBN 10: 0-916764-20-6
    1. Nutritionally induced diseases.   2. Nutrition and dental health.
3. Nutritional anthropology.   4. Civilization.   I. Title.
RC622.P7395   1997
616.3'9–dc21   97-41920
                                               CIP

Printed in the United States of America

PRICE ℞ POTTENGER

Corporate Headquarters
7890 Broadway • Lemon Grove, CA 91945
email: info@price-pottenger.org
website: www.price-pottenger.org

TO THE MEMORY OF THAT
KINDRED SOUL

My Wife, Florence

who assisted me so greatly on these
difficult expeditions, this book is
lovingly dedicated.

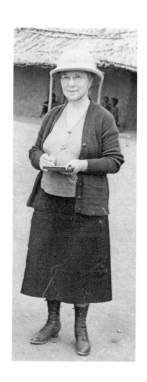

NOTE

Since this invaluable book was first published in 1939, mores and social attitudes have changed to such an extent that some readers may be offended by references to "savages" and other out-of-date nomenclatures, as well as by some of the research studies that are no longer timely. However, in the interest of authenticity and completeness, the publisher feels an obligation to reprint the book exactly as Dr. Price wrote it in 1939.

ACKNOWLEDGMENT

Marion Patricia Connolly
1926–2010

Marion Patricia "Pat" Connolly was a dedicated proponent of the health, nutritional, and environmental values espoused by the nutrition pioneers upon whose work Price-Pottenger is founded. She was both a student and teacher of health and nutrition for over 66 years.

Pat's belief in sound nutrition practices led her to become the foremost authority on the works of Dr. Weston A. Price and Dr. Francis Marion Pottenger, Jr., as well as an author (*The Candida Albicans Yeast-Free Cookbook*) and educator in her own right. She was also a co-author and major contributor to the book *Nourishing Traditions* by Sally Fallon and Mary G. Enig, PhD, when it was first published in 1995. Her desire to positively impact the population's nutritional well-being eventually led to her positions as Executive Director and Curator of the Price-Pottenger Nutrition Foundation.

Because of Pat's work, Price-Pottenger continues to maintain and make available the notes, research, and publications of those dedicated—as she was—to making optimal health an attainable goal.

CONTENTS

LIST OF ILLUSTRATIONS

ix

MAPS

PROLOGUE

Almost seven decades have passed since Weston A. Price began his monumental studies of isolated primitive peoples, studies that led to the publication of this volume, *Nutrition and Physical Degeneration*. In the intervening period, this work—with its fascinating text and unforgettable photographs—has inspired countless readers, some of whom used Price's findings as a springboard for further research, while others applied the principles he discovered to the everyday nourishment of healthy families.

Weston Price's search for isolated, so-called "primitive" groups, living entirely on indigenous foods, took him to remote Swiss villages, windswept islands off the coast of Scotland and idyllic South Sea islands. He visited Eskimos in Alaska, traditional American Indians, African tribes and Australian Aborigines. His studies occurred at a pivotal moment in the history of the world—one in which groups totally isolated from civilized ways could still be found, but which also supplied a key modern invention, the camera, that allowed him to record for future generations the superb physical condition of peoples yet to experience the industrial age.

Price's research proved conclusively that dental decay is caused primarily by nutritional deficiencies, and that those conditions that promote decay also promote disease. Price found fourteen tribal diets that, although radically different, provided almost complete immunity to tooth decay and resistance to illness. Contact with civilization, followed by adoption of what Price termed the "displacing foods of modern commerce" was disastrous for all groups studied. Rampant dental caries was followed by progressive facial deformities in children born to parents consuming refined and devitalized foods. These changes consisted of narrowed facial structure and dental arches, along with crowded teeth, birth defects and increased susceptibility to infectious and chronic disease. Significantly, when some natives returned to their traditional diets, open cavities ceased progressing and children now conceived and born, once again had perfect dental arches and no tooth decay.

The diets of the healthy primitives Price studied were diverse. Some were based on sea foods, some on domesticated animals, some on game and some on dairy products. Some contained almost no plant foods while others contained a variety of fruits, vegetables, grains and legumes. In some mostly cooked foods were eaten, while in others many foods—including animal foods—were eaten raw. However, these diets shared several underlying characteristics. None contained any refined or devitalized foods such as white sugar and flour, canned foods, pasteurized or skimmed milk, and refined and hydrogenated vegetable oils. All the diets contained some form of quality animal proteins and animal fats from animals eating the foods they would naturally find in nature.

Price analyzed the primitive diets and found that all contained at least four times the quantity of minerals and water-soluble vitamins of the American diet of his day. Even more startling was his discovery that these diets contained at least TEN times the amount of fat-soluble vitamins found in animal fats, including vitamin A, vitamin D and the "Price Factor" or "Activator X," discovered by Dr. Price.

Price considered these fat-soluble vitamins to be the key component of healthy diets. He called these nutrients "activators" or "catalysts," upon which the assimilation of all the other nutrients in our food—protein, minerals and water-soluble vitamins—depends. "It is possible to starve for minerals that are abundant in the foods eaten because they cannot be utilized without an adequate quantity of the fat-soluble activators," wrote Price. "The amounts [of nutrients] utilized depend directly on the presence of other substances, particularly the fat-soluble vitamins. It is at this point probably that the greatest breakdown in our modern diet takes place, namely in the ingestion and utilization of adequate amounts of the special activating substances including the vitamins needed for rendering the minerals in the food available to the human system."

The foods that supplied the vital fat-soluble activators included butterfat, marine oils, organ meats, fish and shellfish, eggs and animal tallows—most of which our modern pundits of diet and nutrition have unfairly condemned as unhealthful. Price Factor/Activator X, an extremely powerful catalyst to mineral absorption, occurred in foods considered sacred to the various primitive groups—liver and other organ meats, fish liver oils, fish eggs, and butter from cows eating rapidly growing grass from spring and fall pasturage. These valuable foodstuffs have almost completely disappeared from the American food supply; at the same time the toll of suffering and economic hardship engendered by our modern civilized diseases increases relentlessly.

Weston Price noted that all the groups he studied provided special foods to prospective parents—to both mother and father before conception and to women during their pregnancy—as well as to growing children. They practiced the spacing of children so that mothers could replenish nutrient stores for subsequent children. Above all, they took care to impart their nutritional wisdom to young, thereby ensuring the health of future generations. Such wisdom stands in sharp contrast to the practices of modern parents who approach childbearing with insouciance and who indulge their children in refined and highly sweetened foods from infancy.

The implication of the Price research is profound. If civilized man is to survive, he must somehow incorporate the fundamentals of primitive nutritional wisdom into his modern lifestyle. He must turn his back on the allure of civilized foodstuffs that line his supermarket shelves and return to the whole, nutrient-dense foods of his ancestors. He must restore the soil to health through nontoxic and biological farming methods. And he must repair that "greatest breakdown in our modern civilized diet" which is the gradual replacement of foods rich in fat-soluble activators with substitutes and imitations compounded of vegetable oils, fillers, stabilizers and additives.

The task of preserving Price's research so that it is available to modern men and women, and of assisting them in its practical application, belongs to Price-Pottenger. A charitable educational corporation, Price-Pottenger has the mandate to preserve the precious slides and notes of Weston Price, along with his research into other aspects of dentistry. In addition, Price-Pottenger archives the research of a number of other pioneers in the field of nutrition and serves the public by making this information available through their library of books, a quarterly journal, a catalog of carefully chosen titles, and online access to the archives, past journals, Dr. Price's Radio Interviews, and other helpful information.

Most importantly, Price-Pottenger supplies resources and materials that can assist those individuals who wish to begin the highly satisfying process of reversing the adulteration of our food supply and the perversion of our eating habits, both of which hasten the process of physical degeneration. Price-Pottenger is dedicated to the practical application of the principles enumerated by Weston Price and those who followed in his footsteps in the fields of soil improvement, humane animal husbandry, nontoxic farming and gardening, pollutant free housing, holistic medical therapies, nontoxic dentistry and, above all, proper food choices and preparation techniques that promote optimal health generation after generation.

Like Weston Price, who refused all requests to ally himself with any commercial products, Price-Pottenger is completely independent of any commercial interest or government agency, relying on the generous support of its members, as well as on grants and bequests, to preserve the information entrusted to its care, and to continue to make it available to those who can benefit therefrom. We urge you to join Price-Pottenger so that you can enjoy the services it offers and support its vital mission. Your membership and financial support can make all the difference between a future in which mankind enjoys optimal, vibrant health—or no future at all.

Price-Pottenger
7890 Broadway
Lemon Grove, CA 91945
www.price-pottenger.org
info@price-pottenger.org

PREFACE

THE gracious reception given to my several reports of field studies among primitive racial groups and the many requests for copies of those brief reports and for further data, together with the need for providing interpretations and applications of the data, have induced me to consolidate my investigations. There have also been many requests from my patients and from members of the medical and dental professions for concise statements as to what I have found that would be useful as preventive procedures. In addition I have been conscious of an opportunity for helpfulness to the members of the various primitive races that I have studied and who are so rapidly declining in health and numbers at their point of contact with our modern civilization. Since they have so much accumulated wisdom that is passing with them, it has seemed important that the elements in the modern contacts that are so destructive to them should be discovered and removed.

There has been a deep sense of obligation to the officials of many countries for the great kindness and assistance that they have so cheerfully given by providing the opportunity for these investigations. The list of these individuals is much too long to mention them all by name. One of the joys of my work has been the privilege of knowing the magnificent characters that are at the outposts earnestly striving to better the welfare of the natives whom they are ministering to, but who are distraught with the recognition that under the modernization program the natives decline in health and become afflicted by our modern types of degenerative diseases. It would be fortunate if each of these field workers could be provided with a copy of this report which they have helped to make possible.

In order to make this information available to as wide a group as possible, I have avoided technical language and will ask the indulgence of professional readers.

There are some individuals whose assistance I must acknowledge specifically: Reverend Father John Siegen and Doctor Alfred Gysi of Switzerland; Mrs. Lulu Herron and Doctor J. Romig of Alaska; the Indian Department at Ottawa; the Department of Indian Affairs at Washington, D. C.; the officials of the eight archipelagos studied in the Pacific; Colonel J. L. Saunders of New Zealand; the Minister of Health, New Zealand; Dr. W. Stewart Ziele of Sydney, Australia; Sir Herbert Gepp of Melbourne, Australia; Doctor William M. Hughes, Minister of Health, Canberra; Dr. Cummiston, Director-General of Health, Australian Commonwealth, Canberra; Doctor Rapael Cilento of

Queensland, Australia; Mr. E. W. Saranealis, Thursday Island; the Department of Health of Kenya, Africa; the Department of Health for Belgian Congo, Brussells; the Department of National Parks, Belgian Congo; Minister of the Interior, Peru; Doctor Albert Giesecke and Esther Giesecke of Peru; the Directors of Museums in Sydney and Canberra, Australia; Auckland, New Zealand; Vancouver and Toronto, Canada; Washington, New York and Chicago, the United States; Juneau, Alaska; Rome, Italy; and Cairo, Egypt; the publishers of the *Ohio State Medical Journal*, the *Journal of the American Dental Association*, the *Dental Digest* and the *Dental Items of Interest*; my faithful secretary, Mrs. Ruth MacMaster; Professor W. G. Garnett who so kindly provided the critical reading of the manuscript, and the publishers who furnished constructive suggestions and cooperation. To these and a host of others I am deeply indebted and profoundly grateful.

WESTON A. PRICE

8926 Euclid Avenue
Cleveland, Ohio, 1938.

FOREWORD

THERE is nothing new in the observation that savages, or peoples living under primitive conditions, have, in general, excellent teeth. This fact is a matter of record based upon casual examinations of contemporary primitives made by travellers, explorers, and scientists, and established with better documentation by the studies of teeth preserved in skeletal collections of savages recently or more remotely extinct. Nor is it news that most civilized populations possess wretched teeth which begin to decay almost before they have erupted completely, and that dental caries is likely to be accompanied by periodontal disease with further reaching complications. Indeed this has been a matter of grave concern to the dental profession for more than a generation, and rightly so. A great deal of elaborate and patient research and experimentation has been expended upon this problem of the etiology and control of dental caries, but I do not suppose that anyone would claim that it has been solved. At any rate, the dentists are still busily engaged in drilling our cavities and in plugging them. A quantity of excellent evidence has been amassed which indicates that dental caries is, to a great extent, connected with malnutrition and with deficient diets.

Since we have known for a long time that savages have excellent teeth and that civilized men have terrible teeth, it seems to me that we have been extraordinarily stupid in concentrating all of our attention upon the task of finding out why our teeth are so poor, without ever bothering to learn why savage teeth are good. Dr. Weston Price seems to be the only person who possesses the scientific horse sense to supplement his knowledge of the probable causes of dental disease with a study of the dietary regimens which are associated with dental health. In other words, Dr. Price has accomplished one of those epochal pieces of research which make every other investigator desirous of kicking himself because he never thought of doing the same thing. This is an exemplification of the fact that really gifted scientists are those who can appreciate the obvious.

So Dr. Price has found out why primitive men have good teeth and why their teeth go bad when they become "civilized." But he has not stopped there: he has gone on to apply his knowledge acquired from savages to the problems of their less intelligent civilized brothers. For I think that we must admit that if savages know enough to eat the things which keep their teeth healthy, they are more intelligent in dietary matters than we are. So I consider that Dr. Price has written what is often called "a profoundly significant book." The principal difference between Dr. Price's work and many others so labelled is that in the present instance the designation happens to be correct. I salute Dr. Price with the sincerest admiration (the kind that is tinged with envy) because he has found out something which I should like to have discovered for myself.

EARNEST A. HOOTON

Harvard University
November 21, 1938.

FOREWORD TO THE SECOND EDITION, 1945

WHEN we speak of "good health," we are using terms which thus far have not yielded to exact definition. Information has not yet been tabulated completely enough to tell us just exactly what good health is.

The absence of good health, on the other hand, is recognized by many bodily ills and conditions which we describe volubly and with precision. What is known as disease is made manifest by myriads of variations from the regular structures and functions of the organs.

It was an early belief by Dr. Price that defective and diseased teeth are a manifestation of ill health. Although dentists were studying such teeth for years, there was all the while an apparent increase in dental maladies. To Dr. Price it seemed clear that it would be far more fruitful to search out and study those peoples and places where toothache is unknown.

This was a positive approach to health and to the knowledge or definition of it. It was a decided contrast to the negative way of studying the body in the absence of health. It was this philosophy that carried the author of this work to many parts of the world to observe and study not only the teeth of many peoples, but also to learn what kinds of foods they ate, and whether these were eaten raw or processed. It was necessary to examine the habits of living and other behaviors of many people in order to establish the validity of the belief that defective teeth are evidence of malnutrition. This travel with its many observations was supplemented by chemical studies of foods, by tests of these foods with animals, and numerous other researches. It is the record of these efforts and the well ripened mental experiences by an able dentist, scientist, and humanitarian intent on the positive aspects of good health, that the reader will find in these printed pages.

Gathered through the eyes and mind of a careful thinker, and faithfully recorded by camera and pen, these studies have made it possible to superimpose the geographic picture and pattern of health upon the fertility pattern of the soils. They have made possible the correlation of the health of the native peoples with the types of soils. This soil pattern varies as the areas are less humid and the soils mineral-rich in their production of proteinaceous crops of high growth values for animals and peoples, or as the areas are more humid and the soils grow carbonaceous crops of mainly fuel and fattening values. Dr. Price has made excellent contributions to help us see the health pattern as it is a reflection of the soil fertility pattern that is determining or controlling our nutrition by way of the food plants the soil produces. By that means, the soil is determining the pattern of all life forms.

Not only the dentists, doctors, clinicians, diagnosticians, and others professionally responsible for the treatment of clients' maladies will find interest in this volume, but also all who are intelligently interested in health for its own sake. Those who are scientists in a broader way and hopeful for a better understanding of their own body nourishment and well-being will find this volume of help. It is particularly essential that those in public positions with humanitarian responsibilities get some glimpses of Dr. Price's philosophy as it points to good nutrition as prevention of abnormalities of body, mind, and spirit that have, according to him, been provoking the increase of juvenile delinquencies. Good nutrition from foods grown with an understanding of their greater body services to prevent delinquencies, puts health in a positive position and will relieve us of the increasing struggle for additional medical services and hospitalization.

Nutritious foods and thereby good physical condition and excellent health with its feeling of well-being that generates fellowship—rather than improper foods, physical degeneration, diseases and human strife—are Dr. Price's suggestions for us as individuals and as a nation.

WM. A. ALBRECHT, PHD

FOREWORD TO THE FOURTH EDITION, 1970

To fully understand the implications of Dr. Price's work, and the supporting evidence of others, one must think in terms of ecology and cellular metabolism—for our era of synthetic chemicals has complicated his observations. A simple definition of ecology is the relationship of man, beast, fish, fowl, vegetation and all other forms of life to each other, to the living soil, and to the total environment. Over many centuries the relatively simple life of primitive man and beast has gradually changed to a complex, artificial and chemicalized civilization posing new and difficult problems of adaptation. Food—fresh from fertile soil or the sea—has been replaced, for the most part, by refined, processed and preserved produce of far different nutritional qualities. (The industrial revolution started a migration to the cities, which, in turn, created a demand for foods that could be transported long distances and stored without spoilage.)

In the past two hundred years the natural fertility of our soil has rapidly declined. At first, when crop failures appeared, settlers simply abandoned their farms and moved west to virgin areas. Later, the application of manure, composed of animal or crop residues, and the rotation of crops were effective in maintaining fertility. More recently, the increasing availability of artificial fertilizers of high nitrogen content has enabled the grower to harvest one crop after another without allowing the land to lie fallow—a custom which encouraged the multiplication of soil organisms that, in turn, would release soil nutrients as needed by plants. Often against his better judgment, the modern farmer has been forced to use monoculture, artificial fertilization, pesticides, herbicides and mechanization in order to keep ahead of ruinous taxation, inflation and ever-increasing costs of production. The result has been production for "quantity" rather than "quality," and the gradual destruction of our precious top soil and mineral reserves, in or beneath the soil. This has been well documented by Dr. Wm. Albrecht of the University of Missouri. Our markets are flooded with attractive, but relatively tasteless, vegetables and fruits. The protein content of wheat and other grains has steadily declined; this being a reliable index of soil fertility. Animal foods such as fowl and meat reflect similar changes. Fowl are usually raised in cramped quarters and their food limited to that prescribed by man. As a result cirrhotic livers are common and egg quality is inferior. Both groups are frequently treated with antibiotics, anti-thyroid drugs and hormones which produce castration, myxedema and water-logged tissues. These practices are designed to stimulate more weight gain on less feed. The advantages to the producer are obvious; to the consumer, they are indeed questionable.

Moreover, in this day and age, human beings are increasingly exposed to thousands of chemicals in air, food and water. They are also dosing themselves—or being dosed—with a multitude of drugs. Chemical contacts include food additives, pesticides, herbicides, nitrates, and the effluents from modem industry. Many of these are coal tar products or their derivatives and other synthetic compounds completely foreign to the experience of man's biochemical makeup.

Long-lasting, chlorinated hydrocarbon pesticides, such as DDT, have even penetrated our food chain. In some areas at least, herbicides such as 2,4-D and 2,4,5-T—contaminated by the highly toxic and teratogenic 3,4,6,7-tetra-chloro-p-dibenzodioxin—have entered our food and water supplies. This is also true of other chlorinated diphenyls which are products of modern industry. These compounds may pose even more of a threat than DDT: even 2,4-D and 2,4,5-T have recently been shown to produce birth deformities in animals.

Residues of DDT and related chemicals are now found in most living creatures from the Arctic to the Antarctic, including phytoplankton which not only furnish the basic food for fish, but produce much of the oxygen essential for our survival. Through biological magnification the amounts tend to increase in vertebrates high in the food chain. Pelicans and the bald eagle are threatened with extinction, for DDT interferes with the production of hard egg shells. Abnormal softness seems to follow pathologically rapid destruction of sex hormones by liver enzymes whose actions are speeded up by DDT. (As a result, nesting mothers crush their eggs before they hatch.) Many other birds may share the same fate. Similar mechanisms could be operative in mammals, with different but conceivably bizarre and possibly irreversible changes related to propagation. Perhaps our current alarm about the "population explosion" is premature.

Nutritional surveys in the United States and Canada have indicated that malnutrition is just as prevalent on this continent as in the "backward countries." Since individuals in all walks of life are affected, the problem would seem to be primarily one of neglect in the production of truly nourishing foods, together with ignorance regarding the selection, preparation and use of those available in the market place. In addition, since most of us, through poor inheritance, are nutritional cripples, our need for nutrients is often greater than normal. Therefore some individuals need larger amounts of vitamins, metals, trace elements, fatty acids and amino acids than can be obtained from even the best foods and will never be well until these are supplied as supplements.

At last we are faced with the inevitable consequences of our profligate use and abuse of natural resources. The laws of God and nature are immutable: They cannot long be broken without retribution. As the author has aptly stated: "Life in all its fullness is Mother Nature obeyed."

The observations of Dr. Price graphically portray what happened to primitives in all parts of the world, once they abandoned the tribal wisdom which had kept them physically sound for many generations. In our increasingly urbanized society, we have almost completely lost track of the fundamentals of good nutrition. Unless we mend our ways we may be headed for oblivion.

Hopefully, this Heritage edition of Dr. Price's work will again stimulate private practitioners in medicine and dentistry to apply his findings at the clinical level. They will find the public more receptive than in the past. We cannot turn back the clock: we cannot return completely to the ways of our forefathers, wherein they always had access to fresh food from fertile soil. However, we can—and we must—do everything possible to use this basic knowledge in a modified form. Perhaps we can compensate to some extent for the mischief that has been done. In this respect, the following suggestions, based on thirty-five years of clinical experience, are submitted for consideration:

(1) Reduce the volume of industrial effluents, including fluorides, now contaminating our air, water and food as rapidly as possible, through federal, state and local controls.

(2) Ban the use of untested food additives immediately. Reduce the number of those tested, considered harmless, and approved for use to an absolute minimum.

(3) Rapidly phase out the use of long-acting pesticides and herbicides, unless proven harmless, except for emergency situations such as malaria control. Ban the sale of these pesticides for household use. Seek control of insect pests and weeds through other means, including soil improvement. Well nourished plants are most resistant to insects and fungi than deficient ones.

(4) Warn the public that all petrochemicals, whether in food, water, air, pesticides, cosmetics, detergents, drugs and other environmental contacts, are potentially dangerous to many, and probably to all, individuals. Tell them that the least contact is the best.

(5) Give the public access to fundamental knowledge of good nutrition. If we are to survive, this must be taught in every school grade from kindergarten through college. Primitive wisdom tells us that the production of healthy, normal babies depends upon optimum parental nutrition *before conception*, as

well as during pregnancy. Breast feeding is most important and should be followed by a diet high in raw and unprocessed foods. Most birth deformities are unnecessary. Good bones, good muscles, attractive skin, normal endocrines, a healthy liver, good reproductive capacity, good intelligence and good looks depend upon good food. Our people must know food values—and nourishing food is not necessarily expensive. (Even now, many Russian peasants subsist primarily on vegetable soup, hard rye bread and occasional bits of meat. Their teeth and health are reported to be superior.)

(6) Compost city wastes for use as fertilizers: return organic materials, minerals and trace elements to help rebuild our plundered soil; and reduce the use of synthetic fertilizers high in nitrogen content which are contaminating our water and food supplies. Demonstrate to farmers that this approach is economically feasible.

(7) Raise foods for quality rather than quantity. High-protein, high-vitamin and high-mineral foods have much higher survival value than those with more calories but less of the essential nutrients. Calories alone are not enough.

(8) In line with the concept of "biochemical individuality," as expressed by Dr. Roger Williams, which postulates the inheritance of acquired partial enzyme blocks, many patients need vitamin and mineral supplements for optimal health, and even for normal metabolism. These must be prescribed, along with a basic diet, as deemed necessary by the experience and knowledge of the individual practitioner.

(9) Aside from a study of nutritional values of food—which most people will not undertake—there are a few simple steps available to everyone. If these were to be publicized and universally followed, the immediate and long-term benefits could be incalculable; and the results would certainly be obvious in six months. They are as follows:

(a) Reduce the consumption of sugar in all forms to an absolute minimum.
(b) Avoid white or ordinary whole wheat bread. Eat only whole grain breads made from freshly ground flour, free of chemical preservatives. (The production of such bread would require a mill and adequate bakeries in every community.) Use brown in place of white, polished rice. These simple changes in food production and habits would result in a much higher intake of protein, Vitamin B complex, minerals and Vitamin E. The latter has only recently been recognized as essential for man. (It is appalling to think of the millions of tons of these vital nutrients that have been extracted from our foods and fed to animals over the past century.)

(c) When available, use only fresh fruits, vegetables, dark green leaves of lettuce and other greens such as watercress that have been raised in fertile soil without the use of insecticides. Ordinary fruits should be peeled because of possible pesticide residues and vegetables thoroughly washed for the same reason. Home gardens are to be encouraged. Frozen or canned vegetables and fruits are nourishing but less desirable. Steam or lightly cook all vegetables which are not eaten raw and save any cooking water for tomato juice cocktails or soup.

(d) Sprouted beans, alfalfa and other seeds contain desirable nutrients and are free of contamination. They can be sprouted in every kitchen. The consumption of sixty percent, or more, of food in the uncooked state seems logical.

(e) Avoid stale fats and foods cooked in reused fats, such as ordinary potato chips, french fried potatoes, etc. Recent, preliminary evidence adduced by Robert S. Ford suggests that partially rancid fats, rather than animal fat per se, may be one of the real villains responsible for atherosclerosis. Sources of stale fats include products such as bread, crackers, pastries and commercial cereals made from stored processed flour.

Elimination of the "empty calories" in (a) and (b) alone would result in increased resistance to infection, a marked reduction in the bizarre and disabling symptoms of reactive hypoglycemia, fewer attacks of so-called "viruses," a renewed supply of energy, more zest for life and a gradual reduction in the incidence of degenerative diseases, which seem to be the hallmark of our civilization. In the absence of serious pathology, the results are predictable—even though not based upon "one thousand controlled cases." A healthy body should have increased resistance to chemicals—as well as to invasion by viruses and bacteria.

The Price-Pottenger Nutrition Foundation is indebted to Dr. Price's widow, Monica Price, R.N., whose dedication and help were invaluable to Dr. Price, and to the Pottenger family for entrusting to this organization the scientific works of these pioneers in nutrition, not only for their preservation but for the dissemination of their findings to the public. The Foundation is also grateful for the devoted work of our Curator, Alfreda F. Rooke, M.P.H., who shared Dr. Price's dream; for the unselfish services of our Board of Directors; and for the substantial and loyal help of hundreds of individuals, many of whom have personally experienced the benefits which accompany the application of sound nutritional principles.

We hope to be worthy of this trust and seek the support of others who may now, or in the future, realize the vital importance of this fundamental approach to the survival of our civilization.

GRANVILLE F. KNIGHT, MD

(*Editor's Note:* Founding president (for 17 years) of The Weston A. Price Memorial Foundation, now Price-Pottenger.)

REMINISCENCES FROM
DR. WESTON A. PRICE'S GRAND-NEPHEW

By Donald Delmage Fawcett, Grand-Nephew

MOST folks become acquainted with Dr. Price through his professional writings, books and research papers. I knew him through a close family relationship, as a grand-nephew living in the home of Weston's sister, Minetta Emily Price. My grandmother, Minetta, was the eldest of the twelve children. Weston Andrew Valleau Price was the ninth child of Andrew Valleau Price, a Canadian farmer and Methodist lay preacher, and Adelaide DeMille, a far-sighted mother who sincerely desired the best possible education for her brood.

Of Welsh origin, Weston Andrew Valleau Price was born in 1870 and raised on the family's 200-acre tract in Southern Ontario, affectionately known as Eagle Rock Farm. There were two dentists, one medical doctor, an inventor, a Methodist minister, and a farmer in their family. I was named for Dr. Price's only child, who had died a year before my birth. The child's death had resulted from an infected root canal; this led Dr. Price into the research delineated in 1,174 pages of *Dental Infections Oral and Systemic* and *Dental Infections and the Degenerative Diseases*.

In a pioneering adventure against great odds, the homestead had been carved out of a virgin forest wilderness by Weston's great-grandfather, John Price, and his young Quaker wife, Esther Lyons. Weston's grandfather, Thomas Price, a carpenter, had built a sawmill where a creek tumbled over an outcropping of rocks into a natural pond. With an ample supply of good hardwood lumber on the place, Thomas built the fine home in which Andrew and Adelaide, a generation later, reared their children.

Year around, there were farm chores for everyone, and much to be done in Ontario's short summer. But, apparently there was a little time for diversions, too. I have heard Uncle Weston tell how he sometimes saved meat scraps from his evening meal and once outside would toss them in the air for his dog to gulp down. Occasionally, giving in to a mischievous whim, Weston would vary the fare with a piece of pickle saturated with vinegar. To say the least, the dog was definitely not pleased with the switch but learned a bit of Weston's philosophy that to get the good stuff he had to endure the sour taste along with it.

One lesson Weston really took to heart was the resourceful and determined way his forbearers had overcome the hardships they faced. In a boyhood essay written for his teacher he told of being taken advantage of by an older boy and, because he would not be "beat," had outwitted his challenger. Weston attended a typical little red brick schoolhouse presided over by a strict maiden lady who welcomed the children on their first day with a kiss and showed no mercy or favoritism from then on.

In addition, Adelaide's family received much instruction at home since her education had been in preparation for a teaching career.

Thirty years before Weston's birth, some forward-looking citizens of the village of Newburgh, Ontario, a few miles south of Eagle Rock Farm, had established the Newburgh Academy on the high school level. At that time only five other communities in the province had such a facility. Under a capable and qualified teaching staff the Academy developed an enviable reputation and all of the Price family who attended were well prepared for advancement to college level institutions.

Weston and his brother, Frank, had both decided to go into dentistry, and, one day, they were sitting on a curb in front of the University of Toronto, discussing the pros and cons of which college to choose. The outcome was that Frank decided to enroll in Toronto and Weston was dead set on going to the University of Michigan at Ann Arbor.

Upon completion of his DDS and MS degrees, Weston elected to open an office in Grand Forks, North Dakota, an adventurous plan in any event. Disaster struck within a very short time when he developed typhoid fever and nearly died. His eldest brother, Albert, an inventor and businessman living in Cleveland, Ohio, immediately went out West to shepherd him home to Eagle Rock as soon as Weston's emaciated condition would permit. Once home, he slowly began to rebuild his health.

Minetta's husband, William Delmage, a man of great intuitive wisdom, took Weston to Lake Massanoga (now called Mazinaw), forty miles or so north of Eagle Rock where they camped and fished. The fresh air, sunshine, good water, the salmon, trout, huckleberries, wild raspberries and probably small game, did Weston a world of good. William was a very religious, Christian man and we can be sure that he and Weston prayed for the return of robust health. In any case, the great natural beauty of Massanoga Lake and the sheer granite rock face rising majestically from the water's edge opposite a crescent beach impressed Weston as a place God had chosen to teach man a lesson in humility.

Resolving to someday return and build a Shangri-la retreat with a rustic hotel and cabins so that other people might share such an experience, he did, in fact, later accomplish his mission. Today the site is within the pristine Bon Echo Provincial Park north of Cloyne, Ontario, and enjoyed by thousands of visitors annually. He acknowledged on many occasions his love for this place and felt strongly that it inspired the mind and rejuvenated the body.

When Weston married Florence Anthony of Brampton, Ontario, their honeymoon was, of all the possible places, at Bon Echo! Now, a young bride might be a wee bit apprehensive about jumping off a train at the backwoods whistle-stop crossroads of Kaladar, bouncing around on a rough twenty mile wagon ride to the south end of the lake, followed by a six mile launch trip to a rugged forest campsite. But Aunt Flo was game and was well prepared by experiences such as this to later accompany Weston on his world travels in search of people with good teeth and sturdy bodies.

A converted three-story home in Cleveland, Ohio, served as Weston's office during most of his active practice. It had high ceilings, a wide central staircase and in addition to his private office and the reception room, there were four rooms with dental chairs. Upstairs was a large laboratory and the x-ray machine. As his practice grew he employed other dentists to work with him, but always did the preliminary examinations and prescribed the treatment for each patient. Three of Minetta's daughters, including my mother, worked in his office as dental assistants.

In fact, Weston's life is closely interwoven with his family. He and Albert had persuaded Minetta to come and live in Cleveland after William passed away. Often, Weston and Flo would "drop in" at Minetta's on a Sunday afternoon to take everyone for a ride through the countryside or a hike through one of the vast parks in Cleveland's Metropolitan system. Afterwards, all would return to Minetta's for a light supper and "kin club" talk fest. This is when we learned about Uncle Weston's latest research and discoveries. Aunt Flo would tell about their unusual experiences and the interesting people they had encountered. When they were away on travels we had fascinating letters from faraway places. I frequently assisted Uncle Weston at his local lectures by setting up and operating his slide projector to show some of the thousands of photographs which gave so much clarity and meaning to his spoken words.

As *Nutrition and Physical Degeneration* was being written we had frequent progress reports. Weston wanted the book to be understandable by lay people as well as professionals. He felt the information could and should be applied by anyone in their own individual situation, not necessarily by adopting one of the very different diets of the primitives but by having the enlightened knowledge of how and why to make a wise selection of available food sources. Rejecting all proffered aid and commercial pressure, his independent and unbiased research was entirely financed by the income from his own practice. He steadfastly held to a conviction that it was the only way to follow the trail to the true facts with integrity.

Weston Price may well have been the messenger of the future in his time. By studying groups of people whose teeth and bodies came close to perfection, he showed how we could learn from their extraordinary wisdom. He was appalled at the deterioration which occurred when people of the same genetic background adopted modern ways. In seeking the answers to those very vital questions he advanced the science of human nutrition in a way that is only beginning to be appreciated today. The renewed interest in his book may well serve to improve the quality of life for at least another fifty years.

He would like that and feel that it was worth a lifetime of effort.

COMMENTS FROM PROMINENT HEALTH PRACTITIONERS

DAVID J. GETOFF, CTN, CCN, FAAIM

Nutrition and Physical Degeneration, remains, I believe, the single most important treatise on human nutrition and dietary health ever written. While thousands of new health and nutrition books are written each year, this work stands alone. It is the only book that clearly shows the basics of what a healthy diet truly encompasses. Dr. Price details numerous food variations that have existed around the world while still supporting exemplary health, as well as some of the changes that have been shown to initiate poor health and chronic disease. Unlike the news reports on radio and TV and unlike the "current" dietary information that appears to change every year or two, this information remains both correct and unchanged since its original publication by Dr. Weston Price in 1939. Important and correct, yet this information, known around the world by interested researchers and health professionals, is mostly unknown by the general public and medical professionals. This lack of knowledge continues to plague society as the public's health remains on its current slide in the wrong direction. Many conditions that were rare 100 years ago are now common, while new and terrible conditions such as SARS, MRSA, West Nile and others continue to emerge every few years.

Although I attend numerous scientific nutritional medicine conferences every year, I cannot remember a single one where some researcher did not make reference to either this book, Dr. Price's research, or some of his thousands of photographs. These references were always made in order to depict good health practices and to show how we have forgotten the important findings of these master nutritional pioneers. Often, Dr. Francis M. Pottenger, Jr.'s phenomenal cat study is referenced or discussed as well, due to the many parallels to Dr. Price's observations.

The research of Weston Price represents what is very possibly the origin of many of today's newer dietary ideas and variations such as those proposed by the Paleo diet, the Atkins diet and others. Our population continues to suffer from more frequently occurring chronic diseases which get treated with increasing amounts of pharmaceutical drugs. If only this book and Dr. Price's simple and clear research findings were taught in our schools, it would probably only take 10 years for our national health care crisis to be reduced by more than 50%. No drug or medical discovery will ever accomplish the task that heeding Weston Price's research and changing the way we eat, can accomplish. In my private practice, I see examples of these benefits every day.

I am continually asked, as my patients' health improves and their lives turn back to how they felt before their problems occurred, why so few people understand this information. The only answer I can give is that money and politics, not facts and unbiased research (such as Dr. Price's) determine what the public and the medical profession are taught. Prevention and cure of disease is not nearly as profitable as the treatment (without cure) of disease.

Wouldn't it be nice if the public's health could come before power and profit? Researchers continue to contact Price-Pottenger to study the original works of many of the nutritional pioneers that are archived at Price-Pottenger's library. I deeply thank Dr. Price for this book, as it has been instrumental in giving me the foundation required to help me teach my patients, my students and the physicians to whom I lecture. I hope that his work will someday be recognized in the public eye and by mainstream medicine as it so aptly deserves. I also thank Price-Pottenger for continuing to publish this book and for keeping this information available to heath seekers and researchers around the world.

David J. Getoff, CTN, CCN, FAAIM
                    March 30, 2006

Traditional Naturopath
Board Certified Clinical Nutritionist
Fellow of the American Association of Integrative Medicine
Producer of the video course, *Attaining Optimal Health in the 21st Century*
Co-author of *Reduce Blood Pressure Naturally*
Lecturer and educator.

COMMENTS FROM PROMINENT HEALTH PRACTITIONERS
PATRICK QUILLIN, PhD, RD, CNS

Nutrition and Physical Degeneration is, arguably, the most important nutrition book of the 20th century. Dr. Price traveled the world with his wife, Florence, a la "Indiana Jones" style in the 1930s on prop planes, steamships, canoes, automobiles, and on foot, visiting 14 countries on 5 continents. He was troubled with the dramatic increase in dental problems among his patients. His travels proved his theory: if you eat your native ethnic diet in an unprocessed form you will have good mental, physical, and dental health. If you eat highly processed foods, which adds questionable agents and removes essential nutrients, your health deteriorates. All of the 21st century nutrition controversies can be put to rest in Dr. Price's invaluable book that should be required reading for all health care professionals who profess competency in clinical nutrition, and for anyone who wants to improve their health.

Patrick Quillin, PhD, RD, CNS, former Vice President of Nutrition for Cancer Treatment Centers of America. Author of 14 books, including *Beating Cancer with Nutrition*.

INTRODUCTION

THIS text provides a new approach to some problems of modern degeneration. Instead of the customary procedure of analyzing the expressions of degeneration, a search has been made for groups to be used as controls who are largely free from these affections.

After spending several years approaching this problem by both clinical and laboratory research methods, I interpreted the accumulating evidence as strongly indicating the absence of some essential factors from our modern program, rather than the presence of injurious factors. This immediately indicated the need for obtaining controls. To accomplish this it became necessary to locate immune groups which were found readily as isolated remnants of primitive racial stocks in different parts of the world. A critical examination of these groups revealed a high immunity to many of our serious affections so long as they were sufficiently isolated from our modern civilization and living in accordance with the nutritional programs which were directed by the accumulated wisdom of the group. In every instance where individuals of the same racial stocks who had lost this isolation and who had adopted the foods and food habits of our modern civilization were examined, there was an early loss of the high immunity characteristics of the isolated group. These studies have included a chemical analysis of foods of the isolated groups and also of the displacing foods of our modern civilization.

These investigations have been made among the following primitive racial stocks including both isolated and modernized groups: the Swiss of Switzerland, the Gaelics in the Outer and Inner Hebrides, the Eskimos of Alaska, the Indians in the far North, West and Central Canada, Western United States and Florida, the Melanesians and Polynesians on eight archipelagos of the Southern Pacific, tribes in eastern and central Africa, the Aborigines of Australia, Malay tribes on islands north of Australia, the Maori of New Zealand and the ancient civilizations and their descendants in Peru both along the coast and in the Sierras, also in the Amazon Basin. Where available the modernized whites in these communities also were studied. There have been many important unexpected developments in these investigations. While a primary quest was to find the cause of tooth decay which was established quite readily as being controlled directly by nutrition, it rapidly became apparent that a chain of disturbances developed in these various primitive racial stocks starting even in the first generation after the adoption of the

1

modernized diet and rapidly increased in severity with expressions quite constantly like the characteristic degenerative processes of our modern civilization of America and Europe. While tooth decay has proved to be almost entirely a matter of the nutrition of the individual at the time and prior to the activity of that disease, a group of affections have expressed themselves in physical form. These have included facial and dental arch changes which, heretofore, have been accounted for as results of admixtures of different racial stocks. My investigations have revealed that these same divergencies from normal are reproduced in all these various racial stocks while the blood is still pure. Indeed, these even develop in those children of the family that are born after the parents adopted the modern nutrition.

Applying these methods of study to our American families, we find readily that a considerable percentage of our families show this same deterioration in the younger members. The percentage of individuals so affected in our American communities in which I have made studies varies through a wide range, usually between 25 percent and 75 percent. A certain percentage of this affected group has not only these evidences of physical injury, but also personality disturbances, the most common of which is a lower than normal mental efficiency and acuteness, chiefly observed as so-called mental backwardness which includes the group of children in the schools who are unable to keep up with their classmates. Their I.Q.'s are generally lower than normal and they readily develop inferiority complexes growing out of their handicap. From this group or parallel with it a certain percentage develop personality disturbances which have their expression largely in unsocial traits. They include the delinquents who at this time are causing so much trouble and concern because of evidence of increase in their numbers. This latter group has been accounted for largely on the basis of some conditioning experience that developed after the child had reached an impressionable age. My investigations are revealing a physical structural change and therefore, an organic factor which precedes and underlies these conditioning influences of the environment. The fact that a government survey has shown that 66 percent of the delinquents who have been treated in the best institutions and released as cured, later have developed their unsocial or criminal tendencies, strongly emphasizes the urgent necessity that if preventive methods are to be applied these must precede and forestall the primary injuries themselves.

While it has been known that certain injuries were directly related to an inadequate nutrition of the mother during the formative period of the child, my investigations are revealing evidence that the problem goes back still further to defects in the germ plasms as contributed by the two parents. These injuries, therefore, are related directly to the physical condition of one or of both of these individuals prior to the time that conception took place.

A very important phase of my investigations has been the obtaining of information from these various primitive racial groups indicating that they were conscious that such injuries would occur if the parents were not in excellent physical condition and nourishment. Indeed, in many groups I found that the girls were not allowed to be married until after they had had a period of special feeding. In some tribes a six months period of special nutrition was required before marriage. An examination of their foods has disclosed special nutritional factors which are utilized for this purpose.

The scope of this work, accordingly, becomes of direct interest in many fields including the various branches of the healing arts, particularly medicine and dentistry, and the social organizations that are concerned with betterment of the racial stock. Similarly, the educational groups are concerned directly since, if we are to stem the tide by passing new information on to the parents of the new generation, it must be done prior to the time the emergency shall arise. This involves a system of education directed particularly to the high school age pupils.

The data that are being presented in the following chapters suggest the need for reorientation in many problems of our modern social organization. The forces involved in heredity have in general been deemed to be so powerful as to be able to resist all impacts and changes in the environment. These data will indicate that much that we have interpreted as being due to heredity is really the result of intercepted heredity. While great emphasis has been placed on the influence of the environment on the character of the individual, the body pattern has generally been supposed to require a great number of impacts of a similar nature to alter the design. The brain has been assumed to be similarly well organized in most individuals except that incidents in the life of the individual such as disappointments, fright, etc., are largely responsible for disturbed behavior. Normal brain functioning has not been thought of as being as biologic as digestion. The data provided in the succeeding chapters indicate that associated with disturbances in the development of the bones of the head, disturbances may at the same time occur in the development of the brain. Such structural defects usually are not hereditary factors even though they appear in other members of the family or parents. They are products of the environment rather than hereditary units transmitted from the ancestry.

In the light of these data important new emphasis is placed on the quality of the germ cells of the two parents as well as on the environment provided by the mother. The new evidence indicates that the paternal contribution may be an injured product and that the responsibility for defective germ cells may have to be about equally divided between the father and mother. The blending of races has been blamed for much of the distortion and defects in body form in our modern generation. It will be seen that these face changes occur in all the pure blood races studied in even the first generation, after the nutrition of the parents has been changed.

The origin of personality and character appear in the light of the newer data to be biologic products and to a much less degree than usually considered pure hereditary traits. Since these various factors are biologic, being directly related to both the nutrition of the parents and to the nutritional environment of the individuals in the formative and growth period, any common contributing factor such as food deficiencies due to soil depletion will be seen to produce degeneration of the masses of people due to a common cause. Mass behavior therefore, in this new light becomes the result of natural forces, the expression of which may not be modified by propaganda but will require correction at the source. Nature has been at this process of building human cultures through many millenniums and our culture has not only its own experience to draw from but that of parallel races living today as well as those who lived in the past. This work, accordingly, includes data that have been obtained from several of Nature's other biologic experiments to throw light on the problems of our modern white civilization.

In presenting the evidence I am utilizing photographs very liberally. A good illustration is said to be equivalent to a thousand words of text. This is in keeping too with the recent trend in journalism. The pictures are much more convincing than words can be, and since the text challenges many of the current theories, the most conclusive evidence available is essential.

Owing to the many requests received for slides or the loan of my negatives, provision is being made for supplying a limited number of slides of the illustrations in either black and white or in color. Slides of other subjects are available.

Chapter 1

WHY SEEK WISDOM FROM PRIMITIVE PEOPLES

SOME of the primitive races have avoided certain of the life problems faced by modernized groups and the methods and knowledge used by the primitive peoples are available to assist modernized individuals in solving their problems. Many primitive races have made habitual use of certain preventive measures in meeting crucial life problems.

Search for controls among remnants of primitive racial stocks has been resorted to as a result of failure to find them in our modernized groups or to find the controlling factors by applying laboratory methods to the affected clinical material. Only the primitive groups have been able to provide adequate normal controls.

In the following chapters, I have presented descriptions of certain peoples and their environments in primitive state, and, for comparative study, descriptions of members of the primitive tribes who have been in contact with modernized white races. I have recorded the effects of that contact as expressed in physical and character changes, and have given a survey of the factors in the environment which have changed. It has been necessary to study in this way a wide variety of primitive groups and physical environments. It will, accordingly, be advisable for the reader to keep in mind the comparative effects of different altitudes, latitudes, temperatures and races, and to note the similarity of the reactions of these primitive groups when contact is made with our modern civilization. The purpose is to glean data that will be applicable for use in correcting certain tragic expressions of our modern degeneration, including tooth decay, general physical degeneration, and facial and dental-arch deformities, and character changes. These data will be useful in preventing race decay and deformities, in establishing a higher resistance to infective diseases, and in reducing the number of prenatal deficiency injuries. These latter include such expressions as mental deficiencies caused by brain defects in the formative period, which result in mental disturbances ranging from moderate backwardness to character abnormalities.

The data presented show the level of susceptibility to dental caries (tooth decay) in each isolated primitive group and, contrasted with that, the level of susceptibility in the modernized natives of the same stock. A résumé of the changes in the environment that are associated with the changes in immunity and susceptibility will be presented. These data reveal an average increase in susceptibility of thirty-five fold. Similar contrasts are shown in relation to the relative incidence of facial and dental arch deformities among primitive natives and modernized natives.

It will be easy for the reader to be prejudiced since many of the applications suggested are not orthodox. I suggest that conclusions be deferred until the new approach has been used to survey the physical and mental status of the reader's own family, of his brothers and sisters, of associated families, and finally, of the mass of people met in business and on the street. Almost everyone who studies the matter will be surprised that such clear-cut evidence of a decline in modern reproductive efficiency could be all about us and not have been previously noted and reviewed.

It is important to preface the observations by constructing a mental pattern of physical excellence from the pictures of the various primitive groups and, with this yardstick or standard of normalcy, observe our modern patterns. Certain preconceived ideas may have to be modified, as for example, that based on the belief that what we see is due to heredity or that deformity is due to mixing of races. If so, why should the last child in a large family generally suffer most, and often be different in facial form; or why should there be these changes in the later children, even in pure racial stocks, after the parents have adopted our modern types of nutrition?

Although the causes of physical degeneration that can be seen easily have been hard to trace, the defects in the development of the brain, which affect the mind and character, are much more obscure, and the causes of mental degeneration are exceedingly difficult to trace. Much that formerly has been left to the psychiatrist to explain is now rapidly shifting to the realm of the anatomist and physiologist.

Those contributions of the past cultures which have blended agreeably into our modern experience have been accepted with too little questioning. Much ancient wisdom, however, has been rejected because of prejudice against the wisdom of so-called savages. Some readers may experience this reaction to the primitive wisdom recorded in these chapters.

The writer is fully aware that his message is not orthodox; but since our orthodox theories have not saved us we may have to readjust them to bring them into harmony with Nature's laws. Nature must be obeyed, not orthodoxy. Apparently many primitive races have understood her language better than have our modernized groups. Even the primitive races share our blights when they adopt our conception of nutrition. The supporting evidence for this statement is voluminous and as much of it as space permits is included in this volume. The illustrative material used is taken from the many thousands of my negatives which are available. Photographs alone can tell much of the story, and one illustration is said to be worth as much as one thousand words.

Since the problem of applying the wisdom of the primitives to our modern needs concerns not only health workers and nutritionists, but also educators and social workers, the data are presented without technical details.

While many of the primitive races studied have continued to thrive on the same soil through thousands of years, our American human stock has declined rapidly within a few centuries, and in some localities within a few decades. In the regions in which degeneration has taken place the animal stock has also declined. A decadent individual cannot regenerate himself, although he can reduce the progressive decadence in the next generation, or can vastly improve that generation, by using the demonstrated wisdom of the primitive races. No era in the long journey of mankind reveals in the skeletal remains such a terrible degeneration of teeth and bones as this brief modern period records. Must Nature reject our vaunted culture and call back the more obedient primitives? The alternative seems to be a complete readjustment in accordance with the controlling forces of Nature.

Thinking is as biologic as is digestion, and brain embryonic defects are as biologic as are club feet. Since both are readily produced by lowered parental reproductive capacity, and since Nature in her large-scale human demonstration reveals that this is chiefly the result of inadequate nutrition of the parents and too frequent or too prolonged child bearing, the way back is indicated. Like the successful primitive racial stocks, we, too, can make, as a first requisite, provision for adequate nutrition both for generation and growth, and can make provision for the regulation of the overloads. We, like the successful primitives, can establish programs of instruction for growing youth and acquaint it with Nature's requirements long before the emergencies and stresses arise. This may require a large-scale program of home and classroom instruction, particularly for the high school girls and boys. This would be in accordance with the practice of many of the primitive races reported upon in the following chapters.

If the individuals in our modern society who are sufficiently defective to require some supervision are in part or largely the product of an injured parentage, who should be held responsible? Is it just for society to consign these unsocial individuals which it has made to a life of hard labor or confinement in depressing environments? Is it just for society to permit production of physical and mental cripples?

Many primitive races apparently have prevented the distortions which find expressions in unsocial acts. If so, cannot modern society do this by studying and adopting the programs developed through centuries of experience by the primitives? Nature uses a written language which, without the keys, is made up of meaningless hieroglyphics, but which, with the proper keys, becomes a clear story of racial and individual history. The hieroglyphics indicate racial and individual disaster for modernized groups who heed not the warning story. The primitive races have some of these keys and have used them successfully in avoiding many of the disasters of our modern society. The following chapters record many of the excellent practices of the primitives and they are presented here with the hope that they will be helpful in a program designed to relieve mankind of some of the misfortunes common in the present social order and to prevent disorders for future generations of civilized peoples.

Chapter 2

THE PROGRESSIVE DECLINE OF MODERN CIVILIZATION

THAT modern man is declining in physical fitness has been emphasized by many eminent sociologists and other scientists. That the rate of degeneration is progressively accelerating constitutes a cause for great alarm, particularly since this is taking place in spite of the advance that is being made in modern science along many lines of investigation.

Dr. Alexis Carrel in his treatise "Man, the Unknown" states:

> Medicine is far from having decreased human sufferings as much as it endeavors to make us believe. Indeed, the number of deaths from infectious diseases has greatly diminished. But we still must die in a much larger proportion from degenerative diseases.

After reviewing the reduction in the epidemic infectious diseases he continues as follows:

> All diseases of bacterial origin have decreased in a striking manner. . . . Nevertheless, in spite of the triumphs of medical science, the problem of disease is far from solved. Modern man is delicate. Eleven hundred thousand persons have to attend the medical needs of 120,000,000 other persons. Every year, among this population of the United States, there are about 100,000,000 illnesses, serious or slight. In the hospitals, 700,000 beds are occupied every day of the year. . . . Medical care, under all its forms, costs about $3,500,000,000 yearly. . . . The organism seems to have become more susceptible to degenerative diseases.

The present health condition in the United States is reported from time to time by several agencies representing special phases of the health program. The general health problem has been thoroughly surveyed and interpreted by the Surgeon General of the United States Public Health Service, Dr. Parran. Probably no one is so well informed in all of the phases of health as is the head of this important department of the government. In his recent preliminary report[1] to state and local officers for their information and guidance, he presented data that have been gathered by a large group of government workers. The report includes a census of the health conditions of all the groups constituting the population of the United States—records of the health status and of the economic status of 2,660,000 individuals living in various sections, in various types of communities, on various economic levels. The data

9

include records on every age-group. He makes the following interpretations based upon the assumption that the 2,660,000 offer a fair sampling of the population, and he indicates the conclusions which may be drawn regarding conditions of status for the total population of some 130,000,000 people.

> Every day one out of twenty people is too sick to go to school or work, or attend his customary activities.

> Every man, woman and child (on the average) in the nation suffers ten days of incapacity annually.

> The average youngster is sick in bed seven days of the year, the average oldster 35 days.

> Two million five hundred thousand people (42 percent of the 6,000,000 sick every day) suffer from chronic diseases—heart disease, hardening of the arteries, rheumatism, and nervous diseases.

> Sixty-five thousand people are totally deaf; 75,000 more are deaf and dumb; 200,000 lack a hand, arm, foot or leg; 300,000 have permanent spinal injuries; 500,000 are blind; 1,000,000 more are permanent cripples.

> Two persons on the Relief income level (less than $1,000 yearly income for the entire family) are disabled for one week or longer for every one person better off economically.

> Only one in 250 family heads in the income group of more than $2,000 yearly cannot seek work because of chronic disability. In Relief families one in every 20 family heads is disabled.

> Relief and low-income families are sick longer as well as more often than better-financed families. They call doctors less often. But the poor, especially in big cities, get to stay in hospitals longer than their better-off neighbors.

Concluded Dr. Parran:

> It is apparent that inadequate diet, poor housing, the hazards of occupation and the instability of the labor market definitely create immediate health problems.

It will be seen from this report that the group expressed as oldsters, who spend on an average thirty-five days per year in bed, are sick in bed one-tenth of the time. Those of us who are well, who may have been so fortunate as to spend very little time in bed, will contemplate this fact with considerable concern since it expresses a vast amount of suffering and enforced idleness. It is clear that so great an incidence of morbidity must place a heavy load upon those who at the time are well. The problem of the progressive increase in percentage of individuals affected with heart disease and cancer is adequate cause for alarm. Statistics have been published by the Department of Public Health in New York City which show the increase in the incidence of heart disease to have progressed steadily during the years from 1907 to 1936. The figures provided in their report reveal an increase from 203.7 deaths per 100,000 in 1907 to 327.2 per 100,000 in 1936. This constitutes an increase of 60 percent. Cancer increased 90 percent from 1907 to 1936.

That this problem of serious degeneration of our modern civilization is not limited to the people of the United States has been commented on at length by workers in many countries. Sir Arbuthnot Lane, one of England's distinguished surgeons, and a student of public welfare, has made this comment:[2]

> Long surgical experience has proved to me conclusively that there is something radically and fundamentally wrong with the civilized mode of life, and I believe that unless the present dietetic and health customs of the White Nations are reorganized, social decay and race deterioration are inevitable.

The decline in white population that is taking place in many communities throughout several countries illustrates the widespread working of the forces that are responsible for this degeneration. In discussing this matter in its relation to Australia, S. R. Wolstenhole,[3] lecturer in economics at Sydney University, predicts that:

> A decline in Australia's population is inevitable within 40 years because of the absence of a vigorous population policy.

Students of our modern social problems are recognizing that these problems are not limited to health conditions which we have been accustomed to think of as bodily diseases. This is illustrated in a recent discussion by Will Durant:[4]

> . . . The American people are face to face with at least 4 major and militant problems that have to do with the continuity and worthwhile progress of modern civilization:
>
> 1. The threatened deterioration of our stock.
> 2. The purchasing power of our people must rise as fast as the power to procure. . . .
> 3. The third problem is moral. A civilization depends upon morals for a social and governmental order. . . .
> 4. The sources of statesmanship are drying up. . . .

Dental caries or tooth decay is recognized as affecting more individuals throughout the so-called civilized world today than any other affection. In the United States, England and Europe examinations of highly modernized groups, consisting of several million individuals, reveal the fact that from 85 to 100 percent of the individuals in various communities are suffering from this affection. As a contributing factor to absence from school among children it leads all other affections. From the standpoint of injury to health, it has been estimated by many to be the most serious contributing factor through its involvement of other organs of the body. The Honorable J. A. Young, Minister of Health of New Zealand, strongly emphasized that the insidiousness of the effect of dental disease lies in the fact that it is the forerunner of other far-reaching disturbances and he has referred to the seriousness with which it is viewed in England as follows: "Sir George Newman, Principal Medical Officer of the Ministry of Health in Great Britain, has said that 'dental disease is one of the chief, if not the chief, cause of the ill health of the people.'"

Dr. Earnest A. Hooton, of Harvard University, has emphasized the importance of oral asepsis and the task of stopping tooth decay. In closing Chapter VII of his recent book *Apes, Men and Morons*,[5] he states the case as follows:

> I firmly believe that the health of humanity is at stake, and that, unless steps are taken to discover preventives of tooth infection and correctives of dental deformation, the course of human evolution will lead downward to extinction. . . . The facts that we must face are, in brief, that human teeth and the human mouth have become, possibly under the influence of civilization, the foci of infections that undermine the entire bodily health of the species and that degenerative tendencies in evolution have manifested themselves in modern man to such an extent that our jaws are too small for the teeth which they are supposed to accommodate, and that, as a consequence, these teeth erupt so irregularly that their fundamental efficiency is often entirely or nearly destroyed.

In discussing the strategic situation of dental science, Dr. Hooton states.

> In my opinion there is one and only one course of action which will check the increase of dental disease and degeneration which may ultimately cause the extinction of the human species. This is to elevate the dental profession to a plane on which it can command the services of our best research minds to study the causes and seek for the cures of these dental evils. . . . The dental practitioner should equip himself to become the agent of an intelligent control of human evolution, insofar as it is affected by diet. Let us go to the ignorant savage, consider his way of eating, and be wise. Let us cease pretending that tooth-brushes and tooth-paste are any more important than shoe-brushes and shoe-polish. It is store food which has given us store teeth.

Students of history have continually commented upon the superior teeth of the so-called savages including the human types that have preceded our modernized groups. While dental caries have been found occasionally in several animal species through the recent geologic ages, the teeth of the human species have been comparatively free from dental caries. Primitive human beings have been freer from the disease than has contemporary animal life. This absence of tooth decay among primitive races has been so striking a characteristic of human kind that many commentators have referred to it as a strikingly modern disease.

Dryer,[6] in discussing dental caries in pre-historic South Africans, makes this comment:

> In not one of a very large collection of teeth from skulls obtained in the Matjes River Shelter (Holocene) was there the slightest sign of dental caries. The indication from this area, therefore, bears out the experience of European anthropologists that caries is a comparatively modern disease and that no skull showing this condition can be regarded as ancient.

In connection with the studies reported in this volume, it is of particular importance that a desire to find the cause of dental caries was the primary reason for undertaking these investigations. Since it was exceedingly difficult to find in our modern social organization any large group with relatively high immunity to dental caries, a search was made for such control groups among remnants of primitive racial stocks that could also be examined at the point of contact with modern civilization in order that the changes associated with their racial loss of immunity might be noted. Probably few problems with which our modern social groups are concerned have been so inadequately understood not only by the laity, but by the members of the medical and dental professions as has this problem of the cause of dental caries.

The problem of correcting dental arch deformities and thereby improving facial form has developed a specialty in dentistry known as "orthodontia." The literature dealing with the cause of facial deformities is now voluminous. The blending of racial stocks that differ radically in facial form has been said by many to be the chief factor contributing to the creation of deformities of the face. Crowded teeth have been said to be due to the inheritance of the large teeth of one parent and the small bone formation of the other and that such inheritances would provide dental arches that are too small for the teeth that have been made for them. A more general explanation for certain types of deformity, particularly for the protruding of the upper teeth over the lower, is that they result from thumb-sucking, which tends to bring the upper arch forward and to depress the lower. Among the other contributing factors named have been faulty sleeping and breathing habits. To these has been assigned much of the blame. This problem of facial form, as well as that of bodily design, including dental arch design, is so directly a problem of growth, not only of individuals, but of races themselves, that certain laws have been very definitely worked out by physical anthropologists as laws of development. They have assumed that changes in physical type can occur only through the impact of changes in the environment which have affected a great number of generations. It is important to keep this viewpoint in mind as the succeeding chapters are read, for they contain descriptions of many changes in physical form that have occurred routinely in the various racial groups, even during the first generation after the parents have adopted the foods of modern civilization.

Many of our modern writers have recognized and have emphasized the seriousness of mental and moral degeneration. Laird has made a splendid contribution under the title "The Tail That Wags the Nation,"[7] in which he states:

> The country's average level of general ability sinks lower with each gen-
> eration. Should the ballot be restricted to citizens able to take care of them-
> selves? One out of four cannot. . . . The tail is now wagging Washington, and
> Wall St. and LaSalle Street. . . . Each generation has seen some lowering of
> the American average level of general ability.

In Laird's analysis of our present situation he has stressed a very important phase. While emphasizing that the degeneration is not limited to restricted areas, he raises the question as to whether local conditions in certain areas play important roles in the rate and extent to which degeneration has taken place. He says further,

> Although we might cite any one of nearly two dozen states, we will first
> mention Vermont by name because that is the place studied by the late Dr.
> Pearce Bailey. "It would be," he wrote, "safe to assume that there are at least
> 30 defectives per 1000 in Vermont of the eight-year-old mentality type, and
> 300 per 1000 of backward or retarded persons, persons of distinctly inferior
> intelligence. In other words, nearly one-third of the whole population of
> that state is of a type to require some supervision."

The problem of lowered mentality and its place in our modern conception of bodily diseases has not been placed on a physical basis as have the better understood degenerative processes, with their direct relationship to a diseased organ, but has generally been assigned to a realm entirely outside the domain of disease or injury of a special organ or tissue. Edward Lee Thorndike,[8] of Columbia University, says that "thinking is as biological as digestion." This implies that a disturbance in the capacity to think is directly related to a defect in the brain.

Another of the distinguished students of mental capacity, J. B. Miner,[9] states:

> If morality and intellect are finally demonstrated to be correlated through-
> out the whole range of individual differences, it is probably the most
> profoundly significant fact with which society has to deal.

The origin of backwardness in a child seems to have been assigned very largely to some experience in that child's life which becomes a conditioning factor and which thereafter strongly influences his behavior. The problem of the relation of physical defects to delinquency in its various phases, including major crime, constitutes one of the most alarming aspects of our modern prob-lems in social degeneration. Chassell[10] has made an exhaustive study of the reports from workers in different fields in several countries and summarizes her finding as follows: "The correlation between delinquency and mental inferiority as found in the case of feeble-minded groups is clearly positive, and tends to be marked in degree."

Burt,[11] who had made an extensive study, over an extended period, of the problems of the backward child and the delinquent child in London, states in his summary and conclusion with regard to the origin of backwardness in the child:

> Both at London and at Birmingham between 60 and 70 percent belong to the (innately) "dull" category. . . . In the majority the outstanding cause is a general inferiority of intellectual capacity, presumably inborn and frequently hereditary.

In discussing the relationship between general physical weakness and the mentally backward, he writes:

> Old and time-honoured as it must seem to the schoolmaster, the problem of the backward child has never been attacked by systematic research until quite recently. We know little about causes, and still less about treatment. . . . Thirdly, though the vast majority of backward children—80 percent in an area like London—prove to be suffering from minor bodily ailments or from continued ill-health, nevertheless general physical weakness is rarely the main factor.

Among the many surveys made in the study of the forces that are responsible for producing delinquency and criminality, practically all the workers in this field have testified to the obscure nature of those forces. Burt[12] says that, "it is almost as though crime were some contagious disease, to which the constitutionally susceptible were suddenly exposed at puberty, or to which puberty left them peculiarly prone." He emphasizes a relationship between delinquency and physical deficiency:

> Most repeated offenders are far from robust; they are frail, sickly, and infirm. Indeed, so regularly is chronic moral disorder associated with chronic physical disorder that many have contended that crime is a disease, or at least a symptom of disease, needing the doctor more than the magistrate, physic rather than the whip.

· · · · · · ·

> The frequency among juvenile delinquents of bodily weakness and ill health has been remarked by almost every recent writer. In my own series of cases nearly 70 percent were suffering from such defects; and nearly 50 percent were in urgent need of medical treatment. . . . Of all the psychological causes of crime, the commonest and the gravest is usually alleged to be defective mind. The most eminent authorities, employing the most elaborate methods of scientific analysis, have been led to enunciate some such belief. In England, for example, Dr. Goring has affirmed that "the one vital mental constitutional factor in the etiology of crime is defective intelligence." In Chicago, Dr. Healy has likewise maintained that among the

personal characteristics of the offender "mental deficiency forms the largest single cause of delinquency." And most American investigators would agree.

The assertion of the obscurity of the fundamental causative factors of delinquency constitutes one of the most striking aspects of the extensive literature that has been accumulated through the reporting of intensive studies made by workers in many countries.

Thrasher,[13] in discussing the nature and origin of gangs, expresses this very clearly:

> Gangs are gangs, wherever they are found. They represent a specific type or variety of society, and one thing that is particularly interesting about them is the fact that they are, in respect to their organization, so elementary, and in respect to their origin, so spontaneous.
>
> Formal society is always more or less conscious of the end for which it exists, and the organization through which this end is achieved is always more or less a product of design. But gangs grow like weeds, without consciousness of their aims, and without administrative machinery to achieve them. They are, in fact, so spontaneous in their origin, and so little conscious of the purposes for which they exist, that one is tempted to think of them as predetermined, foreordained, and "instinctive," and so, quite independent of the environment in which they ordinarily are found.

No doubt, many cities have been provided, as has Cleveland, with a special school for delinquent boys. The institution there has been given the appropriate title, the "Thomas A. Edison School." It usually has an enrollment of 800 to 900 boys. Dr. Watson,[14] who has been of outstanding service in the organization of this work, makes an important comment on the origin of the student population there:

> The Thomas A. Edison student population consists of a group of truant and behavior boys, most of them in those earlier stages of mal-adjustment which we have termed predelinquency. . . . In general, they are the products of unhappy experiences in school, home and community. They are sensitive recorders of the total complex of social forces which operate in and combine to constitute what we term their community environment.

It will be seen from these quotations that great emphasis has been placed upon the influence of the environment in determining factors of delinquency.

Hooton, the distinguished physical anthropologist of Harvard, has made important observations regarding our modern physical degeneration. As an approach to this larger problem of man's progressive degeneration, he has proposed the organization and establishment of an Institute of Clinical Anthropology,[15] the purpose of which he has indicated:

> . . . for finding out what man is like biologically when he does not need a doctor, in order to further ascertain what he should be like after the doctor has finished with him. I am entirely serious when I suggest that it is a very

myopic medical science which works backward from the morgue rather than forward from the cradle.

Very important contributions have been made to the forces that are at work in the development of delinquents through an examination of the families in which affected individuals have appeared. Sullenger,[16] in discussing this phase, states:

> Abbott and Breckinridge found in their Chicago studies that a much higher percentage of delinquent boys than girls were from large families. However, Healy and Bronner found in their studies in Chicago and Boston that the large family is conducive to delinquency among children in that the larger the family the greater percentage of cases with more than one delinquent. They were unable to detect whether or not this fact was due to parental neglect, poverty, bad environmental conditions, or the influence of one child on another. In each of the series in both cities the number of delinquents in families of different sizes showed general similarity.

As the investigations outlined in this study are reviewed, many problems not anticipated by the writer when these investigations were undertaken will be presented. These new problems were not, at first, generally thought of as related directly or indirectly to our modern racial degeneration, but have been found recently to be so related.

Since it will be seen that the size and shape of the head and sinuses, including the oral cavity and throat, are directly influenced by forces that are at work in our modern civilization, we shall consider the speaking and singing voice. In traveling among several of the primitive races, one is frequently impressed with the range and resonance of many of the voices—in fact, by almost every voice. We are quite familiar with the high premium that is placed on singing voices of exceptional quality in our modern social order. This is illustrated by the following comment:[17]

> Tip-top Italian-style tenors have always been a scarce commodity, and for the past two decades they have been growing scarcer and scarcer. Opera impresarios count on the fingers of one hand the lust-high-voice Latins. . . . Since the death of Enrico Caruso (1921) opera houses have shown a steady decline.

Important light will be thrown on this phase of the problem—the cause of fewer good voices in Italy today than of old—as we note the narrowing of the face and of the dental arches and as we see the change in the form of the palate of the various primitive races. These changes occur even in the first generation after the parents have adopted the foods of modern white civilizations.

As we study the primitives we will find that they have had an entirely different conception of the nature and origin of the controlling forces which have molded individuals and races.

Buckle,[18] in writing his epoch-making *History of Civilization* about the middle of the last century, summed up his years of historical studies with some very important conclusions, some of which are as follows:

> 2. It is proved by history, and especially by statistics, that human actions are governed by laws as fixed and regular as those which rule in the physical world.
> 3. Climate, soil, food, and the aspects of Nature are the principal causes of intellectual progress.
> 6. Religion, literature, and government are, at best, but the products, and not the cause of civilization.

This important view was not orthodox and was met by very severe criticism. The newer knowledge strongly corroborates his view.

My early studies of the relation of nutrition to dental problems were related chiefly to growth defects in the teeth produced long before the eruption of the permanent teeth, chiefly from one year of age to the time of eruption. These often appeared as lines across the teeth. I was able to trace these lines directly to the use of a few highly processed baby foods. I published an extensive report on this phase of the problem, together with illustrations, in 1913.[19] These injuries are disclosed with the x-ray long before the teeth erupt. These disturbances occur much less frequently in connection with the baby foods used today.

The problems of modern degeneration can in general be divided into two main groups, those which relate to the perfection of the physical body and those which relate to its function. The latter include character as expressed in behavior of individuals and of groups of individuals which thus relate to national character and to an entire culture.

In an enumeration of the phases in which there is a progressive decline of modern civilization, it is essential that we keep in mind that in addition to an analysis of the forces responsible for individual degeneration, the ethical standards of the whole group cannot be higher than those of the individuals that compose it. That recent mass degeneration is in progress is attested by daily events throughout the world. The current interpretation for individual character degeneration largely places the responsibility on a conditioning factor which exerts an influence during early childhood and therefore is directly related to the environment of the child. These, therefore, are postnatal conditioning factors. An important contribution to this phase comes directly from the experience of primitive races and indicates that a more fundamental conditioning factor had developed in the prenatal period. If, therefore, large groups of individuals suffer from such a prenatal conditioning influence, new light will be thrown upon the larger problems of group deterioration. History seems to provide records of such mass degeneration as, for example, those which culminated in the so-called "dark ages." That some such mass degeneration is now in progress is suggested by leading students of human welfare. The regius professor of Greek at Oxford in his inaugural lecture in 1937 made the following observation:[20]

> In the revolution of thought through which we are living, the profoundest and most disturbing element is the breakdown of that ethical system which, since the days of Constantine, has imposed upon European culture at least the semblance of moral unity.

In commenting on this important statement Sir Alfred Zimmern in his address on the decline of international standards said that "Recent events should convince the dullest mind of the extent to which international standards have deteriorated and the anarchy which threatens the repudiation of law and order in favor of brute force."

The problem of progressive decline in individual and group ethical standards is commanding the attention of great international organizations. In discussing this problem before the International Rotary at its meeting in San Francisco in June, 1938, one of the leaders in mass reform, Mayor Harold Burton of Cleveland, stressed very important phases. He stated that the American boys "are making irrevocable choices" between good and bad citizenship which "may make or wreck the nation. It may be on the battlefield of crime prevention that the life of democracy will be saved." He described great industrial cities as battlefields where "the tests of democracy are the newest and sharpest."[21] . . . "For centuries," he said:

> . . . we have fought crime primarily by seeking to catch the criminal after the crime has been committed and then through his punishment to lead or drive him and others to good citizenship. Today the greater range of operation and greater number of criminals argue that we must deal with the flood waters of crime. We must prevent the flood by study, control and diversion of the waters at their respective sources. To do this we must direct the streams of growing boys in each community away from fields of crime to those of good citizenship.

If the "flood waters" that must be controlled lie farther back than the cradle, in order to safeguard individual character and individual citizenship from prenatal conditioning factors which have profound influence in determining the reaction of the individuals to the environment, it is essential that programs that are to be efficient in maintaining national character reach back to those forces which are causing the degeneration of increasing numbers of the population in succeeding generations of our modern cultures.

That the problem of mass degeneration constitutes one of the most alarming problems of our modernized cultures is demonstrated by the urgency of appeals that are being made by students in national and international affairs. The discussion of "An Ethical Declaration for the Times,"[22] a declaration of faith, is accompanied by a pledge. This pledge reads:

> I pledge myself to use every opportunity for action to uphold the great tradition of civilization to protect all those who may suffer for its sake, and to pass it on to the coming generations. I recognized no loyalty greater than that to the task of preserving truth, toleration, and justice in the coming world order.

The author emphasizes the great danger of taking for granted that the cultural progress that has been attained will continue. There is probably no phase of this whole problem of modern degeneration that is so brilliantly illuminated by the accumulated wisdom of primitive races as group degeneration. They have so organized the life of the family and the individual that the nature of the forces which established individual behavior and character are controlled.

Our problem of modern degeneration involves both individual and group destiny. Our approach to this study will, accordingly, involve first a critical examination of the forces that are responsible for individual degeneration.

In my search for the cause of degeneration of the human face and the dental organs I have been unable to find an approach to the problem through the study of affected individuals and diseased tissues. In my two volume work on "Dental Infections," Volume I, entitled *Dental Infections, Oral and Systemic*, and Volume II, entitled *Dental Infections and the Degenerative Diseases*,[23] I reviewed at length the researches that I had conducted to throw light on this problem. The evidence seemed to indicate clearly that the forces that were at work were not to be found in the diseased tissues, but that the undesirable conditions were the result of the absence of something, rather than of the presence of something. This strongly indicated the need for finding groups of individuals so physically perfect that they could be used as controls. In order to discover them, I determined to search out primitive racial stocks that were free from the degenerative processes with which we are concerned in order to note what they have that we do not have. These field investigations have taken me to many parts of the world through a series of years. The following chapters review the studies made of primitive groups, first, when still protected by their isolation, and, second, when in contact with modern civilization.

REFERENCES

[1] PARRAN, T. Sickness survey. *Time*, Vol. 31, No. 4, Jan. 31, 1938, p. 22.
[2] LANE, A. Preface to *Maori Symbolism* by Ettie A. Rout. London: Paul Trench Trubner, 1926.

[3] WOLSTENHOLE, S. R. Proposes Stork Derby. *Cleveland Press*, March 12, 1937.

[4] DURANT, W. A. Crisis in civilization. *Speakers Library Magazine*, p. 2, Jan. 15, 1938.

[5] HOOTON, E. A. *Apes, Men and Morons*. New York: Putnam, 1937.

[6] DRYER, T. F. Dental caries in prehistoric South Africans. *Nature*, 136:302, 1935.

[7] LAIRD, D. The tail that wags the nation. *Rev. of Revs.*, 92:44, 1935.

[8] THORNDIKE, E. L. Big Chief's G. G. *Time*, Vol. 30, Dec. 13, 1937, p. 25.

[9] MINER, J. B. *Proc. Am. Ass. for Feeble-Minded*, p. 54, 1919.

[10] CHASSELL, C. F. Relation between morality and intellect. N. Y., Columbia, 1935.

[11] BURT, C. L. *The Backward Child*. New York: Appleton, 1937.

[12] BURT, C. L. *The Young Delinquent*. London: University of London Press, 1925.

[13] THRASHER, F. M. *The Gang*. Chicago: University of Chicago Press, 1936.

[14] WATSON, M. P. Organization and administration of a public school for pre-delinquent boys in a large city. Thesis, Cleveland, Western Reserve University.

[15] HOOTON, E. A. An Anthropologist Looks at Medicine. Reviewed in *Time*, Vol. 27, Mar. 30, 1936, p. 73.

[16] SULLENGER, T. E. *Social Determinants in Juvenile Delinquency*. London: Chapman and Hall, 1936.

[17] TENOR. *Time*, Vol. 30, Dec. 13, 1937, p. 50.

[18] BUCKLE, H. T. *History of Civilization in England*. New York: Appleton, 1910.

[19] PRICE, W. A. Some contributions to dental and medical science. *Dental Summary*, 34:253, 1914.

[20] ZIMMERN, A. Scientific research in international affairs. *Nature*, 141:947, 1938.

[21] Burton Tells of Crime Drive. *Cleveland Press*, June 22, 1938.

[22] WHYTE, L. L. An ethical declaration for the times. *Nature*, 141:827, 1938.

[23] PRICE, W. A. *Dental Infections, Oral and Systemic*. Cleveland: Penton, 1923.

Chapter 3

ISOLATED AND MODERNIZED SWISS

IN ORDER to study the possibility of greater nutritive value in foods produced at a high elevation, as indicated by a lowered incidence of morbidity, including tooth decay, I went to Switzerland and made studies in two successive years, 1931 and 1932. It was my desire to find, if possible, groups of Swiss living in a physical environment such that their isolation would compel them to live largely on locally produced foods. Officials of the Swiss Government were consulted as to the possibility of finding people in Switzerland whose physical isolation provided an adequate protection. We were told that the physical conditions that would not permit people to obtain modern foods would prevent us from reaching them without hardship. However, owing to the completion of the Loetschberg Tunnel, eleven miles long, and the building of a railroad that crosses the Löetschental Valley, at a little less than a mile above sea level, a group of about 2,000 people had been made easily accessible for study, shortly prior to 1931. Practically all the human requirements of the people in that valley, except a few items like sea salt, have been produced in the valley for centuries.

A bird's-eye view of the Löetschental Valley, looking toward the entrance, is shown in Fig. 1. The people of this valley have a history covering more than a dozen centuries. The architecture of their wooden buildings, some of them several centuries old, indicates a love for simple stability, adapted to expediency and efficiency. Artistically designed mottoes, many of them centuries old, are carved deep in the heavy supporting timbers, both within and without the buildings. They are always expressive of devotion to cultural and spiritual values rather than to material values. These people have never been conquered, although many efforts have been made to invade their valley. Except for the rugged cleft through which the river descends to the Rhone Valley, the Löetschental Valley is almost completely enclosed by three high mountain ranges which are usually snow-capped. This pass could be guarded by a small band against any attacking forces since artificial landslides could easily be released. The natural occurrence of these landslides has made passage through the gorge hazardous, if not impossible, for months of the year. According to early legends of the valley these mountains were the parapets of the universe, and the great glacier of the valley, the end of the universe. The

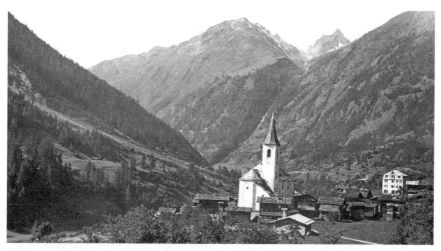

FIG. 1. Beautiful Löetschental Valley about a mile above sea level. About two thousand Swiss live here. In 1932 no deaths had occurred from tuberculosis in the history of the valley.

glacier is a branch of the great ice field that stretches away to the west and south from the ice-cap of the Jungfrau and Monch. The mountains, however, are seldom approached from this direction because of the hazardous ice fields. The gateway to them with which the traveling world is familiar is from Interlaken by way of the Lauterbrunnen or Grindelwald valleys.

At the altitude of the Löetschental Valley the winters are long, and the summers short but beautiful, and accompanied by extraordinarily rapid and luxuriant growth. The meadows are fragrant with Alpine flowers, with violets like pansies, which bloom all summer in deepest hues.

The people of the Löetschental Valley make up a community of two thousand who have been a world unto themselves. They have neither physician nor dentist because they have so little need for them; they have neither policeman nor jail, because they have no need for them. The clothing has been the substantial homespuns made from the wool of their sheep. The valley has produced not only everything that is needed for clothing, but practically everything that is needed for food. It has been the achievement of the valley to build some of the finest physiques in all Europe. This is attested to by the fact that many of the famous Swiss guards of the Vatican at Rome, who are the admiration of the world and are the pride of Switzerland, have been selected from this and other Alpine valleys. It is every Löetschental boy's ambition to be a Vatican guard. Notwithstanding the fact that tuberculosis is the most serious disease of Switzerland, according to a statement given me by a government official, a recent report of inspection of this valley did not reveal a single case.

I was aided in my studies in Switzerland by the excellent cooperation of the Reverend John Siegen, the pastor of the one church of this beautiful valley.

The people live largely in a series of villages dotting the valley floor along the river bank. The land that is tilled, chiefly for producing hay for feeding the cattle in the winter and rye for feeding the people, extends from the river and often rises steeply toward the mountains which are wooded with timber so precious for protection that little of it has been disturbed. Fortunately, there is much more on the vast area of the mountain sides than is needed for the relatively small population. The forests have been jealously guarded because they are so greatly needed to prevent slides of snow and rocks which might engulf and destroy the villages.

The valley has a fine educational system of alternate didactic and practical work. All children are required to attend school six months of the year and to spend the other six months helping with the farming and dairying industry in which young and old of both sexes must work. The school system is under the direct supervision of the Catholic Church, and the work is well done. The girls are also taught weaving, dyeing and garment making. The manufacture of wool and clothing is the chief homework for the women in the winter.

No trucks nor even horses and wagons, let alone tractors, are available to bear the burdens up and down the mountain sides. This is all done on human backs for which the hearts of the people have been made especially strong.

We are primarily concerned here with the quality of the teeth and the development of the faces that are associated with such splendid hearts and unusual physiques. I made studies of both adults and growing boys and girls, during the summer of 1931, and arranged to have samples of food, particularly dairy products, sent to me about twice a month, summer and winter. These products have been tested for their mineral and vitamin contents, particularly the fat-soluble activators. The samples were found to be high in vitamins and much higher than the average samples of commercial dairy products in America and Europe, and in the lower areas of Switzerland.

Hay is cut for winter feeding of the cattle, and this hay grows rapidly. The hay proved, on chemical analysis made at my laboratory, to be far above the average in quality for pasturage and storage grasses. Almost every household has goats or cows or both. In the summer the cattle seek the higher pasturage lands and follow the retreating snow which leaves the lower valley free for the harvesting of the hay and rye. The turning of the soil is done by hand, since there are neither plows nor draft animals to drag the plows, in preparation for the next year's rye crop. A limited amount of garden stuff is grown, chiefly green foods for summer use. While the cows spend the warm summer on the verdant knolls and wooded slopes near the glaciers and fields of perpetual snow, they have a period of high and rich productivity of milk. The milk constitutes an important part of the summer's harvesting. While the men and boys gather in the hay and rye, the women and children go in large numbers with the cattle to collect the milk and make and store cheese for the following winter's use. This cheese contains the natural butterfat and minerals of the splendid milk and is a virtual storehouse of life for the coming winter.

From Dr. Siegen, I learned much about the life and customs of these people. He told me that they recognize the presence of Divinity in the life-giving qualities of the butter made in June when the cows have arrived for pasturage near the glaciers. He gathers the people together to thank the kind Father for the evidence of his Being in the life-giving qualities of butter and cheese made when the cows eat the grass near the snow line. This worshipful program includes the lighting of a wick in a bowl of the first butter made after the cows have reached the luscious summer pasturage. This wick is permitted to burn in a special sanctuary built for the purpose. The natives of the valley are able to recognize the superior quality of their June butter, and, without knowing exactly why, pay it due homage.

The nutrition of the people of the Löetschental Valley, particularly that of the growing boys and girls, consists largely of a slice of whole rye bread and a piece of the summer-made cheese (about as large as the slice of bread), which are eaten with fresh milk of goats or cows. Meat is eaten about once a week. In the light of our newer knowledge of activating substances, including vitamins, and the relative values of food for supplying minerals for body building, it is clear why they have healthy bodies and sound teeth. The average total fat-soluble activator and mineral intake of calcium and phosphorus of these children would far exceed that of the daily intake of the average American child. The sturdiness of the child life permits children to play and frolic bareheaded and barefooted even in water running down from the glacier in the late evening's chilly breezes, in weather that made us wear our overcoats and gloves and button our collars. Of all the children in the valley still using the primitive diet of whole rye bread and dairy products the average number of cavities per person was 0.3. On an average it was necessary to examine three persons to find one defective deciduous or permanent tooth. The children examined were between seven and sixteen years of age.

If one is fortunate enough to be in the valley in early August and witness the earnestness with which the people celebrate their national holiday, he will be privileged to see a sight long to be remembered. These celebrations close with the gathering together of the mountaineers on various crags and prominences where great bonfires are lighted from fuel that has been accumulated and built into an enormous mound to make a huge torchlight. These bonfires are lighted at a given hour from end to end of the valley throughout its expanse. Every mountaineer on a distant crag seeing the lights knows that the others are signaling to him that they, too, are making their sacred consecration in song which says, "one for all and all for one." This motive has been crystallized into action and has become a part of the very souls of the people. One understands why doors do not need to be bolted in the Löetschental Valley.

How different the level of life and horizon of such souls from those in many places in the so-called civilized world in which people have degraded themselves until life has no interest in values that cannot be expressed in gold or pelf, which they would obtain even though the life of the person being cheated or robbed would thereby be crippled or blotted out.

One immediately wonders if there is not something in the life-giving vitamins and minerals of the food that builds not only great physical structures within which their souls reside, but builds minds and hearts capable of a higher type of manhood in which the material values of life are made secondary to individual character. In succeeding chapters we will see evidence that this is the case.

Our quest has been for information relative to the health of the body, the perfection of the teeth, and the normality of development of faces and dental arches, in order that we might through an analysis of the foods learn the secret of such splendid body building and learn from the people of the valley how the nutrition of all groups of people may be reinforced, so that they, too, may be free from mankind's most universal disease, tooth decay and its sequelae. These studies included not only the making of a physical examination of the teeth, the photographing of subjects, the recording of voluminous data, the obtaining of samples of food for chemical analysis, the collecting of detailed information regarding daily menus; but also the collecting of samples of saliva for chemical analysis. The chemical analysis of saliva was used to test out my newly developed procedure for estimating the level of immunity to dental caries for a given person at a given time. This procedure is outlined in following chapters. The samples of saliva were preserved by an addition of formalin equivalent in amount to one percent of the sample of saliva.

These children will, it is hoped, be reexamined in succeeding years in order to make comparative studies of the effect of the changes in the local nutritional programs. Some of these changes are already in progress. There is now a modern bakery dispensing white bread and many white-flour products which was in full operation in 1932.

I inquired of many persons regarding the most favorable districts in which to make further studies of groups of people living in protected isolation because of their physical environment, and decided to study some special high Alpine valleys between the Rhone Valley and Italy, which I included in 1932. The Canton of Wallis is bordered by French-speaking people on the west, by Italian-speaking people on the south, and by German-speaking people on the east and north. I had as guides and interpreters in Wallis, Dr. Alfred Gysi and also Dr. Adolf Roos through part of the territory.

Our first expedition was into the valley of the Visp which is a great gorge extending southward from the Rhone River, dividing into two gorges, one going to the Saas Fee country, and the other to the vicinity of the Matterhorn with its almost spirelike pinnacle lifting itself above the surrounding snow-capped mountains and visible from eminences in all directions as one of the mightiest and most sublime spectacles in the world. It was one of the last mountains of Europe to be scaled by man. One has not seen the full majesty of the Alps if he has not seen the Matterhorn.

We left the mountain railroad, which makes many of the grades with the cog system, at the town of St. Nicholas, and climbed the mountain trail to an isolated settlement on the east bank of the Mattervisp River, called Grachen, a five-hour journey. The settlement is on a shelf high above the east side of the river where it is exposed to southern sunshine and enjoys a unique isolation because of its physical inaccessibility. An examination made of the children in this community showed that only 2.3 teeth out of every hundred had been attacked by tooth decay.

The hardihood of the people was splendidly illustrated by a woman of 62 years who carried an enormous load of rye on her back at an altitude of about 5,000 feet. We met her later and talked to her, and found that she was extraordinarily well developed and well preserved. She showed us her grandchildren who had fine physiques and facial developments.

The rye is so precious that while being carried the heads are protected by wrapping them in canvas so that not a kernel will be lost. The rye is thrashed by hand and ground in stone mills which were formerly hand-turned like the one shown in Fig. 2. Recently water turbines have been installed. Water power

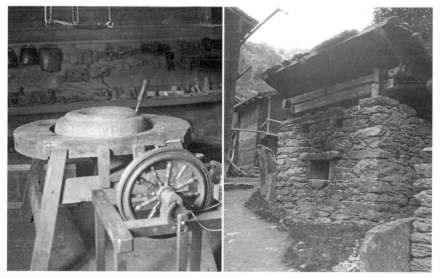

FIG. 2. For centuries the natives ground their rye in this type of hand mill. This community bake-oven for whole rye bread is passing.

is abundant and the grinding is done for the people of the mountain side in these water-driven mills. Only whole rye flour is available. Each household takes turns in using the community bake-oven, which is shown in Fig. 2. A month's supply of whole rye bread is baked at one time for a given family.

Here again the cows were away in the midsummer, pasturing up near the glaciers. Grachen has an altitude of about 5,000 feet. The church at Grachen was built several hundred years ago. We were shown an embossed certificate of honor and privilege extended to a group of about 120 people who had originally built the edifice. We were given valued assistance by the local priest, and were provided with facilities in his spacious and well-kept rooms for making our studies of the children.

From Grachen we returned to St. Nicholas and proceeded from there by train down the valley and up another steep ascent, requiring several hours, to the hamlet of Visperterminen, on the east side of the mountain above the Visp River, and below the junction of the Mattervisp and Saaservisp. This community is made up of about 1,600 people living on a sheltered shelf high above the river valley. The view from this position is indescribably beautiful. It is a little below the timber line of this and the surrounding mountains. Majestic snow-clad peaks and precipitous mountains dot the horizon and shade off into winding gorges which mark the course of wandering streams several thousand feet below our vantage point. It is a place to stop and ponder.

The gradations in climate range in the summer from a tropical temperature in protected nooks during the daytime to sub-zero weather with raging blizzards at night on the high mountains. It is a place where human stamina can be tempered to meet all the vicissitudes of life.

The village consists of a group of characteristically designed Swiss chalets clustered on the mountain side. The church stands out as a beacon visible from mountains in all directions. Visperterminen is unique in many respects. Notwithstanding its relative proximity to civilization—it is only a few hours' journey to the thoroughfare of the Rhone Valley—it has enjoyed isolation and opportunity for maintaining its characteristic primitive social and civil life. We were greeted here by the president of the village who graciously opened the school house and sent messengers to have the children of the community promptly come to the school building in order that we might make such studies as we desired. This study included a physical examination of the teeth and of the general development of the children, particularly of the faces and dental arches, the making of photographic records, the obtaining of samples of saliva, as in other places, and also the making of a detailed study of the nutrition. In addition, we obtained samples of foods for chemical analysis.

The people of Visperterminen have the unique distinction of owning land in the lower part of the mountain on which they maintain vineyards to supply wine for this country. They have the highest vineyards of Europe. They are grown on banks that are often so steep that one wonders how the tillers of the soil or the gatherers of the fruit can maintain their hold on the precarious and shifting footing. Each terrace has a trench near its lower retaining wall to catch the soil that is washed down, and this soil must be carried back in baskets to the upper boundary of the plot. This is all done by human labor. The vineyards afforded them the additional nutrition of wine and of fruit minerals and vitamins which the two groups we studied at Löetschental and Grachen did not have.

This additional nutrition was of importance because of the opportunity for obtaining through it vitamin C. It is of particular interest in the study of the incidence of tooth decay in Visperterminen that these additional factors had not created a higher immunity to tooth decay, nor a better condition of health in gingival tissues than previously found. In each one hundred teeth examined 5.2 were found to have been attacked at some time by tooth decay. Here again the nutrition consisted of rye, used almost exclusively as the cereal; of dairy products; of meat about once a week; and also some potatoes. Limited green foods were eaten during the summer. The general custom is to have a sheep dressed and distributed to a group of families, thus providing each family with a ration of meat for one day a week, usually Sunday. The bones and scraps are utilized for making soups to be served during the week. The children have goat's milk in the summer when the cows are away in the higher pastures near the snow line. Certain members of the families go to the higher pastures with the cows to make cheese for the coming winter's use.

The problem of identifying goats or cattle for establishing individual ownership is a considerable one where the stock of all are pastured in common herds. It was interesting to us to observe how this problem was met. The president of the village has what is called a "tessel" which is a string of manikins in imitation of goats or cattle made of wood and leather. Every stock owner must provide a manikin to be left in the safekeeping of the president of the village with whom it is registered. It carries on it the individual markings that this member of the colony agrees to put on every member of his animal stock. The marking may be a hole punched in the left ear or a slit in the right ear, or any combination of such markings as is desired. Thereafter all animals carrying that mark are the property of the person who registered it; similarly, any animals that have not this individual symbol of identification cannot be claimed by him.

As one stands in profound admiration before the stalwart physical development and high moral character of these sturdy mountaineers, he is impressed by the superior types of manhood, womanhood, and childhood that Nature has been able to produce from a suitable diet and a suitable environment. Surely, here is evidence enough to answer the question whether cereals should be avoided because they produce acids in the system which, if formed, will be the cause of tooth decay and many other ills including the acidity of the blood or saliva. Surely, the ultimate control will be found in Nature's laboratory where man has not yet been able to meddle sufficiently with Nature's nutritional program to blight humanity with abnormal and synthetic nutrition. When one has watched for days the childlife in those high Alpine preserves of superior manhood; when one has contrasted these people with the pinched and sallow, and even deformed, faces and distorted bodies that are produced by our modern civilization and its diets; and when one has contrasted the unsurpassed beauty of the faces of these children developed on Nature's primitive foods with the varied assortment of modern civilization's children with their defective facial development, he finds himself filled with an earnest desire to see that this betterment is made available for modern civilization.

Again and again we had the experience of examining a young man or young woman and finding that at some period of his life tooth decay had been rampant and had suddenly ceased; but, during the stress, some teeth had been lost. When we asked such people whether they had gone out of the mountain and at what age, they generally replied that at eighteen or twenty years of age they had gone to this or that city and had stayed a year or two. They stated that they had never had a decayed tooth before they went or after they returned, but that they had lost some teeth in the short period away from home.

At this point of our studies Dr. Roos found it necessary to leave, but Dr. Gysi accompanied us to the Anniviers Valley, which is also on the south side of the Rhone. The river of the valley, the Navisence, drains from the high Swiss and Italian boundary north to the Rhone River. Here again we had the remarkable experience of finding communities near to each other, one blessed with high immunity to tooth decay, and the other afflicted with rampant tooth decay.

The village of Ayer lies in a beautiful valley well up toward the glaciers. It is still largely primitive, although a government road has recently been developed, which, like many of the new arteries, has made it possible to dispatch military protection when and if necessary to any community. In this beautiful hamlet, until recently isolated, we found a high immunity to dental caries. Only 2.3 teeth out of each hundred examined were found to have been attacked by tooth decay. Here again the people were living on rye and dairy products. We wonder if history will repeat itself in the next few years and if there, too, this enviable immunity will be lost with the advent of the highway. Usually it is not long after tunnels and roads are built that automobiles and wagons enter with modern foods, which begin their destructive work. This fact has been tragically demonstrated in this valley since a roadway was extended as far as Vissoie several years ago. In this village modern foods have been available for some time. One could probably walk the distance from

Ayer to Vissoie in an hour. The number of teeth found to be attacked with caries for each one hundred children's teeth examined at Vissoie was 20.2 as compared with 2.3 at Ayer. We had here a splendid opportunity to study the changes that had occurred in the nutritional programs. With the coming of transportation and new markets there had been shipped in modern white flour; equipment for a bakery to make white-flour goods; highly sweetened fruit, such as jams, marmalades, jellies, sugar and syrups—all to be traded for the locally produced high-vitamin dairy products and high-mineral cheese and rye; and with the exchange there was enough money as premium to permit buying machine-made clothing and various novelties that would soon be translated into necessities.

Each valley or village has its own special feast days of which athletic contests are the principal events. The feasting in the past has been largely on dairy products. The athletes were provided with large bowls of cream as constituting one of the most popular and healthful beverages, and special cheese was always available. Practically no wine was used because no grapes grew in that valley, and for centuries the isolation of the people prevented access to much material that would provide wine. In the Visperterminen community, however, the special vineyards owned by these people on the lower level of the mountain side provided grape juice in various stages of fermentation, and their feasts in the past have been celebrated by the use of wines of rare vintage as well as by the use of cream and other dairy products. Their cream products took the place of our modern ice cream. It was a matter of deep interest to have the President of Visperterminen show us the tankards that had been in use in that community for nine or ten centuries. The care of these was one of the many responsibilities of the chief executive of the hamlet.

It is reported that practically all skulls that are exhumed in the Rhone valley, and, indeed, practically throughout all of Switzerland where graves have existed for more than a hundred years, show relatively perfect teeth; whereas the teeth of people recently buried have been riddled with caries or lost through this disease. It is of interest that each church usually has associated with it a cemetery in which the graves are kept decorated, often with beautiful designs of fresh or artificial flowers. Members of succeeding generations of families are said to be buried one above the other to a depth of many feet. Then, after a sufficient number of generations have been so honored, their bodies are exhumed to make a place for present and coming generations. These skeletons are usually preserved with honor and deference. The bones are stacked in basements of certain buildings of the church edifice with the skulls facing outward. These often constitute a solid wall of considerable extent. In Naters there is such a group said to contain 20,000 skeletons and skulls. These were studied with great interest as was also a smaller collection in connection with the cathedral at Visp. While many of the single straight-rooted teeth had been lost in the handling, many were present. It was a matter of importance to find that only a small percentage of teeth had had caries. Teeth that had been attacked with deep caries had developed apical abscesses with consequent destruction of the alveolar processes. Evidence of this bone change was readily visible. Sockets of missing teeth still had continuous walls, indicating that the teeth had been vital at death.

The reader will scarcely believe it possible that such marked differences in facial form, in the shape of the dental arches, and in the health condition of the teeth as are to be noted when passing from the highly modernized lower valleys and plains country in Switzerland to the isolated high valleys can exist. Fig. 3 shows four girls with typically broad dental arches and regular arrangement of the teeth. They have been born and raised in the Löetschental Valley or other isolated valleys of Switzerland which provide the excellent nutrition that we have been reviewing. They have been taught little regarding the use of tooth brushes. Their teeth have typical deposits of unscrubbed mouths; yet they are almost completely free from dental caries, as are the other individuals of the group they represent. In a study of 4,280 teeth of the children of these high valleys, only 3.4 percent were found to have been attacked by tooth decay. This is in striking contrast to conditions found in the modernized sections using the modern foods.

In Löetschental, Grachen, Visperterminen and Ayer, we have found communities of native Swiss living almost exclusively on locally produced foods consisting of the cereal, rye, and the animal product, milk, in its various forms. At Vissoie, with its available modern nutrition, there has been a complete change in the level of immunity to dental caries. It is important that studies be made in other communities which correspond in altitude with the first four places studied in which there was a high immunity to dental caries. Modern foods should be available in the new communities selected for comparative study. To find such places one would naturally think of those that are world-famed as health resorts providing the best things that modern science and industry can assemble. Surely St. Moritz would be such a place. It is situated in the southeastern part of the Republic of Switzerland near the headwaters of the Danube in the upper Engadin. This world-famous watering place attracts people of all continents for both summer and winter health building and for the enjoyment of the mountain lakes, snow-capped peaks, forested mountain sides, and crystal clear atmosphere with abundance of sunshine.

The journey from the Canton of Wallis (Valais) to the upper Engadin takes one up the Rhone valley, climbing continually to get above cascades and beautiful waterfalls until one comes to the great Rhone glacier which blocks the end of the valley. The water gushes from beneath the mountain of ice to become the parent stream of the Rhone river which passes westward through

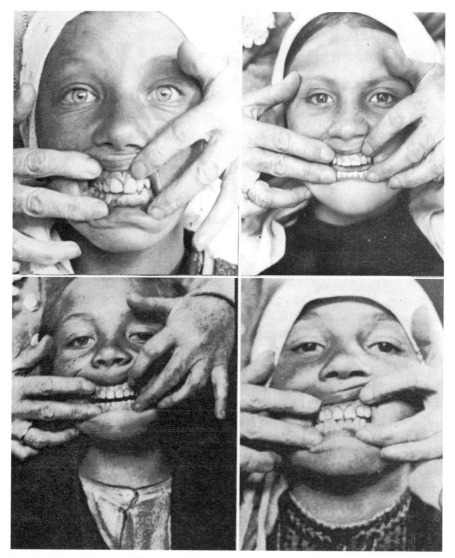

FIG. 3. Normal design of face and dental arches when adequate nutrition is provided for both the parents and the children. Note the well-developed nostrils.

the Rhone valley receiving tributaries from snow-fed streams from both north and south watersheds, as it rolls westward to the beautiful Lake Geneva and then onward west and south to the Mediterranean.

It is of significance that a study of the child life in the Rhone valley, as made by Swiss officials and reported by Dr. Adolf Roos and his associates, shows that practically every child had tooth decay and the majority of the children had decay in an aggravated form. People of this valley are provided with adequate railroad transportation for bringing them the luxuries of the world. As we pass eastward over the pass through Andermatt, we are reminded that the trains of the St. Gotthard tunnel go thundering through the mountain a mile below our feet en route to Italy. To reach our goal, the beautiful modern city and summer resort of St. Moritz, we enter the Engadin country famed for its beauty and crystal-clear atmosphere. We already know something of the beauty that awaits us which has attracted pleasure seekers and beauty lovers of the world to St. Moritz. One would scarcely expect to see so modern a city as St. Moritz at an altitude of a little over a mile, with little else to attract people than its climate in winter and summer, the magnificent scenery, and the clear atmosphere. We have passed from the communities where almost everyone wears homespuns to one of English walking coats and the most elegant of feminine attire. Everyone shows the effect of contact with culture. The hotels in their appointments and design are reminiscent of Atlantic City. Immediately one sees something is different here than in the primitive localities: the children have not the splendidly developed features, and the people give no evidence of the great physical reserve that is present in the smaller communities.

Through the kindness of Dr. William Barry, a local dentist, and through that of the superintendent of the public schools, we were invited to use one of the school buildings for our studies of the children. The summer classes were dismissed with instructions that the children be retained so that we could have them for study. Several factors were immediately apparent. The teeth were shining and clean, giving eloquent testimony of the thoroughness of the instructions in the use of the modern dentifrices for efficient oral prophylaxis. The gums looked better and the teeth more beautiful for having the debris and deposits removed. Surely this superb climate, this magnificent setting, combined with the best of the findings of modern prophylactic science, should provide a 100-percent immunity to tooth decay. But in a study of the children from eight to fifteen years of age, 29.8 percent of the teeth had already been attacked by dental caries. Our study of each case included careful examining of the mouth; photographing of the face and teeth; obtaining of samples of saliva for chemical analysis; and a study of the program of nutrition followed by the given case. In most cases, the diet was strikingly modern, and the only children found who did not have tooth decay proved to be children who were eating the natural foods, whole rye bread and plenty of milk.

In Chapter 15, a detailed discussion of the chemical differences in the food constituents is presented for both the districts subject to immunity, and for those subject to susceptibility.

I was told by a former resident of this upper Engadin country that in one of the isolated valleys only a few decades ago the children were still carrying their luncheons to school in the form of roasted rye carried dry in their pockets. Their ancestors had eaten cereal in this dry form for centuries.

St. Moritz is a typical Alpine community with a physical setting similar to that in the Cantons of Bern and Wallis (Valais). It is, however, provided with modern nutrition consisting of an abundance of white-flour products, marmalades, jams, canned vegetables, confections, and fruits—all of which are transported to the district. Only a limited supply of vegetables is grown locally. We studied some children here whose parents retained their primitive methods of food selection, and without exception those who were immune to dental caries were eating a distinctly different food from those with high susceptibility to dental caries.

Few countries of the world have had officials so untiring in their efforts to study and tabulate the incidence of dental caries in various geographic localities as has Switzerland. In the section lying to the north and east, and near Lake Constance, there is a considerable district where it is reported that 100 percent of the people are suffering from dental caries. In almost all the other parts of Switzerland in which the population is large 95 to 98 percent of the people suffer from dental caries. Of the two remaining districts, in one there is from 90 to 95 percent and in the other from 85 to 90 percent individual susceptibility to dental caries. Since in the district in the vicinity of Lake Constance the incidence of dental caries is so high that it is recorded as 100 percent, it seemed especially desirable to make a similar critical study there and to obtain samples of saliva and detailed information regarding the food, and to make detailed physical examinations of growing children in this community, and through the great kindness of Dr. Hans Eggenberger, Director of Public Health for this general district, we were given an opportunity to do so.

Arrangements were made by Dr. Eggenberger so that typical groups of children, some in institutions, could be studied. He is located at Herisau in the Canton of St. Gall. We found work well organized for building up the health of these children in so far as outdoor treatment, fresh air, and sunshine were concerned. As dental caries is a major problem, and probably nutritional, it is treated by sunshine. The boys' group and girls' group are both given suitable athletic sports under skillfully trained directors. These groups are located in different parts of the city. Their recreation grounds are open lawns adjoining wooded knolls which give the children protection and isolation in which to play in their sunsuits and build vigorous appetites, and thus to prepare for their institutional foods which were largely from a modern menu. Critical dental examinations were made and an analysis of the data obtained revealed that one-fourth of all teeth of these growing boys and girls had already been attacked by dental caries, and that only 4 percent of the children had escaped from the ravages of tooth decay, which disease many of them had in an aggravated form.

In the Herisau group 25.5 percent of the 2,065 teeth examined had been attacked by dental caries and many teeth were abscessed. The upper photographs in Fig. 4 are of two girls with typically rampant tooth decay. The one to the left is sixteen years of age and several of her permanent teeth are decayed to the gum line. Her appearance is seriously marred, as is also that of the girl to the right.

Another change that is seen in passing from the isolated groups with their more nearly normal facial developments, to the groups of the lower valleys, is the marked irregularity of the teeth with narrowing of the arches and other facial features. In the lower half of Fig. 4 may be seen two such cases. While in the isolated groups not a single case of a typical mouth-breather was found, many were seen among the children of the lower-plains group. The children studied were from ten to sixteen years of age.

Many individuals in the modernized districts bore on their faces scars which indicated that the abscess of an infected tooth had broken through to the external surface where it had developed a fistula with resultant scar tissue, thus producing permanent deformity.

Bad as these conditions were, we were told that they were better than the average for the community. The ravages of dental caries had been strikingly evident as we came in contact with the local and traveling public. As we had at St. Moritz, we found an occasional child with much better teeth than the average. Usually the answer was not far to seek. For example, in one of the St. Moritz groups, in a class of sixteen boys, there were 158 cavities, or an average of 9.8 cavities per person (fillings are counted as cavities). In the cases of three other children in the same group, there were only three cavities, and one case was without dental caries. Two of these three had been eating dark bread or entire-grain bread, and one was eating dark bread and oatmeal porridge. All three drank milk liberally.

When looking here for the source of dairy products one is impressed by the absence of cows at pasture in the plains of Switzerland, areas in which a large percentage of the entire population resides. True, one frequently sees large laiteries or creameries, but the cows are not in sight. On asking the explanation for this, I found that a larger quantity of milk could be obtained from the cows if they were kept in the stables during the period of high production. Indeed, this was a necessity in most of these communities since there were so few fences, and during the time of the growth of the crops, including the stock feed for the winter's use, it was necessary that the cows be kept enclosed. About the only time that cows were allowed out on pasture was in the fall after the crops had been harvested and while the stubble was being plowed.

Among the children in St. Moritz and Herisau, those groups with the lower number of cavities per person were using milk more or less liberally. Of the

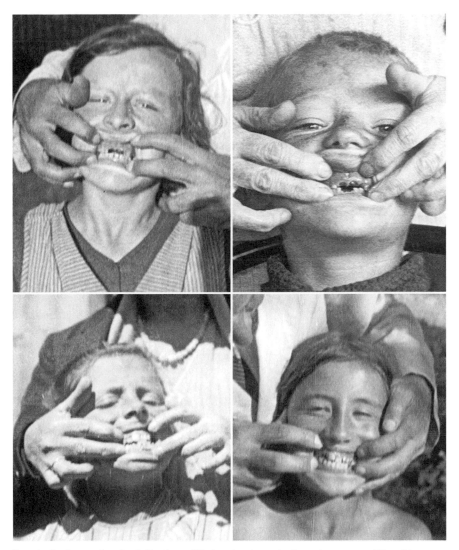

FIG. 4. In the modernized districts of Switzerland, tooth decay is rampant. The girl, upper left, is sixteen and the one to the right is younger. They use white bread and sweets liberally. The two children below have very badly formed dental arches with crowding of the teeth. This deformity is not due to heredity.

total number of children examined in both places only 11 percent were using milk in their diets, whereas 100 percent of the children in the other districts that provided immunity were using milk. Nearly every child in St. Moritz was eating white bread. In Herisau, all but one of the children examined were eating white bread in whole or in principal part.

Since so many cattle were stall-fed in the thickly populated part of Switzerland, and since so low a proportion of the children used milk even sparingly, I was concerned to know what use was made of the milk. Numerous road signs announcing the brand of sweetened milk chocolate made in the several districts suggested one use. This chocolate is one of the important products for export and as a beverage constitutes a considerable item in the nutrition of large numbers living in this and in other countries. It is recognized as a high source of energy, primarily because of the sugar and chocolate which when combined with the milk greatly reduces the ratio of the minerals to the energy factors as expressed in calories.

It was formerly thought that dental caries which were so rampant in the greater portion of Switzerland was due in part to low iodine content in the cattle feed and in other food because of iodine deficiency in the soil. Large numbers of former generations suffered from clinical goiter and various forms of thyroid disturbances. That this is not the cause seems clearly demonstrated by the fact that dental caries is apparently as extensive today as ever before, if not more so, while the iodine problem has been met through a reinforcement of the diet of growing children and others in stress periods with iodine in suitable form. Indeed the early work done in Cleveland by Crile, Marine, and Kimball was referred to by the medical authorities there as being the forerunner of the control of the thyroid disorder in these communities.

The officials of the Herisau community were so deeply concerned regarding the prevalence of dental caries that they were carrying forward institutional and community programs with the hope of checking this affliction. If dental caries were primarily the result of an inadequate amount of vitamin D, then sunning the patients should provide an adequate reinforcement. This is one of the principal purposes for getting the growing boys and girls of the community into sunsuits for tanning their bodies.

Another procedure to which my attention was called consisted of adding to the bread a product high in lime, which was being obtained in the foothills of the district. This and other types of bread were studied by chemical analyses. Clinically, tooth decay was not reduced.

I made an effort to establish a clinic in a neighboring town for the purpose of demonstrating with a group of children that dental caries can be controlled by a simple nutritional program. An interesting incident developed in connection with the selection of the children for this experimental group. When parents were asked to permit their children to have one meal a day reinforced, according to a program that has proved adequate with my clinical groups in Cleveland, the objection was made that there was no use trying to save the teeth of the girls. The girls should have all their teeth extracted and artificial teeth provided before they were married, because if they did not they would lose them then.

It is of interest that the southern part of Switzerland including the high Alpine country is largely granite. The hills in the northern part of Switzerland are largely limestone in origin. A great number of people live in the plain between these two geologic formations, a plain which is largely made of alluvial deposits which have been washed down from the upper formations. The soil is extraordinarily fertile soil and has supported a thrifty and healthy population in the past.

When I asked a government official what the principal diseases of the community were, he said that the most serious and most universal was dental caries, and the next most important, tuberculosis; and that both were largely modern diseases in that country.

When I visited the famous advocate of heliotherapy, Dr. Rollier, in his clinic in Leysin, Switzerland, I wondered at the remarkable results he was obtaining with heliotherapy in nonpulmonary tuberculosis. I asked him how many patients he had under his general supervision and he said about thirty-five hundred. I then asked him how many of them come from the isolated Alpine valleys and he said that there was not one; but that they were practically all from the Swiss plains, with some from other countries.

I inquired of several clinicians in Switzerland what their observations were with regard to the association of dental caries and tuberculosis among the people of Switzerland. I noted that the reports indicated that the two diseases were generally associated. We will find a corollary to this in many studies in other parts of the world.

These studies in Switzerland, as briefly presented here, seem to demonstrate that the isolated groups dependent on locally produced natural foods have nearly complete natural immunity to dental caries, and that the substitution of modern dietaries for these primitive natural foods destroys this immunity whether in ideally located elevated districts like St. Moritz or in the beautiful and fertile plains of lower Switzerland. The question seems to answer itself in a general way, without much laboratory data, from the results of a critical examination of the foods. The laboratory analyses, however, identify the particular factors in the foods which are primarily responsible by their presence for establishing immunity, and by their absence in inducing susceptibility to dental caries. These chemical data are discussed in Chapter 15.

High immunity to dental caries, freedom from deformity of the dental arches and face, and sturdy physiques with high immunity to disease were all found associated with physical isolation, and with forced limitation in selection of foods. This resulted in a very liberal use of dairy products and whole-rye bread, in connection with plant foods, and with meat served about once a week.

The individuals in the modernized districts were found to have widespread tooth decay. Many had facial and dental arch deformities and much susceptibility to diseases. These conditions were associated with the use of refined cereal flours, a high intake of sweets, canned goods, sweetened fruits, chocolate, and greatly reduced use of dairy products.

Chapter 4

ISOLATED AND MODERNIZED GAELICS (GAELS)

STORIES have long been told of the superb health of the people living in the Islands of the Outer Hebrides. The smoke oozing through the thatched roofs of their "black houses" has added weirdness to the description of their home life and strange environment. These stories have included a description of their wonderfully fine teeth and their stalwart physiques and strong characters. They, accordingly, provide an excellent setting for a study to throw light on the problem of the cause of dental caries and modern physical degeneration. These Islands lie off the northwest coast of Scotland, extending to a latitude nearly as far north as the southern part of Greenland. A typical view of their thatched-roof cottages may be seen in Fig. 5.

The Isle of Lewis has a population of about twenty thousand, made up almost entirely of fisher folk and crofters or sheep raisers. This island has so little lime in its soil that it is said that there are no trees in the entire island except a few which have been planted. The surface of the island is largely covered with peat, varying in thickness from a few inches to twenty feet. This is the fuel. Peat contains the rootlets of the plant life which grew many centuries ago. There is so little bacterial growth that vegetable products undergo very slow decay. The pasturage of the island is so poor that exceedingly few cattle are to be found, largely because they do not properly mature and reproduce. In a few districts some highland cattle with long shaggy hair and wide spread horns are found. Almost all of these are imported. The principal herd of cattle on the island consists of a few dozen head on the government experimental farm.

The basic foods of these islanders are fish and oat products with a little barley. Oat grain is the one cereal which develops fairly readily, and it provides the porridge and oat cakes which in many homes are eaten in some form regularly with each meal. The fishing about the Outer Hebrides is specially favorable, and small sea foods, including lobsters, crabs, oysters and clams, are abundant. An important and highly relished article of diet has been baked cod's head stuffed with chopped cod's liver and oatmeal. The principal port of the Isle of Lewis is Stornoway with a fixed population of about four thousand and a floating population of seamen over week-ends, of an equal or greater number. The Sunday we spent there, 450 large fishing boats were said to be in the port for the week-end. Large quantities of fish are packed here for

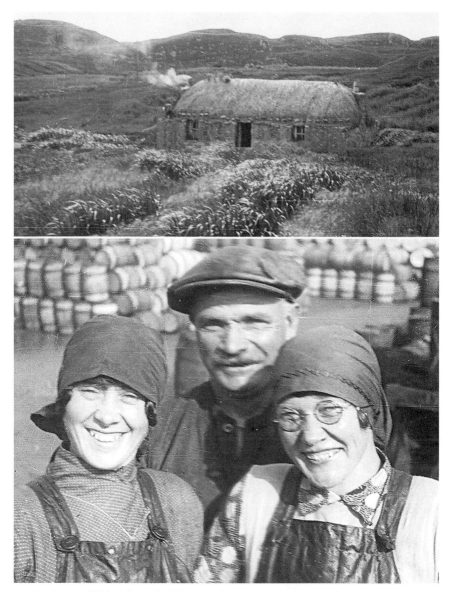

Fig. 5. A typical "black house" of the Isle of Lewis derives its name from the smoke of the peat burned for heat. The splendid physical development of the native Gaelic fisherfolk is characterized by excellent teeth and well-formed faces and dental arches.

foreign markets. These hardy fisherwomen often toil from six in the morning to ten at night. The abundance of fish makes the cost of living very low.

In Fig. 5 may be seen three of these fisher-people with teeth of unusual perfection. We saw them at the fish-cleaning benches from early morning till late at night dressed, as you see them pictured, in their oilskin suits and rubber boots. We met them again in their Sunday attire taking important parts in the leading church. It would be difficult to find examples of womanhood combining a higher degree of physical perfection and more exalted ideals than these weather-hardened toilers. Theirs is a land of frequent gales, often sleet-ridden or enshrouded in penetrating cold fogs. Life is full of meaning for characters that are developed to accept as everyday routine raging seas and piercing blizzards representing the accumulated fury of the treacherous north Atlantic. One marvels at their gentleness, refinement and sweetness of character.

The people live in these so-called black houses. These are thatched-roof dwellings containing usually two or three rooms. The walls are built of stone and dirt, ordinarily about five feet in thickness. There is usually a fireplace and chimney, one or two outside doors, and very few windows in the house. The thatch of the roofs plays a very important role. It is replaced each October and the old thatch is believed by the natives to have great value as a special fertilizer for their soil because of its impregnation with chemicals that have been obtained from the peat smoke which may be seen seeping through all parts of the roof at all seasons of the year. Peat fires are kept burning for this explicit purpose even when the heat is not needed. This means that enormous quantities of peat are required to maintain a continuous smudge. Some of the houses have no chimney because it is desirable that the smoke leave the building through the thatched roof. Not infrequently smoke is seen rolling out of an open door or open window. Fortunately the peat is so abundant that it can be obtained easily from the almost limitless quantities nearby. The sheep that roam the heather-covered plains are of a small black-faced breed, exhibiting great hardihood. They provide wool of specially high quality, which, incidentally, is the source of the famous Harris Tweeds which are woven in these small black houses chiefly on the Isle of Harris.

We are particularly concerned with the people of early Scotch descent who possess a physique that rivals that found in almost any place in the world. They are descendants of the original Gaelic stock which is their language to-day, and the only one which a large percentage of them can speak. This island has only one port which means that most of the shore line still provides primitive living conditions as does the central part of the island. It was a great surprise, and indeed a very happy one, to find such high types of manhood and womanhood as exist among the occupants of these rustic thatched-roof homes, usually located in an expanse of heather-covered treeless plains. It would be hard to visualize a more complete isolation for child life than many of these homes provide, and one marvels at the refinement, intelligence, and strength of character of these rugged people. They resent, and I think justly so, the critical and uncomplimentary references made to their homes in attaching to them the name "black-houses." Several that we visited were artistically decorated with clean wallpaper and improvised hangings.

One would expect that in their one seaport town of Stornoway things would be gay over the week-end, if not boisterous, with between four and five thousand fishermen and seamen on shore-leave from Saturday until midnight Sunday. On Saturday evening the sidewalks were crowded with happy carefree people, but no boisterousness and no drinking were to be seen. Sunday the people went in throngs to their various churches. Before the sailors went aboard their crafts on Sunday evening they met in bands on the street and on the piers for religious singing and prayers for safety on their next fishing expedition. One could not buy a postage stamp, a picture card, or a newspaper, could not hire a taxi, and could not find a place of amusement open on Sunday. Everybody has reverence for the Sabbath day on the Isle of Lewis. Every activity is made subservient to their observance of the Sabbath day. In few places in the world are moral standards so high. One wonders if the bleak winds which thrash the north Atlantic from our Labrador and Greenland coasts have not tempered the souls of these people and created in them higher levels of nobility and exalted human expression. These people are the outposts of the western fringe of the European continent.

Just as one sees in Brittany, on the west coast of France, the prehistoric druidical stone forest marking a civilization which existed so far in the past as to be without historic records except in its monuments; so, too, we find here the forest of granite slabs in which these sturdy prehistoric souls worshipped their divinities before they were crowded into the sea by the westward moving hordes. When one realizes the distance that these heavy stones had to be transported, a distance of probably twenty miles over difficult terrain, we can appreciate the task. Their size can be calculated from the depth to which they must be buried in order to stand erect even to this day.

We are concerned primarily with the physical development of the people, and particularly with their freedom from dental caries or tooth decay. One has only to see them carrying their burdens of peat or to observe the ease with which the fisherwomen on the docks carry their tubs of fish back from the cleaning table to the tiers of packing barrels to be convinced that these people have not only been trained to work, but have physiques equal to the task. These studies included the making of dental examinations, the taking of photographs, the obtaining of samples of saliva for chemical analysis, the gathering of detailed clinical records, and the collecting of samples of food for chemical analysis and detailed nutritional data.

Communication is very difficult among many of these islands. It would be difficult to find more complete isolation than some of them afford. We tried to get to the islands of Taransay and Scarpa on the west coast of the Isle of Harris, but were unable to obtain transportation since the trip can be made only in special, seaworthy crafts, which will undertake the passage only at certain phases of the tide and at certain directions of the winds. On one of these islands, we were told, the growing boys and girls had exceedingly high immunity to tooth decay. Their isolation was so great that a young woman of about twenty years of age who came to the Isle of Harris from Taransay Island had never seen milk in any larger quantity than drops. There are no dairy animals on that island. Their nutrition is provided by their oat products and fish, and by a very limited amount of vegetable foods. Lobsters and flat fish are a very important part of their foods. Fruits are practically unknown. Yet the physiques of these people are remarkably fine.

It was necessary sometimes for us to engage skilled seamen and their crafts to make a special trip to some of these isolated islands. These seamen watch critically the tide, wind and sky, and determine the length of time it will be safe to travel in a certain direction under conditions existing in the speed of the running tide and the periodic change of the wind. Some of the islands are isolated by severe weather conditions for many months of the year.

These islands have been important in the whaling industry, even up to recent years. We visited a whaling station on the Isle of Harris, not active at this time, where monsters of the sea were towed into a deep bay.

In the interior of the Isle of Lewis the teeth of the growing boys and girls had a very high degree of perfection, with only 1.3 teeth out of every hundred examined that had even been attacked by dental caries.

An important part of the study of these islands was the observations made on conditions at the fringe of civilization. A typical cross-section of the residents of the seaport town of Stornoway can be seen assembled on the docks to greet the arrival of the evening boat, the principal event of the community. The group consists largely of adult young people. In a count of one hundred individuals appearing to be between the ages of twenty and forty, twenty-five were already wearing artificial teeth, and as many more would have been more presentable had they too been so equipped. Dental caries was very extensive in the modernized section of Stornoway. Since an important part of these studies involved a determination of the kinds and quantities of foods eaten, it was necessary to visit the sources available for purchasing foods in each town studied. In Stornoway, one could purchase angel food cake, white bread, as snow white as that to be found in any community in the world, many other white-flour products; also, canned marmalades, canned vegetables, sweetened fruit juices, jams, confections of every type filled the store windows and counters. These foods probably made a great appeal both because of their variety and their high sugar content to the pallets of these primitive people. The difference in physical appearance of the child life of Stornoway from that of the interior of the Isle of Lewis was striking. We found a family on the opposite coast of the island where the two boys shown in the upper half of Fig. 6 resided. One had excellent teeth and the other had rampant caries. These boys were brothers eating at the same table. The older boy, with excellent teeth, was still enjoying primitive food of oatmeal and oatcake and sea foods with some limited dairy products. The younger boy, seen to the left, had extensive tooth decay. Many teeth were missing including two in the front. He insisted on having white bread, jam, highly sweetened coffee and also sweet chocolates. His father told me with deep concern how difficult it was for this boy to get up in the morning and go to work.

One of the sad stories of the Isle of Lewis has to do with the recent rapid progress of the white plague. The younger generation of the modernized part of the Isle of Lewis is not showing the same resistance to tuberculosis as their ancestors. Indeed a special hospital has been built at Stornoway for the rapidly increasing number of tubercular patients, particularly for girls between twenty and thirty years of age. The superintendent told me with deep concern of the rapidity with which this menace is growing. Apparently very little consideration was being given to the change in nutrition as a possible explanation for the failure of this generation to show the defense of previous generations against pulmonary tuberculosis. In this connection much blame had been placed upon the housing conditions, it being thought that the thatched-roof house with its smoke-laden air was an important contributing factor, notwithstanding the fact that former generations had been free from the disease. I was told that the incidence of tuberculosis was frequently the same in the modern homes as it was in the thatched-roof homes. It was of special interest to observe the mental attitude of the native with regard to the thatched-roof house. Again and again, we saw the new house built beside the old one, and the people apparently living in the new one, but still keeping the smoke smudging through the thatch of the old thatched-roof house. When I inquired regarding this I was told by one of the clearthinking residents that this thatch collected something from the smoke which when put in the soil doubled the growth of plants and yield of grain. He showed me with keen interest two patches of grain which seemed to demonstrate the soundness of his contention.

I was particularly interested in studying the growing boys and girls at a place called Scalpay in the Isle of Harris. This Island is very rocky and has only small patches of soil for available pasturage. For nutrition, the children of this community were dependent very largely on oatmeal porridge, oatcake and sea foods. An examination of the growing boys and girls disclosed the fact that only one tooth out of every hundred examined had ever been attacked by tooth

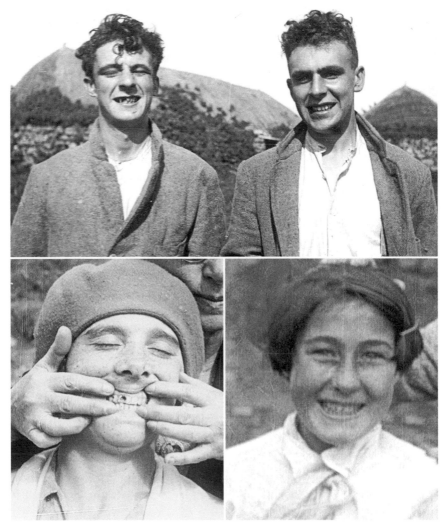

FIG. 6. Above: brothers, Isle of Harris. The younger at left uses modern food and has rampant tooth decay. Brother at right uses native food and has excellent teeth. Note narrowed face and arch of younger brother. Below: typical rampant tooth decay, modernized Gaelic. Right: typical excellent teeth of primitive Gaelic.

decay. The general physical development of these children was excellent, as may be seen in the upper half of Fig. 7. Note their broad faces.

This is in striking contrast with the children of the hamlet of Tarbert which is the only shipping port on the Isle of Harris, and the place of export of most of the famous Harris Tweeds which are manufactured on looms in the various crofters' homes. These Tarbert children had an incidence of 32.4 carious teeth out of every hundred teeth examined. The distance between these two points is not over ten miles and both have equal facilities for obtaining sea foods, being on the coast. Only the latter, however, has access to modern foods, since it supports a white bread bakery store with modern jams, marmalades, and other kinds of canned foods. In studying the tragedy of the rampant tooth decay in the mouth of a young man, I asked him regarding his plans and he stated that he was expecting to go to Stornoway about sixty miles away in the near future, where there was a dentist, and have all his teeth extracted and plates made. He said that it was no use to have any teeth filled, that he would have to lose them anyway since that was everybody's experience in Tarbert. The young women were in just as poor a condition.

Through the department of dental inspection for north Scotland, I learned of a place on the Isle of Skye, Airth of Sleat, in which only a few years ago there were thirty-six children in the school, and not one case of dental caries in the group. My examination of the children in this community disclosed two groups, one living exclusively on modern foods, and the other on primitive foods. Those living on primitive foods had only 0.7 carious teeth per hundred, while those in the group living on modern foods had 16.3, or twenty-three times as many.

This community living near the sea had recently been connected with the outside world by daily steamboat service which delivered to the people modern foods of various kinds, and within this community a modern bakery, and a supply house for purchasing the canned vegetables, jams and marmalades had been established. This district was just in the process of being modernized.

I examined teeth of several people in their seventies and eighties, and except for gingival infections with some loosening of the teeth, nearly all of the teeth were present and there was very little evidence that dental caries had ever existed. The elderly people were bemoaning the fact that the generation that was growing up had not the health of former generations. I asked what their explanation was and they pointed to two stone grinding mills which they said had ground the oats for oatcake and porridge for their families and preceding families for hundreds of years. Though they prized them highly, the plea that they would be helpful in educational work in America induced them to sell the mills to me. They told us with great concern of the recent rapid decline in health of the young people of this district.

This one-time well-populated Island, the misty Isle of Skye, still has one of the finest of the famous old castles, that belonging to the Dunvegan clan. It participated in the romantic life of Prince Charlie. The castle equipment still boasts the grandeur of a past glory. Among the relics is a horn which measured the draft to be drunk by a prospective chieftain before he could aspire to the leadership of the clan. He must drink its contents of two quarts

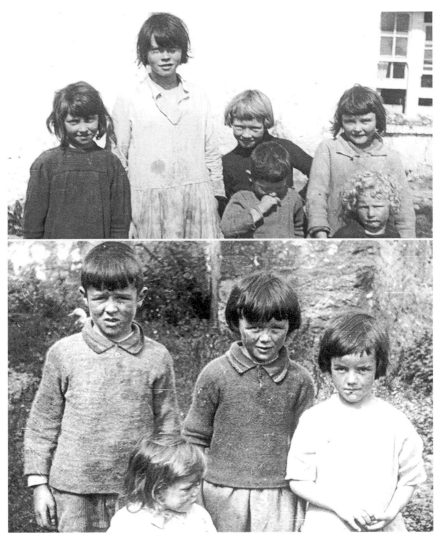

FIG. 7. Above: typical rugged Gaelic children, Isle of Harris, living on oats and sea food. Note the breadth of the faces and nostrils. Below: typical modernized Gaelics, Isle of Bardsey. Note narrowed faces and nostrils.

without stopping. Again the character of that manhood is reflected in the fact that although a bounty of thirty thousand pounds was placed upon the head of Prince Charlie, none of the many who knew his place of hiding betrayed it.

On my return from the Outer Hebrides to Scotland, I was concerned to obtain information from government officials relative to the incidence of tooth decay and the degenerative diseases in various parts of north Scotland.

I was advised that in the last fifty years the average height of Scotch men in some parts decreased four inches, and that this had been coincident with the general change from high immunity to dental caries to a loss of immunity in a great part of this general district. A study of the market places revealed that a large part of the nutrition was shipped into the district in the form of refined flours and canned goods and sugar. There were very few herds of dairy cattle to be seen. It was explained that even the highland cattle did not do as well as formerly on the same ranges.

As one proceeds from the north of Scotland southward to England and Wales, there is a marked increase in the percentage of individuals wearing artificial restorations or in need of them. In several communities this reached fifty percent of adults over thirty years of age. An effort was made to find primitive people in the high country of Wales, but without success. We were advised that about the only place that we would be likely to find people living under primitive conditions would be on the Island of Bardsey off the northwest coast of Wales. This is a rock and storm-bound island with the decadent walls of an old castle and a community made up largely of recently imported colonists whom we were advised had been taken to the Island to re-populate it. There is considerable good farm land, but very limited grazing stock. Formerly the Island had produced the foods for its inhabitants with the assistance of the sea. These sources of natural foods have been largely displaced with imported white flour, marmalades, sugar, jams and canned goods. We found the physical condition of the people very poor, particularly that of the growing boys and girls. Tooth decay was so wide-spread that 27.6 out of every hundred teeth examined in the growing boys and girls had already been attacked by dental caries. It was even active in three year olds. From a conference with the director of public health of this district I learned that tuberculosis constituted a very great problem, not only for the people on this island, but for those of many districts of northern Wales. This was ascribed to the lowered defense of the people due to causes unknown. It had been noted that individuals with rampant tooth decay were more susceptible to pulmonary tuberculosis.

While on the Island of Bardsey, I inquired as to what they thought was the cause of such extensive tooth decay as we found, and was told that they were familiar with the cause and that it was due to close contact with the salt water and salt air. When I asked why many of the old people who had lived by the sea all their lives in some districts still had practically all their teeth and had never had tooth decay, no explanation was available. This they said was the reason that had been given in answer to their inquiries.

There is a very remarkable history written in the ruins of the island, and in the faces of the people who live on the Island of Bardsey. The rugged walls of ancient castles bespeak the glory and power of the people who lived proudly in past centuries. They are testified to also by the monuments in the cemeteries; but a new era has come to this island. The director of public health, of this district of Wales, including Bardsey Island, told me the story of the decline and almost complete extinction of the population due to tuberculosis. He also told how the government had re-populated the Island with fifty healthy young families, and then the sad story of how these new settlers were breaking down as rapidly as the former occupants.

The lower photograph in Fig. 7 is of a family of four children in whose faces the tragic story is deeply written. Everyone is a mouth-breather and everyone has rampant tooth decay. These people are products of modernization on this island which one time produced vigorous children and stalwart men and women. It is important to compare the faces of the children of the Isle of Bardsey shown in Fig. 7 below with those shown in Fig. 7 above living in an isolated district in the Isle of Harris. As we will see later, the facial deformity does not reach its maximum severity until the eruption of the second dentition and the development of the adult face, usually at from nine to fourteen years of age. In cases of extreme injury, however, we find it appearing in the childhood face during the period of temporary or deciduous dentition. These children will, doubtless, be much more seriously deformed when their permanent dentitions and adult faces develop. It is important for us to keep this picture in mind in its relation to the high incidence of tuberculosis as we read succeeding chapters and find the part played by modernization in breaking down the defense of individuals to infective processes including tuberculosis.

In Fig. 6 (lower left) is a young girl from the Isle of Bardsey. She is about seventeen years of age. Her teeth were wrecked with dental caries, the disease involving even the front teeth. We ate a meal at the home in which she was living. It consisted of white bread, butter and jam, all imported to the island. This is in striking contrast with the picture of the girl shown in Fig. 6 (lower right) living in the Isle of Lewis, in the central area. She has splendidly formed dental arches and a high immunity to tooth decay. Her diet and that of her parents was oatmeal porridge and oatcake and fish which built stalwart people. The change in the two generations was illustrated by a little girl and her grandfather on the Isle of Skye. He was the product of the old régime, and about eighty years of age. He was carrying the harvest from the fields on his back when I stopped him to take his picture. He was typical of the stalwart product raised on the native foods. His granddaughter had pinched nostrils and narrowed face. Her dental arches were deformed and her teeth crowded. She was a mouth-breather. She had the typical expression of the result of modernization after the parents had adopted the modern foods of commerce, and abandoned the oatcake, oatmeal porridge and sea foods.

Since a fundamental part of this study involves an examination of the accumulated wisdom of the primitive racial stocks, it is important that we look further into the matter of the smoked thatch. I was advised by the old

residents that a serious conflict existed between them and the health officials
who came from outside to their island. The latter blamed the smoke for the
sudden development of tuberculosis in acute form, and they insisted that the
old procedure be entirely discontinued. For this purpose the government
gave very substantial assistance in the building of new and modern homes.
The experienced natives contended that the oat crop would not mature in
that severe climate without being fertilized with the smoked thatch. While
they were willing to move into the new house, they were not willing to give
up the smoking of the oat straw used for the thatch to prepare it for fertilizing the ground. I brought some of this smoked thatch with me both for
chemical analysis and for testing for the influence on plant growth. This was
done by adding different quantities of the smoked thatch to a series of pots
in which oat seeds were planted. In Fig. 8 will be seen the result. The pot to
the right shows the result of planting the oats in a sandy soil almost like that
of the Islands of the Outer Hebrides. The oats only grew to the fuzzy limited condition shown. As increasing amounts of this thatch were added to the
soil, there was an increase in the ruggedness of the plants so that in the last
pot to the left tall stalks were developed heavily loaded with grain which

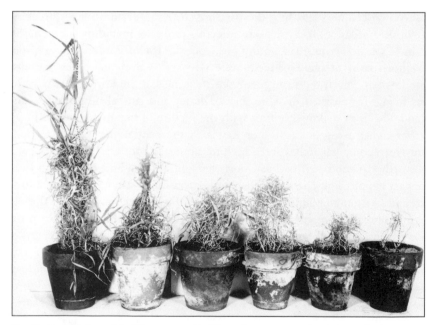

FIG. 8.   From left to right. These pots of soil growing oats contained decreasing amounts
of smoke-thatch. Only the first produced mature grain. This is in accord with the belief
and practice of the native Gaelics.

ripened by the time the growth shown in the other pots had occurred. The chemical analysis of the thatch showed that it contained a quantity of fixed nitrogen and other chemicals resulting from the peat smoke circulating through the thatch. This explains the confidence of the hardy old natives who insisted on being permitted to continue the smoking of the thatch even though they did not live in the house.

A dietary program competent to build stalwart men and women and rugged boys and girls is provided the residents of these barren Islands, with their wind and storm-swept coasts, by a diet of oats used as oatcake and oatmeal porridge; together with fish products, including some fish organs and eggs. A seriously degenerated stock followed the displacement of this diet with a typical modern diet consisting of white bread, sugar, jams, syrup, chocolate, coffee, some fish without livers, canned vegetables, and eggs.

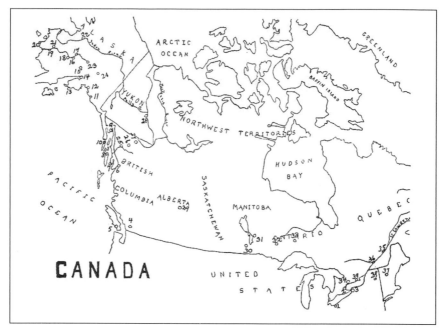

Key to Location of Indian and Eskimo Groups Examined in Canada

1. (Cleveland, Ohio)
2. Six Nation Indian Reservations, Ontario
3. Tuscarora Indian Reservations, New York
4. No. Vancouver Indian Reservation, British Columbia
5. Craigflower Indian Reservation, Victoria, British Columbia
6. Skeena River, British Columbia
7. Ketchikan, Alaska
8. Wrangell, Alaska
9. Juneau, Alaska
10. Sitka, Alaska
11. Cordova, Alaska
12. Valdez, Alaska
13. Seward, Alaska
14. Anchorage, Alaska
15. Stoney River, Alaska
16. Sleet Mute, Alaska
17. Crooked Creek, Alaska
18. Napaimute, Alaska
19. Bethel, Alaska
20. Kokamute, Alaska
21. Bethel Island, Alaska
22. Holy Cross, Alaska
23. McGrath, Alaska
24. Eklutna, Alaska
25. Telegraph Creek, British Columbia
26. Dease Lake Indian Reservation, British Columbia
27. McDames, British Columbia
28. Liard, British Columbia, Yukon Border
29. Edmonton, Alberta
30. Winnipeg, Manitoba
31. Broken Head Indian Reservation, Manitoba
32. Sioux Lookout, No. Ontario
33. Ombabika, No. Ontario
34. Toronto, Ontario
35. Loretteville Reservation, Quebec
36. Caughnawaga Reservation, Quebec
37. Vergennes, Vermont
38. Saranac Tuberculosis Sanitarium, New York
39. Mohawk Reservation, Ontario

Chapter 5

ISOLATED AND MODERNIZED ESKIMOS

DURING the rise and fall of historic and prehistoric cultures that have often left their monuments and arts following each other in succession in the same location, one culture, the Eskimo, living on until today, brings us a robust sample of the Stone Age people. The Maya race is gone, but has left its monuments. The Indian race is rapidly changing or disappearing in North America. The Eskimo race has remained true to ancestral type to give us a living demonstration of what Nature can do in the building of a race competent to withstand for thousands of years the rigors of an Arctic climate. Like the Indian, the Eskimo thrived as long as he was not blighted by the touch of modern civilization, but with it, like all primitives, he withers and dies.

In his primitive state he has provided an example of physical excellence and dental perfection such as has seldom been excelled by any race in the past or present. We are concerned to know the secret of this great achievement since his circumscribed life greatly reduces the factors that may enter as controlling units in molding this excellence. While we are primarily concerned in this study with the characteristics of the Eskimo dentition and facial form and the effect upon it of his contact with modern civilization, we are also deeply concerned to know the formula of his nutrition in order that we may learn from it the secrets that will not only aid the unfortunate modern or so-called civilized races, but will also, if possible, provide means for assisting in their preservation.

It is a sad commentary that with the coming of the white man the Eskimos and Indians are rapidly reduced both in numbers and physical excellence by the white man's diseases. We have few problems more urgent or more challenging than that means shall soon be found for preventing the extermination of the primitive Americans.

Many reports have been made with regard to the condition of the teeth of the Eskimos. Doubtless, all have been relatively authentic for the groups studied, which have been chiefly along the routes of commerce. Clearly those people would not represent the most primitive groups, which could only be located beyond the reach of contact with modern civilization. The problems involved strongly suggested the desirability of locating and studying Eskimos in isolated districts. While dog teams could furnish means of approach in the winter season, they would not be available for summer travel.

Through the kindness of Dr. Alexis Hrdlička, who has made anthropological studies of the Eskimos in many of the districts of Alaska, I learned that the most primitive groups were located south of the Yukon in the country between it and Bristol Bay including the Delta and mouth of the Kuskokwim River. A government station has been established on the Kuskokwim River for which a government boat enters the mouth of the Kuskokwim to deliver supplies. It carries officials, but not passengers. This contact with civilization has made available modern foods for a limited district, chiefly at the point at which the boat lands, namely, Bethel. A portion of these supplies is transported by a stern-wheel river boat to settlements farther up the river. A great number, however, of Eskimos live between the mouth of the Kuskokwim and the mouth of the Yukon River, on the mainland and islands, a distance of several hundred miles, and have little or no contact with this food.

Accordingly, our program for making these field studies among the Eskimos in 1933 required transportation over long distances and into districts where travelling facilities were practically non-existent by other means than by modern aeroplane. Mrs. Price accompanies and assists me with my records. Our itinerary included steamship service to Seward in western Alaska and railway to Anchorage, where an aeroplane was chartered which carried us to various districts in western and central Alaska. This plane carried our field equipment, and travelled to the points selected. The great Alaska mountain range, culminating in the magnificent Mt. McKinley, stretches across Alaska from the Aleutian Peninsula at the southwest far into the heart of this vast territory. The highest mountain in the United States proper is Mt. Whitney, 14,502 feet. The highest mountain in Canada is Mt. Logan, 19,539 feet. Alaska, however, boasts many mountains that are higher than any of these, many of which are in this range. Mt. McKinley is 20,300 feet. It was necessary for us to surmount this magnificent range to reach the territory in which our investigations were to be made. The special aeroplane selected was equipped with radio for both sending and receiving, and was in touch, or could be in touch at all times, with the Signal Service Corps, as well as with the headquarters and branches of the Company. Owing to clouds in the selected pass, the pilot found it necessary to go one hundred fifty miles out of his course to find one that was clear enough to fly through. Beyond these mountains were vast areas of bare wilderness with no signs of human life. Moose were frequently seen.

Our first objective was to find, if possible, a band of Indians reported to live on Stony River. They had been described as being very primitive. Our pilot, who was well informed about this region, said this was the first time he had even landed in this district. All the people were busy catching and storing the running salmon. After drying the fish they are smoked for a few hours and then stored for winter use. These thrifty people have physical features quite unlike the Indians of central, southern and eastern Alaska. Of the twelve individuals studied here, ten had lived entirely on the native foods or practically so. In their 288 teeth only one tooth was found that had ever been attacked by tooth decay, or 0.3 percent. Two had come up from the Kuskokwim River, of which the Stony River is a branch. There, they had received a considerable quantity of the "store grub" that had been shipped up the Kuskokwim from Bethel. Twenty-seven percent of the teeth of these two had been attacked by dental caries.

We then proceeded to Sleet Mute, on the Kuskokwim River, where three individuals were found who had lived entirely on native foods. None of them had ever had a tooth attacked by tooth decay. Seven others had lived partly on native foods and partly on "store grub," and they had dental caries in 12.2 percent of their teeth.

At Crooked Creek, the next settlement, eight individuals were examined and of their 216 teeth forty-one, or 18.9 percent, had caries. All but one of these were living in considerable part on "store grub," and this individual had no dental caries.

At Napimute, 16 percent of the teeth had been attacked by dental caries, but no individuals studied here were living entirely on native foods.

Bethel is the largest settlement on the Kuskokwim, and contains in addition to the white residents many visiting Eskimos from the nearby Tundra country surrounding it. Eighty-eight individuals studied here were largely Eskimos and mixed-bloods. Of their 2,490 teeth, 11.6 percent, or 281 teeth, had been attacked by tooth decay. Of these eighty-eight individuals twenty-seven with 796 teeth had lived almost exclusively on natural foods, and in this group only one tooth was found with dental caries, or 0.1 percent. Forty individuals were living almost exclusively on modern foods as shipped in by the government supply boat. Of their 1,094 teeth, 252, or 21.1 percent, had been attacked by tooth decay. Twenty-one individuals were living partly on native foods and partly on "store grub," and of their 600 teeth thirty-eight, or 6.3 percent, had been attacked by tooth decay.

At Kokamute, on the Bering Sea at the mouth of the Kuskokwim River, a large band of very primitive Eskimos was studied. They had come from the vicinity of Nelson Island, a district which has had exceedingly little contact with modern civilization. In this group twenty-eight individuals with 820 teeth showed only one tooth, or 0.1 percent, that had ever been attacked by dental caries.

Bethel Island is situated in the Kuskokwim River. It is visited in the summer by Eskimos from the Tundra Country for laying in their store of fish for winter use. Of fifteen individuals here, thirteen, with 410 teeth, had lived exclusively on native foods, and not a single tooth had been attacked by dental caries. Two had come from Bethel, and of their sixty teeth twenty-one or 35 percent had been attacked by tooth decay.

In the various groups in the lower Kuskokwim seventy-two individuals who were living exclusively on native foods had in their 2,138 teeth only two teeth or 0.09 percent that had ever been attacked by tooth decay. In this district eighty-one individuals were studied who had been living in part or in considerable part on modern foods, and of their 2,254 teeth 394 or 13 percent had been attacked by dental caries. This represents an increase in dental caries of 144 fold.

It next became desirable to study a district that had been in contact with the foods of modern commerce for many years, and for this Holy Cross was selected. This community is located on the Yukon River above the Arctic Circle. It has been in contact with the summer commerce of the Yukon for several decades. It has one of the oldest and best organized Catholic Missions of Alaska. The individuals studied were all in the school connected with the Mission. The students had come from as far north as Point Barrow on the Arctic Ocean and west to the Bering Straits. All but one had been in contact with and had used modern foods before coming to the Mission, and were using them while there. This one individual had lived exclusively on native foods before coming to the Mission and he had no carious teeth. In eight individuals with 224 teeth, who had lived very largely on modern foods, forty-two teeth or 18.7 percent had been attacked by tooth decay. Four individuals had lived partly on native foods and partly on modern foods, and of their 112 teeth four, or 3.5 percent, had been attacked by tooth decay.

It is of interest that while the Eskimos and Indians have lived in accord, they have not intermarried. The Eskimos occupy the lower section of the Yukon and Kuskokwim Rivers, and the Bering Sea frontier. The Indians have occupied the Upper waterways of both these rivers. The next place selected for study was McGrath, which is on the Upper Kuskokwim not far distant from the McKinley Mountain Range. It is the upper terminus of navigation on the Kuskokwim River for the stern-wheel river boats. Its chief importance lies in the fact that it is the division point on the Cross Alaska Aeroplane Routes from Anchorage or Fairbanks to Nome and other western points. Its population consists of several white prospectors and miners who have stayed in the country following the gold rush. Some of them have married Indian and Eskimo women. Of twenty-one individuals only one had lived almost exclusively on native foods and she had no dental caries. Twenty had lived chiefly on imported foods, and of their 527 teeth 175, or 33.2 percent, had been attacked by tooth decay.

Among the residents of McGrath there is a remarkable family. The father is an American mining engineer who has spent much of his life in that country. His wife is a charming Eskimo woman of splendid intelligence and fine

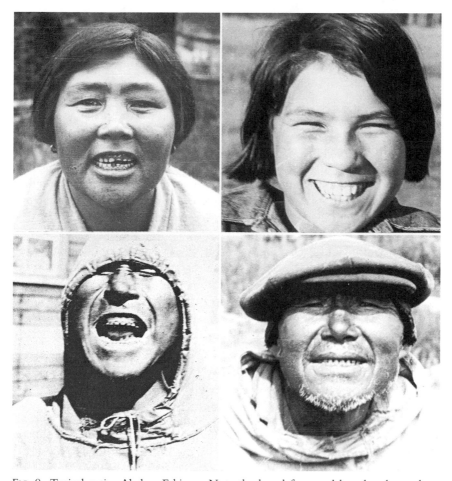

FIG. 9. Typical native Alaskan Eskimos. Note the broad faces and broad arches and no dental caries (tooth decay). Upper left, woman has a broken lower tooth. She has had twenty-six children with no tooth decay.

personality. She had come originally from the lower Kuskokwim and was one of the primitive Eskimo stock. While mining interests had provided food supplies for the family, shipped from the United States, she followed her early training and insisted on catching and storing salmon in season as an important part of her own dietary. The salmon were dried and smoked as was the custom of her people. She is the mother of at least twenty children, for she could give the names of that many. Only eleven were living, however, several having died from tuberculosis. Notwithstanding her many overloads, not a single tooth had ever been attacked by tooth decay. A lower anterior tooth had been broken. A picture of this woman is shown in Fig. 9 (upper, left).

There has been extensive wear of the teeth, as is characteristic of the teeth of many of the Eskimos, a matter which we will presently discuss. It is of interest to note the splendid symmetry of her dental arches. Her children and husband and son-in-law had lived very largely on modern foods and in these eight individuals with 212 teeth eighty-seven, or 41 percent, had been attacked by tooth decay. Her oldest living daughter is twenty-two years of age. She has a narrowing of the upper arch and extensive tooth decay. Another daughter, sixteen, is a beautiful girl except for her narrow dental arches. She was reported by our pilot to have become so deeply interested in the engines of the aircrafts as they stopped at this point for servicing and fuel that she had become expert in tuning up and conditioning aeroplane motors. She, doubtless, inherited some of the genius of her father, who is a mining engineer. Twelve of her teeth had been attacked by dental caries.

One does not get a conception of the magnificent dental development of the more primitive Eskimos simply by learning that they have freedom from dental caries. The size and strength of the mandible, the breadth of the face and the strength of the muscles of mastication all reach a degree of excellence that is seldom seen in other races. This is typically illustrated in Fig. 9. I was told that an average adult Eskimo man can carry one hundred pounds in each hand and one hundred pounds in his teeth with ease for a considerable distance. This illustrates the physical development of other parts of the body as well as the jaws, and suggests that the exercising of the jaws is not the sole reason for their very fine teeth, since the superb development of the musculature includes all parts of the body. It has also been suggested that chewing of tough foods, by building teeth of exceptionally fine quality, has been an important factor in the establishment of immunity to caries. As will be shown presently, the teeth of these individuals with their excellent physical development and fine tooth structure develop caries when they depart from their native foods and adopt our modern foods.

Much has been reported in the literature of the excessive wear of the Eskimos' teeth, which in the case of the women has been ascribed to the chewing of the leather in the process of tanning. It is of interest that while many of the teeth studied gave evidence of excessive wear involving the crowns to a depth that in many individuals would have exposed the pulps, there was in no case an open pulp chamber. They were always filled with secondary dentin. This is important since our newer knowledge indicates that with the chemical characteristics of their food we might expect that secondary dentin would be readily formed within the pulp chambers by a process similar to that which occurs in many individuals under a diet reinforced with mineral and activator-providing foods. One old Eskimo had a scar on his lower lip, which was the result of perforations for carrying a decoration as practiced by his tribe. I have found primitive tribes in several parts of the world with this marking.

The principal outer garment worn by the Eskimo for the more primitive groups consists of a parka carrying a hood which is pulled over the head and closed around the neck with a shirr string, while another shirr string controls the size of the face opening in the hood when it is up. In the summer this is made of cloth or of skin without the fur. A typical case is shown in Fig. 9. It will again be noted that the teeth are excessively worn.

Owing to the bleakness of the winds off the Bering Sea, even in the summer many of the women wear furs. A typical mother and child dressed in their warm clothing are shown in Fig. 10. The Eskimo women are both artistic and skillful in needle work. They use fur of different colors for decorating their garments. These women make artistic decorations by carving ivory from walrus teeth and from the buried tusks of the hairy mammoth that wandered over the Tundra tens of thousands of years ago. The ear decoration of this Eskimo woman is a typical design. This mother's teeth are literally "two rows of pearls." It is important to note the width of the arches. One is continually impressed with the magnificent health of the child life which is illustrated in Fig. 10. In our various contacts with them we never heard an Eskimo child crying except when hungry, or frightened by the presence of strangers. The women are characterized by the abundance of breastfood which almost always develops normally and is maintained without difficulty for a year. The mothers were completely free of dental caries, and I was told that the children of the Eskimos have no difficulties with the cutting of their teeth.

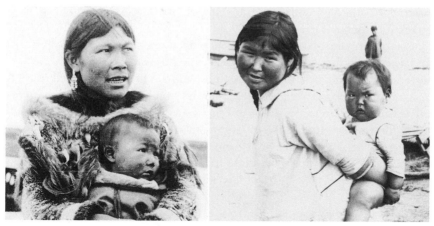

FIG. 10. These primitive Alaskan mothers rear strong, rugged babies. The mothers do not suffer from dental caries.

The excellence of dentitions among the Eskimos has been a characteristic also of the skulls that have been excavated in various parts of Alaska.

It might be expected that such wonderfully formed teeth would maintain so high an immunity to dental caries that their proud possessors would never be troubled with tooth decay. This, unfortunately, is not the case, a fact of great significance in evaluating our modern theories of the causes of dental caries. When these adult Eskimos exchange their foods for our modern foods, which we will discuss in Chapter 15, they often have very extensive tooth decay and suffer severely. This is clearly illustrated in Fig. 11, for these Eskimos' teeth had been seriously wrecked by tooth decay. They had been living on modern foods and were typical of a large number who are in contact with the Bering Sea ports. Their plight often becomes tragic since there are no dentists in these districts.

A typical effect of modernization on a growing girl was shown in a case in which the central incisors and 16 other teeth were attacked by dental caries. Sixty-four percent of her teeth had tooth decay.

There are no dentists in western Alaska, north or west of Anchorage, which is near the southern coast, except at Fairbanks which, like Anchorage, is many hundreds of miles from these Eskimos. It would take months for them to make the journey in winter by dog team, and it would be practically impossible to make it in the summer season by any means of travel except by aeroplane, which clearly these people could not afford. Their dilemma is, accordingly, most tragic when they suddenly become victims of diseases which require hospitalization or skilled medical or dental service. One mining engineer in the interior told me that he had spent two thousand dollars to have a dentist brought in by aeroplane to render dental service. On my examination of his mouth I found twenty-nine of his thirty-two teeth had been attacked by dental caries.

One important phase of modern degeneration, namely, change in facial and dental arch form and other physical expressions, is of interest. It is a matter of great significance that the Eskimos who are living in isolated districts and on native foods have produced uniformly broad dental arches and typical Eskimo facial patterns. Even the first generation forsaking that diet and using the modern diet, presents large numbers of individuals with marked changes in facial and dental arch form. In Fig. 12 will be seen four Eskimo girls who are of the first generation following the adoption of modernized foods by their parents. All have deformed dental arches. It is important to note the pattern of the settling inward of the lateral incisors and the crowding outward of the cuspids. This facial design is currently assigned to a mixing of racial bloods. These girls are pure-blooded Eskimos whose parents have normally formed dental arches.

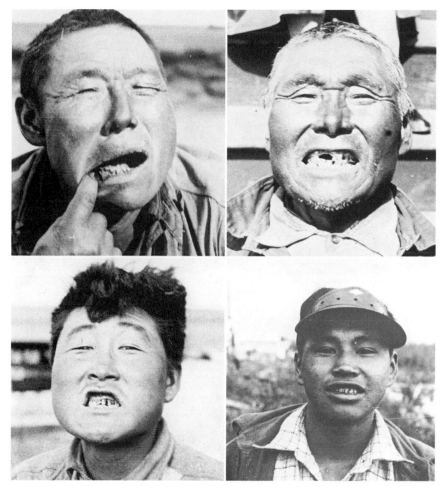

FIG. 11. When the primitive Alaskan Eskimos obtain the white man's foods, dental caries become active. Pyorrhea also often becomes severe. In many districts dental service cannot be obtained and suffering is acute and prolonged.

We are particularly concerned with the foods used by these primitive Eskimos. They almost always have their homes on or near deep water. Their skill in handling their kayaks is most remarkable. During the salmon running season they store large quantities of dried salmon. They spear many of these fish from their kayaks; even young boys are very skillful. They land salmon so large that they can hardly lift them. They are expert in spearing seals from these light crafts. Seal oil provides a very important part of their nutrition. As each piece of fish is broken off, it is dipped in seal oil. I obtained some

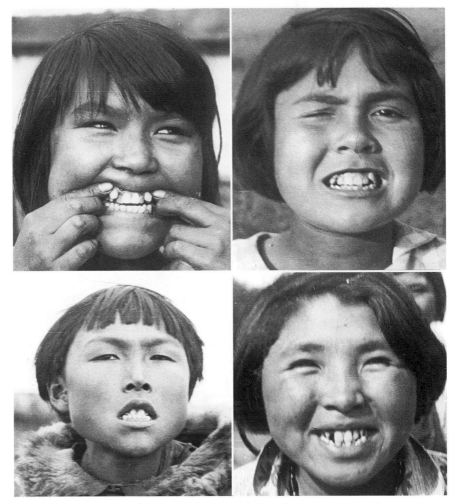

FIG. 12. While dental arch deformities or crowded teeth are practically unknown among many of the primitive groups of Eskimos, they occur frequently in the first generation of children born after the parents have adopted the white man's foods. Note the narrow nostrils and changed facial form of these children. This is not due to thumb-sucking.

seal oil from them and brought it to my laboratory for analyzing for its vitamin content. It proved to be one of the richest foods in vitamin A that I have found.

The fish are hung on racks in the wind for drying. Fish eggs are also spread out to dry, as shown in Fig. 13. These foods constitute a very important part of the nutrition of the small children after they are weaned. Naturally, the drifting sands of the bleak Bering Straits lodge upon and cling to the moist surfaces of the fish that are hung up to dry. This constitutes the principal cause for the excessive wear of the Eskimos' teeth in both men and women.

The food of these Eskimos in their native state includes caribou, ground nuts which are gathered by mice and stored in caches, kelp which is gathered in season and stored for winter use, berries including cranberries which are preserved by freezing, blossoms of flowers preserved in seal oil, sorrel grass preserved in seal oil, and quantities of frozen fish. Another important food factor consists of the organs of the large animals of the sea, including certain layers of the skin of one of the species of whale, which has been found to be very high in vitamin C.

Since contact with our modern civilization, the Eskimo population for Alaska is very rapidly declining. One authority has quoted the reduction of 50 percent in population in seventy-five years.

An important observation has been made relative to the rapid shortening of the average life by Dr. V. E. Levine and Professor C. W. Bauer, of Creighton University, Nebraska, who reported:

> Cordova, Alaska, Oct. 26, 1934—Due to susceptibility to tuberculosis and other diseases the average life span of the Eskimo of Alaska is only 20 years and their race is doomed to extinction within a few generations unless modern medical science comes to their aid.

Unless a very radical change is made in the interference with the native supply of game and sea foods, the Eskimo population seems destined to have a rapid decline and an early extinction. Their primitive fish foods have been largely curtailed by the encroachment on their salmon streams made by modern canneries.

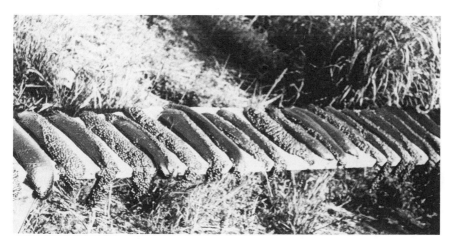

FIG. 13. The eggs of the salmon are dried and stored as an important item of nutrition for both children and adults. They are also used to increase the fertility of the women. From a chemical standpoint they are one of the most nutritious foods I have found anywhere.

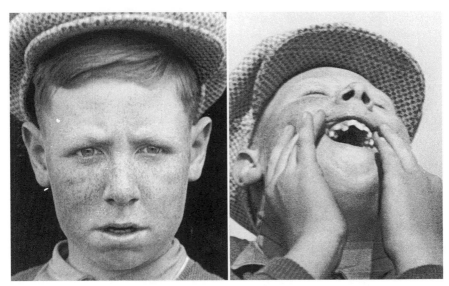

FIG. 14. This white boy was born and raised in Alaska on imported foods. His facial deformity includes a lack of development of the air passages, so that he breathes through his mouth. Lack of bone development creates the crowded condition of the teeth. Note his narrow nostrils.

It is of interest to discuss in connection with the Alaskan Eskimo two white boys (one is shown in Fig. 14), who were sons of a mining engineer. They had been born and raised in a mining camp in Alaska, where their foods had been almost entirely shipped in. I travelled with the mother of these two boys who was bringing them to the United States for operations on their noses, because they were mouth-breathers. It is important to observe the marked underdevelopment of both the middle third and lower third of the face of the boy shown in Fig. 14. The nutrition of the family during their development and growth had been largely provided in package form shipped in from the United States. Their disfiguration is typical of that of large numbers that are developing in our highly modernized communities, and is similar, in general, to the deformities which develop in the primitive races after they adopt the modernized nutrition.

Notwithstanding the very inhospitable part of the world in which they reside, with nine or ten months of winter and only two or three of summer, and in spite of the absence for long periods of plant foods and dairy products and eggs, the Eskimos were able to provide their bodies with all the mineral and vitamin requirements from sea foods, stored greens and berries and plants from the sea.

Chapter 6

PRIMITIVE AND MODERNIZED NORTH AMERICAN INDIANS

NATURE seems to have made one of her large scale demonstrations in the Americas of the power of adaptation of a single racial stock to the scale of climates ranging from torrid jungles of the tropics to the Arctics. The various members of the American Indian race seem clearly to have come from a common origin. The route by which they reached America from Asia as suggested by anthropologists was by way of the Bering Strait. Within a decade a Russian engineer has crossed from Asia to America on the pack ice of the Bering sea, a distance of ninety miles. If this is possible now, how much more likely is it that it has been possible in earlier periods of the world's history, as, for example, during or following the last ice age, or at the time of an earlier ice age. The American Indian, therefore, provides a very remarkable opportunity to study both the capacity for adaptability to different environments and the variations that different environments can produce in a single racial stock. That the Indian of today is not in general a counterpart of the native resident at the time of the discovery of America by Columbus is clearly demonstrated both by the skeletal material and by the early records.

Our problem involved the location and study of groups of the original stock, if such were to be found, who were living in accordance with the tradition of their race and as little affected as might be possible by the influence of the white man. At first thought it might seem impossible that such groups can exist, but as a matter of fact there are still great areas of the American continent inhabited by the original stock living in areas still unexplored. In order to find Indians as little changed as possible by reason of their contact with the white man, particularly with the white man's foods, I went to northern Canada to the region inside the Rocky Mountain range to study the Indians of Northern British Columbia and the Yukon territory. Since an aeroplane could not be used, owing to the lack of a base of supplies for fuel for the return trip; and since the MacKenzie water route was impracticable (an expedition could not go up the waterways through Canada on the MacKenzie River and its branches and return the same season), the route selected was that which enters that territory from Alaska on the large waterway of the Stikine River. This river has cut its channel through the Coast and Cascade Ranges of mountains and has its origin in the high western watershed of the Rockies. It was particularly desirable to reach a group of Indians who could not obtain the animal life of the sea, not even the running salmon. These fish do not enter the waterways draining to the Arctic. We used a high-powered river transport specially designed for going up rapids on the Stikine River to the end of navigation at Telegraph Creek. At this point large quantities of modern foods are stored during the short open navigation season of the summer to be exchanged for furs during the long winter. A Hudson Bay Post has been established at this point. Here a truck was chartered which took us over a trail across the Rocky Mountain Divide to the headwaters of the rivers flowing north to the Arctic. At this outpost two guides were engaged and a high powered scow chartered to make the trip down the waterways toward the Arctic on the Diese and Liard Rivers. This made it possible, in the summer of 1933, to make contact with large bands of Indians who had come out of the Pelly mountain country to exchange their catch of furs at the last outpost of the Hudson Bay Company. Most of the Indians of Canada are under treaty with the Canadian Government whereby that government gives them an annual per capita bounty. This arrangement induces the Indians in the interior to come out to the designated centers to obtain the bounty. Since it is based on the number in the family, all of the children are brought. This treaty, however, was never signed by the Indians of the British Columbia and Yukon Territory. And, accordingly, they have remained as nomadic wandering tribes following the moose and caribou herds in the necessary search to obtain their foods.

The rigorous winters reach seventy degrees below zero. This precludes the possibility of maintaining dairy animals or growing seed cereals or fruits. The diet of these Indians is almost entirely limited to the wild animals of the chase. This made a study of them exceedingly important. The wisdom of these people regarding Nature's laws, and their skill in adapting themselves to the rigorous climate and very limited variety of foods, and these often very hard to obtain, have developed a skill in the art of living comfortably with rugged Nature that has been approached by few other tribes in the world. The sense of honor among these tribes is so strong that practically all cabins, temporarily unoccupied due to the absence of the Indians on their hunting trip, were entirely unprotected by locks; and the valuables belonging to the Indians were left in plain sight. The people were remarkably hospitable, and where they had not been taken advantage of were very kind. Many of the women had never seen a white woman until they saw Mrs. Price. Their knowledge of woodcraft as expressed in skill in building their cabins so that they would be kept comfortably warm and protected from the sub-zero weather was remarkable. Their planning ahead for storing provisions and firewood strongly emphasized their community spirit. When an Indian and his family moved to a camp site on a lake or river, they always girdled a few more trees than they would use for firewood so that there would be a plentiful supply of dry standing timber for future visitors to the camp.

They lived in a country in which grizzly bears were common. Their pelts were highly prized and they captured many of them with baited pitfalls. Their knowledge of the use of different organs and tissues of the animals for providing a defense against certain of the affections of the body which we speak of as degenerative diseases was surprising. When I asked an old Indian, through an interpreter, why the Indians did not get scurvy he replied promptly that that was a white man's disease. I asked whether it was possible for the Indians to get scurvy. He replied that it was, but said that the Indians know how to prevent it and the white man does not. When asked why he did not tell the white man how, his reply was that the white man knew too much to ask the Indian anything. I then asked him if he would tell me. He said he would if the chief said he might. He went to see the chief and returned in about an hour, saying that the chief said he could tell me because I was a friend of the Indians and had come to tell the Indians not to eat the food in the white man's store. He took me by the hand and led me to a log where we both sat down. He then described how when the Indian kills a moose he opens it up and at the back of the moose just above the kidney there are what he described as two small balls in the fat. These he said the Indian would take and cut up into as many pieces as there were little and big Indians in the family and each one would eat his piece. They would eat also the walls of the second stomach. By eating these parts of the animal the Indians would keep free from scurvy, which is due to the lack of vitamin C. The Indians were getting vitamin C from the adrenal glands and organs. Modern science has very recently discovered that the adrenal glands are the richest sources of vitamin C in all animal or plant tissues. We found these Indians most cooperative in aiding us. We, of course, had taken presents that we thought would be appreciated by them, and we had no difficulty in making measurements and photographs, nor, indeed, in making a detailed study of the condition of each tooth in the dental arches. I obtained samples of saliva, and of their foods for chemical analysis. A typical Indian family in the big timber forests is shown in Fig. 15.

The condition of the teeth, and the shape of the dental arches and the facial form, were superb. Indeed, in several groups examined not a single tooth was found that had ever been attacked by tooth decay. In an examination of eighty-seven individuals having 2,464 teeth only four teeth were found that had ever been attacked by dental caries. This is equivalent to 0.16 percent. As we came back to civilization and studied, successively, different groups with increasing amounts of contact with modern civilization, we found dental caries increased progressively, reaching 25.5 percent of all of the

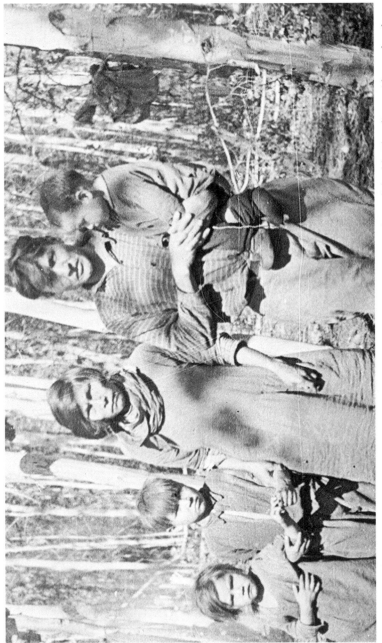

FIG. 15. This typical family of forest Indians of Northern Canada presents a picture of superb health. They live amidst an abundance of food in the form of wild animal life in the shelter of the big timber.

teeth examined at Telegraph Creek, the point of contact with the white man's foods. As we came down the Stikine River to the Alaskan frontier towns, the dental caries problem increased to 40 percent of all of the teeth.

Careful inquiry regarding the presence of arthritis was made in the more isolated groups. We neither saw nor heard of a case in the isolated groups. However, at the point of contact with the foods of modern civilization many cases were found including ten bed-ridden cripples in a series of about twenty Indian homes. Some other affections made their appearance here, particularly tuberculosis which was taking a very severe toll of the children who had been born at this center. In Fig. 16 are seen two typical cases of tubercular involvement of glands of the neck. The suffering from tooth decay was tragic. There were no dentists, no doctors available within hundreds of miles to relieve suffering.

The physiques of the Indians of the far north who are still living in their isolated locations and in accordance with their accumulated wisdom were superb. There were practically no irregular teeth, including no impacted third molars, as evidenced by the fact that all individuals old enough to have the molars erupted had them standing in position and functioning normally for mastication. The excellence of the dental arches is shown in Fig. 17. Where the Indians were using the white man's food tooth decay was very severe, as shown in Fig. 18. In the new generation, after meeting the white civilization

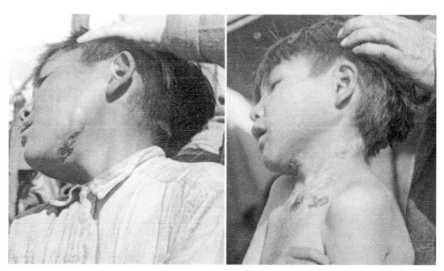

FIG. 16. At the point of modernization including the use of the foods of modern commerce, the health problem of the Indians is very different. These modernized Indian children are dying of tuberculosis which seldom kills the primitives.

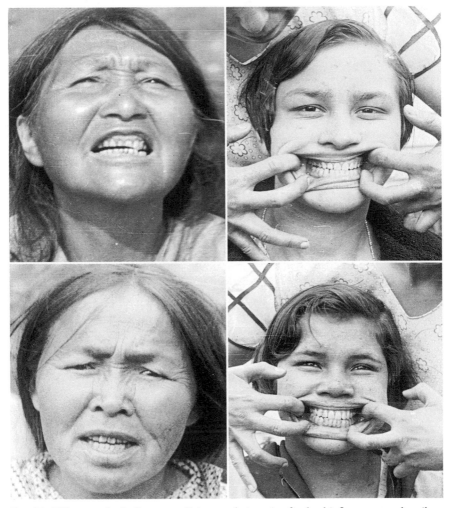

FIG. 17. Wherever the Indians were living on their native foods, chiefly moose and caribou meat, their physical development including facial and dental arch form was superb with nearly complete immunity to dental caries. These two women and two girls are typical.

and using his foods, many developed crooked teeth, so-called, with deformed dental arches, as seen in Fig. 19.

Contact was also made with representatives of relatively isolated primitive Indian stocks in the district south of Hudson Bay. These groups were reached by a newly projected railroad extending eastward and northward from Winnipeg, Manitoba, and we were thus brought into contact with the Indians that had come out of the waterways draining the Hudson Bay and from as

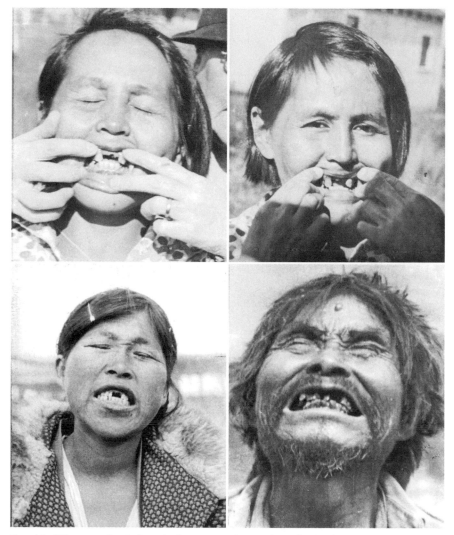

FIG. 18. Wherever the Indians had access to the modern foods of commerce, the dental conditions were extremely bad. These four individuals are typical.

far north as James Bay. They had come down to dispose of their furs in exchange for ammunition, blankets, etc. Since this contact was made only once or twice a year, it was quite impossible for the Indians to carry back a sufficient quantity of the foods of the white man to have great influence on their total diet for the year. They still lived on the wild animal game of the land. As in the northern country just reviewed, their principal large animal was the moose. These are treaty Indians, and many of them come out to this frontier

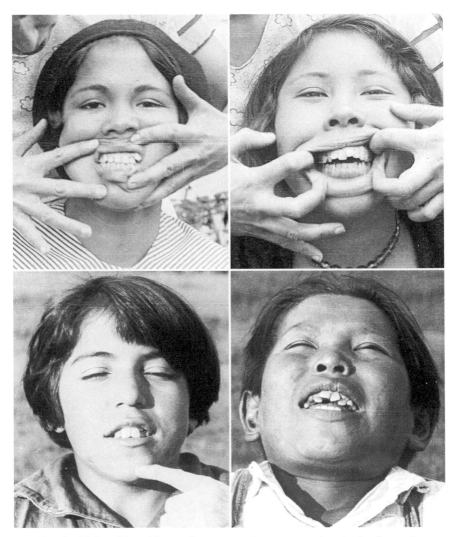

FIG. 19. The blight of the white man's commerce is seen everywhere in the distorted countenances of even the first generation after the adoption by the parents of the foods of modern commerce. These young people with their deformed dental arches are typical. Note the faulty development of the facial bones as evidenced by the narrow nostrils and crowded teeth.

to obtain the government bounty and, accordingly, were obliged to bring their families. The bounty here amounted to five dollars per head, a considerable income in exchange for blankets and other equipment. Some of these contact points were at the height of the land dividing the waters running north and east to James Bay and Hudson Bay, or south to Lake Superior. This was historic country that had been the meeting ground of the tribes of the northern waters with the tribes of the Great Lakes district. Many battles had been fought there. For comparison with these more primitive groups from the Hudson and James Bay watershed, I had the opportunity here of studying families that had taken up residence along the railroad or in its vicinity in order that they might have the advantage of exchanging furs for the modern white man's foods. This gave us an excellent opportunity to study the effects of the modern dietary, of which an example is shown in Fig. 20. This Indian and his wife had built their bodies before the contact with the white man. He is about six feet tall. Both the parents had splendid dental arches and well-formed faces. His teeth are shown in Fig. 20 (upper, left). Their two children shown in the photograph were born after the adoption of the white man's foods brought in by the railroad. Both are mouth-breathers and both have narrow dental arches and marked underdevelopment of the middle third of the face. The older girl has tuberculosis. Another adult man is shown in Fig. 20 (upper, right). He, like the generation he represents, has exceptionally fine dental arches and well-developed face.

At this point we again found many of the younger generation ill with tuberculosis or crippled with arthritis. Two of these are shown in Fig. 21.

For further comparison of the more isolated and more highly modernized groups a study was made of the Indians in the largest single Indian Reservation in Canada, which is located at Brantford, Ontario. In this group there are about 4,700 Indians living under highly modernized conditions provided by the Canadian Government. They live on very fertile land and in close proximity to a modern Canadian city. Each head of a family is provided with a tract of land from which he usually has an income sufficient to permit him to have an automobile. They were able to buy not only necessities and comforts according to the modern standards of the white man, but many of the luxuries as well. The government provides a well-administered hospital and staff. When I asked the director of this hospital, Dr. Davis, what the principal use of the hospital was at that time (1933), he said that the demand for beds had completely changed in the twenty-eight years he had been there. The principal services requested at the hospital in 1933 related to the problems of maternity. He stated that in his period of contact he had seen three generations of mothers. The grandmothers of the present generation would take a shawl and either alone or accompanied by one member of their family retire to the bush and give birth to the baby and return with it to the cabin. A problem of little difficulty or concern, it seemed. He stated that today the young mothers of this last generation are brought to his hospital sometimes after they have been in labor for days. They are entirely different from their grandmothers or even mothers in their capacity and efficiency in the matter of reproduction. He stated that that morning he had had two cases in which surgical interference was necessary in order to make birth possible.

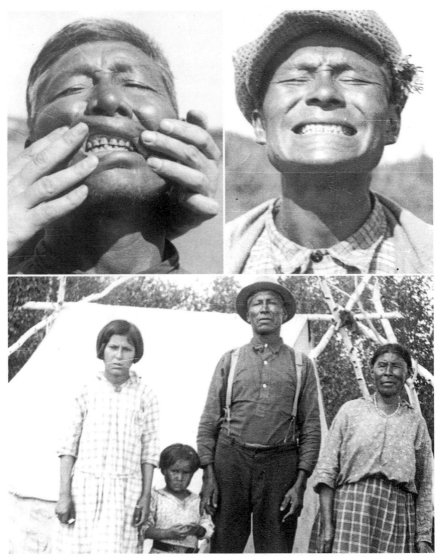

FIG. 20. These primitive Indians are in central Canada. The three parents were developed before their district was reached by modern civilization. Note their good physical and facial form in contrast with the pinched nostrils of the two children. The oldest girl has tuberculosis. They are the product of civilization's contact with their primitive parents.

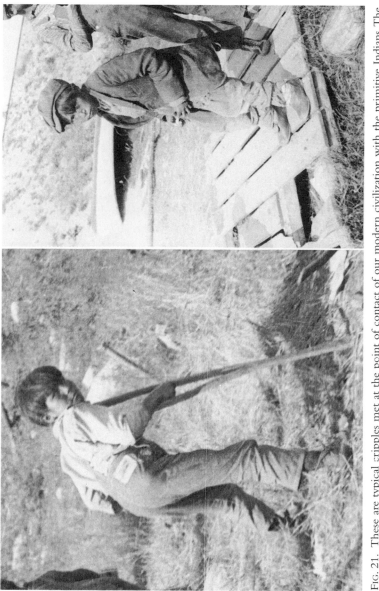

FIG. 21. These are typical cripples met at the point of contact of our modern civilization with the primitive Indians. The boy at the left has arthritis in nearly all of his joints. He has several abscessed teeth. The boy at the right has tuberculosis of the spine.

We had an opportunity here to study the effects of modernization. Indians are great lovers of sports, particularly of their own national game which is lacrosse. We were able to witness one of these contests with a team from another reservation. Indian families came in modern automobiles dressed in modern clothes and purchased pop and candy and modern confections at typical confection stands. These were highly modernized Indians.

The group on this reservation, comprising approximately four thousand seven hundred Indians, belong to the following tribes: Mohawks, Onondagas, Cayugas, Senecas, Oneidas and Delawares making up the Six Nation or Iroquois group. A later addition to this group has been the Tuscaroras from the Carolinas. While there were many mixed-bloods, there were also a goodly number of full-blooded Indian families, so that there was an opportunity to study comparatively the effects of intermingling of the Indians with the whites. As in previous investigations, a special effort was made to study the children from eight to sixteen years of age. Typical cases were selected from different environments. For example, boys and girls selected from a training school called Mohawk Institute, which was near the city of Brantford, represented one type of environment. There are approximately one hundred and sixty students under training here, and we were informed that they study half a day and work half a day. The boys are taught craftsmanship and farming, the girls, home economics and garment making, and such practical training as would prepare them for later home building. While most of the boys and girls come from that reservation, a few are accepted from other reservations. It is of interest that 77 percent of the children in this Institution had suffered from earlier dental caries and that 17 percent of all the teeth examined had already been attacked by dental caries. But this had occurred apparently before their entrance to the Institute, for we did not find a single case of active caries among those examined, and this is particularly important in connection with their excellent nutrition. The Institute maintained a fine dairy herd and provided fresh vegetables, whole wheat bread, and limited the sugar and white flour.

The children of this group were compared with children of approximately the same age in a public school of the reservation where it was found that 90 percent had had dental caries, and that at present in 70 percent of the cases the caries was apparently active. It is important to note that in this group 28.5 percent of all the teeth examined had already been attacked by tooth decay.

A study was made of patients at the reservation hospital where free service of all kinds is provided. We found that 83 percent had suffered from dental caries, and that 23.2 percent of all teeth had already been attacked by caries.

We were particularly interested in the conditions obtaining in the homes, especially with the mothers. A typical young mother had approximately half her teeth attacked by dental caries, as had also her son, aged seven. The middle third of his face was underdeveloped and all of his upper anterior teeth were decayed to the gum line.

A study was made of an Indian reservation in New York State for comparison and for making an estimate of typical modern American Indian life with regard to dental caries and nutrition. For this study a band of 450 in the Tuscarora Reservation northeast of Niagara Falls was visited. Here again we were fortunate to see the people in holiday mood since the study was made on Decoration Day and events of the year had been scheduled, a lacrosse match and a baseball game, between the Indians' teams and white teams from adjacent towns. Several hundred Indians were congregated to exhibit their best in wearing apparel, transportation equipment, and physical prowess. There was evidence of a similarity of features in the older Indians who had not been highly modernized, and a striking deficiency in the facial development of many of the moderns.

A typical mother was studied at her home. She had four children. Her teeth were ravaged by dental caries. She was strictly modern, for she had gold inlays in some of her teeth. The roots of the missing teeth had not been extracted. Twenty of her teeth had active dental caries. Her little girl, aged four, already had twelve very badly carious teeth. Another daughter aged eight had sixteen carious teeth, and her son aged ten had six. The husband was in bed from an acute lung involvement, doubtless tuberculosis. The children were eating their noon day meal when we arrived, which consisted of a white bread and some stewed vegetables. Milk was available for only the small baby in arms. In this Tuscarora group 83 percent of those examined had dental caries and 38 percent of all teeth had already been attacked by dental caries. Every one studied in this reservation was using white-flour products, none was using milk liberally, and only a few in even limited amounts. I was told that in both reservations a few years ago the Indians grew wheat and kept cows to provide a liberal supply of natural cereal and milk for their families, but of late this practice had been discontinued. They were now buying their wheat in the form of white flour and their vegetables largely put up in cans. In both reservations they were using commercial vegetable fats, jams and marmalades, sweetened goods, syrups and confections very liberally. It is remarkable how early the child life adopts modern civilization's confections.

In order to provide a further cross section of the modernized Indians of North America, I made a study in a reservation on Winnipeg Lake in Manitoba. This reservation lies north and east of Winnipeg and is quite highly modernized.

These people were reached with much difficulty because of the natural protection provided by the location of their reservation at the mouth of Brokenhead River. They had been provided with fertile lands and taught modern methods of farming. Their proximity to a great body of water fairly well-stocked with fish gave them an opportunity to secure fish, if they were disposed to make the effort to do so, as their ancestors had done through previous centuries. Their homes were found to be in a dilapidated condition, and while their lands were stocked with cattle and horses, such as we found were in poor condition, and limited in number. The people had been provided with a government school and a government agent to assist in providing for their needs and in giving material assistance when needed. They were within fairly easy distance of hospitals, and had available modern medical service. Notwithstanding all these advantages, their physical condition was very poor. Dental caries was so wide-spread that 39.1 percent of all teeth studied were found to be affected. They were living almost entirely on modern foods, imported white flours, jams, canned vegetables and liberal quantities of sugar. Over 90 percent of the individuals had rampant dental caries. Their physical condition and their supply of necessities was very much lower than was that of either of the two preceding groups. Distress was evident even in late summer.

The Indians so far reported were living inland with access to inland foods only. The Pacific Coast Indians were examined to determine the effect of sea foods. To find evidence relating to the physical, and particularly to the dental condition of the Indians who inhabited the Pacific slope a thousand or more years ago, a visit was made to the Vancouver Museum at Vancouver which fortunately possesses splendidly preserved specimens of prehistoric periods. Some of these skulls were uncovered while cutting through a hill for a street extension in the city of Vancouver. Above was a virgin forest of large size green firs and underneath them in the soil there were preserved fallen trunks of other large trees. Several feet below these, burials were uncovered containing skeletons of an early Indian race. This collection contains also skulls from several places and from prehistoric periods. The teeth are all splendidly formed and free from dental caries. The arches are very symmetrical and the teeth in normal and regular position.

It was important to study the conditions of their successors living in the same general community. Accordingly, we examined the teeth and general physical condition of the Indians in a reservation in North Vancouver, so situated that they have the modern conveniences and modern foods. In this group of children between eight and fifteen years of age, 36.9 percent of all the teeth examined had already been attacked by dental caries. No people were found in this group who were living largely on native foods.

Vancouver Island with its salubrious climate is one of the most favored places of residence on the Pacific Coast. It was of particular interest to study the Indians near Victoria on this island in the Craigflower Indian Reservation. Indeed, the city of Victoria has been partly built on the original Craigflower Indian Reservation. As the need became acute for the territory reserved for them, an arrangement was consummated whereby the Indians were induced to exchange that land for new land in an adjoining district in which a new house was built free for each family. Besides a house, an allotment of land and a sum of money, reported to be ten thousand dollars, was given to each family. This allowed them to become very modern, and, accordingly, many of them owned automobiles and other modern luxuries. The physical effects of the use of food luxuries, resulting from ample funds for purchasing any foods that they might desire, was marked. They were in close proximity to skilled dental service and had practical training in oral prophylaxis. Notwithstanding this, 48.5 percent of all teeth examined had already been attacked by dental caries. Every individual examined was suffering from tooth decay. The original diet of the Indians of the Pacific Coast was, as we shall see, very largely sea foods, which are probably as abundant today as ever before. It would require a real urge to go to catch the fish since they can now be purchased canned in the open market. Like most modern people, they were living on white-flour products, sweet foods and pastries.

Probably few cities of the Pacific Coast have had a greater abundance and variety of edible sea foods, particularly the various kinds of salmon, than Ketchikan. It is beautifully located on an island, and is the most southerly city in Alaska. Among the many fish that are abundant along this part of the Pacific Coast is the oolachan or candle fish. It is a small fish, but very rich in oil; so much so that it gets its name from being burned as a candle for light. This oil is collected in large quantities and used as a dressing for many of their sea foods. It is also traded with the Indians of the interior for furs and other products. An Indian settlement in this city was studied and it was found that 46.6 percent of all teeth examined had already been attacked by tooth decay. In many of the homes individuals were ill with tuberculosis or arthritis. Tuberculosis had robbed many of the homes of one or more of its children.

At Juneau, the capital of Alaska, two groups were studied; one in the government hospital, and the other in an Indian settlement. In the hospital were both Indians and Eskimos, chiefly the former. Seventy-five percent of the patients were reported to have been brought because they had tuberculosis, and some who had come because of accident and other conditions were reported to have tuberculosis also. Approximately 50 percent of the total hospital enrollment was under 21 years of age. The dental conditions were bad, for 39.1 percent of all the teeth examined had been attacked by tooth decay.

In the Indian settlement, a group of elderly primitives was found, every one of whom had complete dentitions in normal arrangement of the arches and without dental caries. In a settlement of modern Indians living principally on modern foods 40 percent of all teeth had been attacked by tooth decay.

At Sitka, the former capital, two important groups were studied. Located here is the Sheldon Jackson School for Eskimos and Indian boys and girls, chiefly Indians. They have come from widely scattered territory throughout Alaska, and represent the finest physical specimens that can readily be secured for giving the advantages of an education. Of necessity they came very largely from the modernized districts. In this group 53.7 percent of all the teeth examined had already been attacked by tooth decay. This gives an indication of the dental conditions in the large number of modernized districts which they represented.

In a settlement at Sitka, a group of Indians of various ages were studied, and it was found that 35.6 percent of all their teeth had already been attacked by dental caries. A well-preserved native Indian, seventy years of age, was found who had come into town from another district. He stated that his diet had consisted chiefly of fish, fish eggs, seaweed and deer. His teeth were of very high excellence and were entirely free from past or present dental caries. He is a splendid example of the product of the native dietary provided for the Pacific Coast people of any period or stage of civilization.

The local physician at Sitka kindly gave very valuable information relative to the attitude of the native Indians in the matter of obtaining fresh sea foods when foods that were very satisfying could be so easily obtained in concentrated form at the various stores. They could go to one of the piers at almost any time of the year and catch fish or secure them as they had been accustomed to do before the arrival of modern foods, but there is a constant striving to be like and live like the white people. They seem to think it is a mark of distinction to purchase their foods and that it is degrading to have to forage for one's foods. They very readily come to depend on white flour and sugar, jams and canned vegetables; and much prefer to have the government or charitable organization supply these when they cannot purchase them, rather than go out and secure their own nutrition. This physician stated that there were about 800 whites living in the town and about 400 Indians, and that notwithstanding this difference in numbers there were twice as many Indian children born as white children, but that by the time these children reached six years of age there were more white children living than Indian and half-breed children. This he stated was largely due to the very high child mortality rate, of which the most frequent cause is tuberculosis. While it does not take many decades to record a distinct physical deterioration, a deteriorating parenthood greatly speeds up this process. While physical defects acquired by the parent will not be transmitted as such, prenatal deficiencies may be established because of the physical defects of the mother resulting from her faulty nutrition, and these deficiencies, together with disturbed nutrition of infancy and early childhood will go far in determining whether there will be for the child a physical breakdown or whether the normal defense of the body will be adequate to protect it from various infections to which it may later be exposed.

Sitka has furnished the longest history of contact with white men of almost any community on the Pacific Coast. Indeed, it was a famous seaport long before any United States Pacific Coast communities had been established. It is of much interest that it was a shipbuilding center for vessels in the Russian trade. Its foundries were developed so efficiently that the bells of the early monasteries of California were cast in this town by the Russians. It contains some of the best examples of the early Russian architecture, particularly in its cathedral.

Anchorage is the principal city of western Alaska, since it is not only a base for the railroad running north to Fairbanks, but a base for aeroplane companies operating throughout various parts of Alaska. It is accordingly a combination of a coast city with its retail activities and a wholesale base for outfitters for the interior. It has an excellent government hospital which probably has been built around the life of one man whom many people told us was the most beloved man in all Alaska. He is Dr. Josef Romig, a surgeon of great skill and with an experience among the Eskimos and Indians, both the primitives and modernized, extending over thirty-six years. I am deeply indebted to him for much information and for assistance in making contacts. He took me, for example, to several typically modernized Indian homes in the city. In one, the grandmother, who had come from the northern shore of Cook Inlet to visit her daughter, was sixty-three years of age, and was entirely free from tooth decay and had lost only one of her teeth. Her son, who had accompanied her, was twenty-four years of age. He had only one tooth that had ever been attacked by tooth decay. Their diet had been principally moose and deer meat, fresh and dried fish, a few vegetables and at times some cranberries. Recently the son had been obtaining some modern foods. Her daughter, twenty-nine years of age, had married a white man and had had eight children. She and they were living on modern foods entirely. Twenty-one of her thirty-two teeth had been wrecked by dental caries. Their diet consisted largely of white bread, syrup and potatoes. Her children whom we examined ranged from five to twelve years of age, and in that family 37 percent of all the teeth have already been attacked by dental caries, notwithstanding the young age of the children. The mother of this family is shown in Fig. 18 (upper, left). It is of great importance that not only was dental caries rampant, but that there were marked deformity of the dental arches and irregularity of teeth in the cases of the children.

Among the many items of information of great interest furnished by Dr. Romig were facts that fitted well into the modern picture of association of modern degenerative processes with modernization. He stated that in his thirty-six years of contact with these people he had never seen a case of malignant disease among the truly primitive Eskimos and Indians, although it frequently occurs when they become modernized. He found similarly that the acute surgical problems requiring operation on internal organs such as the gall bladder, kidney, stomach, and appendix do not tend to occur among the primitive, but are very common problems among the modernized Eskimos and Indians. Growing out of his experience, in which he had seen large numbers of the modernized Eskimos and Indians attacked with tuberculosis, which tended to be progressive and ultimately fatal as long as the patients stayed under modernized living conditions, he now sends them back when possible to primitive conditions and to a primitive diet, under which the death rate is very much lower than under modernized conditions. Indeed, he reported that a great majority of the afflicted recover under the primitive type of living and nutrition.

The institutions that have been organized for the care of orphans and for the education of Eskimo and Indian boys and girls provide an opportunity to study conditions. A particularly favorable institution is located at Eklutna on the railroad north of Anchorage. Many of the individuals in the school had come from districts so remote from transportation facilities that their isolation had compelled them to live mostly on native foods, at least during their early childhood. They had come from districts very widely distributed throughout the Alaskan peninsula. Credit is due to the management of this institution for preparing and storing dried salmon for use throughout the winter. The beneficial effects of their good nutritional program were evident. The percentage of teeth attacked by dental caries was 14.6. A large percentage of these pupils were of mixed blood of native Eskimos or Indians with whites. The white parent had probably been largely responsible for their attendance at this training school. There were several full-blooded Eskimos and Indians from modernized communities where they had been living on modern foods throughout their entire lifetime. This gave an opportunity to study the role of nutritional deficiencies in the development of deformities and irregularities in the facial features, in the arrangement of the teeth, and in the inter-relationship between the dental arches. The typical irregularities and divergences from normal were present in the full-blooded Eskimo and Indian boys and girls in as high percentage as in the mixed-bloods. Some of the young people with parentage of mixed blood have beautiful features.

Another important institutional group was studied at Seward in the Jesse Lee Home which had first been established at Nome and had been moved to Seward to avoid the extreme isolation of that district. This institution is located at Resurrection Bay which is one of the most beautiful harbors in the world. It gives shelter and educational opportunities to Eskimos and Indians, chiefly of mixed blood, from a large area of Alaska, and particularly from the Aleutian Peninsula, the Aleutian Islands and the Bering Sea. These individuals, whether of mixed or pure blood, had come chiefly from homes that were in large part modernized. The incidence of dental caries found here was 27.5 percent for all teeth examined. Here again all individuals were affected. Notwithstanding the unusually fine hygienic conditions and highly trained dietitians of this institution, a medical ward and trained nurses, tuberculosis was reaping a heavy toll. I was told that 60 percent of all those students who had moved with the school from Nome to this location were already dead from tuberculosis. It is common knowledge that tuberculosis has played a very important role in decimating the Indian and Eskimo population in the Pacific Coast towns and villages. A very important phase of these investigations is the development of new light on the role of nutrition in lowering the defense of these individuals so that with their low inheritance of defensive factors they rapidly become susceptible to tuberculosis.

The problem of evaluating the influence of a particular environment on racial and tribal development is relatively simple when studying contemporary remnants of primitive racial stocks. However, groups that have lived and disappeared in the past do not permit of so simple a procedure for making physical estimates. Fortunately, we have in the burial grounds not only the skeletons, but also many of the implements used in daily life. Sometimes these contain samples of the foods. We may find also their art ware and hunting equipment. While the period may not be definitely recorded, the knowledge of the history of the pottery of the tribe often gives an important clue to the dates as will also the method of burial. Burials made before the advent of the Christian era will in many groups show the bodies in a flexed position with the arms in the lap, whereas in the Christian burials the bodies have been laid prone and the arms crossed on the chest. By this sign the pre-Columbian burials can readily be separated from the post-Columbian.

Using these guides, a study of the Indians of Florida, past and present, permits of comparing the pre-Columbians with those living today in that same territory. We will, accordingly, consider the dental caries problem and that of facial and dental arch form in the Florida Indians by comparing three groups: namely, the pre-Columbian, as evidenced from a study of the skull material in the museums; the tribes of Indians living in as much isolation as is possible in the Everglades and Cypress Swamps; and the Indians of the same stock that are living in contact with the foods of modern civilization. This latter group lives along the Tamiami trail and near Miami. In a study of several hundred skulls taken from the burial mounds of southern Florida, the incidence of tooth decay was so low as to constitute an immunity of apparently one hundred percent, since in several hundred skulls not a single tooth was found to have been attacked by tooth decay. Dental arch deformity and the typical change in facial form due to an inadequate nutrition were also completely absent, all dental arches having a form and interdental relationship such as to bring them into

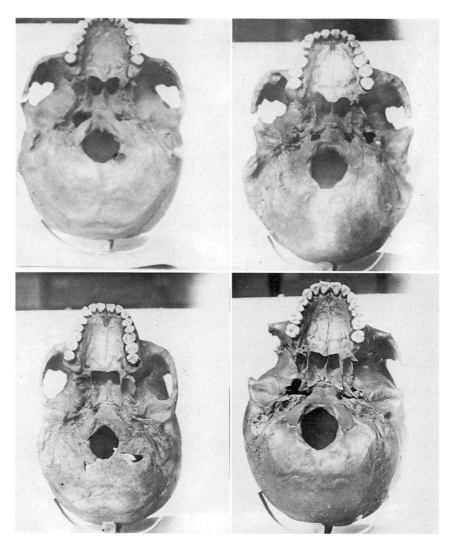

FIG. 22. Skulls of primitive Indians showing superb dental arches typical of Nature's normal plan. Note the splendid position of the third molars which are so frequently defective in position and quality in our modern white civilization. In many districts where I have made studies among primitive Indians and in many collections of their skulls close to a hundred percent of the teeth have been free from dental caries or faulty position.

the classification of normal. These are illustrated in Figs. 22 and 23. The problem of reaching the isolated groups living in the depth of the Cypress Swamps was complicated by the fact that these people had a dread of all whites growing out of their belief that they had been grossly taken advantage of in some of their early efforts to make a treaty with the whites. With the assistance of

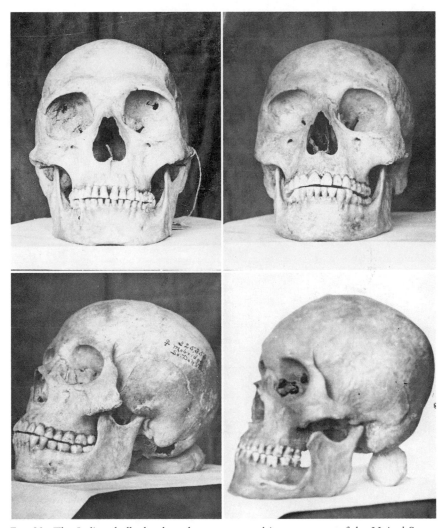

FIG. 23. The Indian skulls that have been uncovered in many parts of the United States and Canada show a degree of excellence comparable to those seen in this Figure. These levels of excellence were the rule with them, not the exception as with us. The parents of these individuals knew what they and their children should eat!

three guides, one, an Indian of their own group, another, a white man whom they trusted, and the third, a government nurse who had been very helpful in case of sickness, we were able to take the desired measurements and records and photographs. A group of these more primitive representatives is shown in Fig. 24. While their hunting territory had been grossly encroached upon

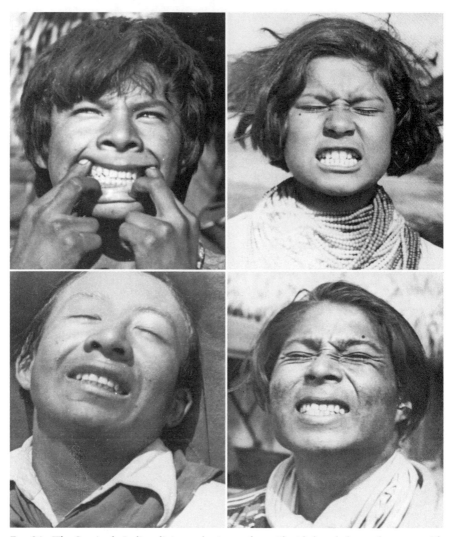

FIG. 24. The Seminole Indians living today in southern Florida largely beyond contact with the white civilization still produce magnificent teeth and dental arches of which these are typical. They live in the Everglade forest and still obtain the native foods.

by the white hunters, they were still able to maintain a very high degree of physical excellence and high immunity to dental caries. Only four teeth in each hundred examined were found to have been attacked by tooth decay.

Practically all of the dental arches were normal in contour with freedom from facial distortion. In contrast with this, the Indians of Florida who are living today in contact with modern civilization present a pathetic picture.

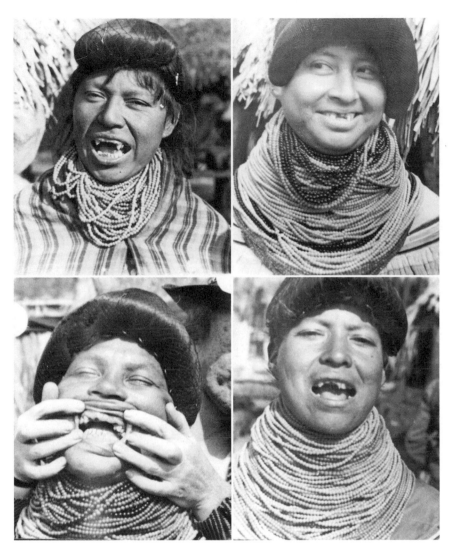

FIG. 25. The Seminole Indians of Florida who are living in contact with our modern civilization and its foods suffer from rampant dental caries.

Forty out of every hundred teeth examined were found to have been attacked by tooth decay, typically illustrated in Fig. 25. In the latest generation, many dental arches showed a typical deformation with crowding of the teeth and narrowing of the face, conditions that have been found in all human stocks when on an inadequate nutrition during the formative and early growth period. A group of these is typically illustrated in Fig. 26.

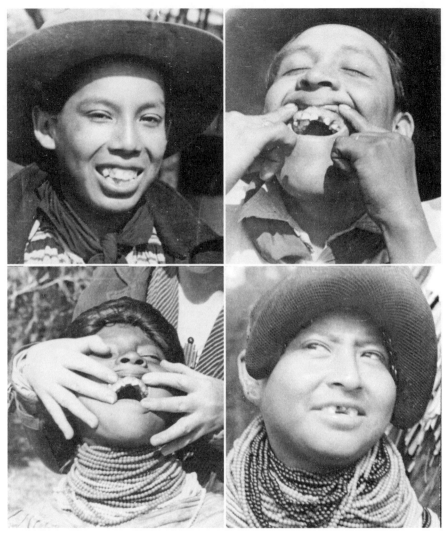

Fig. 26. Seminole Indians. Note the change in facial and dental arch form in the children of this modernized group. They have a marked lack of development of the facial bones with a narrowing of the nostrils and dental arches with crowding of the teeth. Their faces are stamped with the blight which so many often think of as normal because it is so common with us.

It is of interest that the quality of the skeletal material that is taken from the mounds showed unusually fine physical development and freedom from joint involvements. In contrast with this, many of the individuals of the modernized group were suffering from advanced deformities of the skeleton due to arthritic processes.

The effects of the excellent nutrition of the pre-Columbian Indians is indicated in the comparative thickness of the skulls. In Fig. 27 are shown two pieces of a pre-Columbian skull in contrast with a modern skull. The specimen of a trephined lower jaw, shown in Fig. 27 (right) indicates a knowledge of surgery that is very remarkable. The margins show new bone growth. The operation opened a cyst.

For the study of a group of Indians now living in a high western state, Albuquerque, New Mexico, was visited.

Several other Indian studies have been made including studies of living groups, recently opened burials and museum collections, all of which support the findings recorded here. I am indebted to the directors and to the staffs of these institutions for their assistance.

Notwithstanding the wide range of physical and climatic conditions under which primitive Indians had been living, their incidence of tooth decay while on their native foods was always near zero; whereas, the modernized Indians

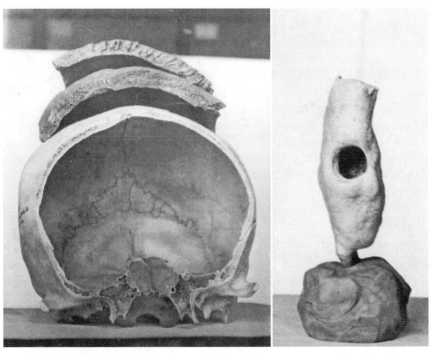

FIG. 27. Left: Example of greater thickness of pre-Columbian Indian skulls in Florida than modern skulls. Right: Illustration of bone surgery of ancient Florida Indians. Note healing of margins of trephined opening into a cyst, of the lower jaw. This is typical of the advanced surgery of the Peruvian Indians.

of these groups showed very high incidence of dental caries. A summary of percentages follows: *Primitive Indians:* Pelly Mountain, 0.16 percent; Juneau, 0.00 percent; Florida Pre-Columbian, 0.00 percent; Florida Seminoles, 4.0 percent. *Modernized Indians:* Telegraph Creek, 25.5 percent; Alaska Frontier, 40.0 percent; Mohawk Institute, 17 percent; Brantford Reservation Public School, 28.5 percent; Brantford Reservation Hospital, 23.2 percent, Tuscarora Reservation, 38.0 percent; Winnipeg Lake Reservation, 39.1 percent; North Vancouver Reservation, 36.9 percent; Craigflower Indian Reservation, 48.5 percent; Ketchikan, 46.6 percent; Juneau Hospital, 39.1 percent; Sheldon Jackson School, 53.7 percent; Sitka, 35.6 percent; Eklutna, 14.6 percent; Jesse Lee Home, Seward, 27.5 percent, and Florida Seminoles, 40.0 percent.

The foods used by the primitives varies according to location and climate. The foods of the modernized groups in all cases were the typical white man's foods of commerce.

While the primitive groups constantly presented well-formed faces and dental arches reproducing the tribal pattern, the new generation, after the adoption of white man's foods, showed marked changes in facial and dental arch form.

The Indians, like several primitive races I have studied, are aware of the fact that their degeneration is in some way brought about by their contact with the white man. The dislike of the American Indian for the modern white civilization has been emphasized by many writers. In my studies among the Seminole Indians of Florida I found great difficulty in communicating with or making examination of the isolated Seminoles living deep in the Everglades and Cypress Swamp. Fortunately, I had the able assistance of one of their own tribe, a government nurse who had been very helpful to them and also a white man who had befriended them and whom they trusted. With their assistance I was able to carry out very detailed studies. It was of interest, however, that when we arrived at a settlement in the bush we practically always found it uninhabited. Our Indian guide would go into the surrounding scrub and call to the people assuring them it was to their advantage to come out, which they finally did. I was told that this attitude had grown out of the belief on their part that their treaties had been violated. These isolated Seminole Indian women had the reputation of turning their backs on all white men.

A United States Press report[1] provides an article with the heading "Tribes 'Fed Up' Seek Solitude, Indians Dislike Civilization, Ask Land Barred to White Men." The article continues:

> The Bureau of Indian Affairs revealed today that five Indian tribes in Oklahoma are "fed up" with white civilization and want new, secluded tribal lands.
>
> So widespread is the discontent among the 100,000 Indians living in Oklahoma, officials said, that serious study is being given to the possibility of providing new lands where the redman may hunt and fish as his ancestors did.

Dissatisfaction has been brewing for a long time as a result of an increasing Indian population, decreasing Indian lands and unsatisfactory economic conditions. It was brought officially to the notice of bureau officials several days ago when a delegation, headed by Jack Gouge, a Creek Indian from Hanna, Oklahoma, told Indian Commissioner John Collier that most of the Oklahoma Indians wanted new tribal lands away from white civilization.

So anxious are his people to escape from the white man and his influences, Jack Gouge said, that an organization of about 1000 Indians has been formed to press the demands. It is known as the "Four Mothers," apparently representing four of the "civilized tribes"—the Creeks, Choctaws, Cherokees and Chickasaws.

The fifth civilized tribe, the Seminoles of Oklahoma, are negotiating with the Mexican government for tribal lands in that country.

These tribes are described as "civilized" because of the high degree of culture they attained in their original tribal lands along the eastern coast. As their eastern lands became valuable the Indians were moved to the area which is now Oklahoma. At the turn of the century, however, with the discovery of oil there the new tribal lands were broken up. The Indians were forcibly removed to small tracts despite their desire to remain together. Indian Bureau officials do not conceal their bitterness over the white man's "treachery." One official pointed out that about 300 treaties have been signed with the Indians and that practically every one has been violated.

It will be most fortunate if in the interest of science and human betterment such a program as this will be carried out in order to permit these Indians to live in accordance with the accumulated wisdom of their various tribes. Their preservation in isolation would preserve their culture. The greatest heritage of the white man today is the accumulated wisdom of the human race.

REFERENCE

[1] Tribes "Fed Up" Seek Solitude. *Cleveland Press*, June 19, 1938.

Chapter 7

ISOLATED AND MODERNIZED MELANESIANS

SINCE our quest was to gather data that will throw light upon the cause of modern physical degeneration among human racial stocks in various parts of the world, it became necessary to include for study various groups living in the hot sultry climates of the tropics. Again it was desirable to obtain contact with both highly isolated and, therefore, relatively primitive stocks for comparison with modernized groups of the same stock. In order to accomplish this an expedition was made in 1934 to eight archipelagos of the Southern Pacific to study groups of Melanesians and Polynesians. The Melanesians described here were living in New Caledonia and the Fiji Islands.

If the causative factors for the physical degeneration of mankind are practically the same everywhere, it should be possible to find a common cause operating, regardless of climate, race, or environment.

Owing to the vast extent of the Pacific waters and the limited number of transportation lines, it became very difficult to arrange a convenient itinerary. This, however, was finally accomplished satisfactorily by going southward through the more easterly archipelagos; namely, the Marquesas Islands, Society Islands and Cook Islands, then westward to the Tongan Islands in the southern central Pacific near New Zealand, and then westward to New Caledonia near Australia. From this group we went northward to the Fiji Islands, also in the western Pacific, then to the Samoan Islands in the central Pacific south of the equator, and then to the Hawaiian Islands north of the equator. These island groups were all populated by different racial stocks speaking different languages. The movements from archipelago to archipelago were made on the larger ships, and between the islands of the group in small crafts, except in the Hawaiian Islands where an aeroplane was used.

The program in each group consisted in making contact with local guides and interpreters. They had generally been arranged for in advance by correspondence with government officials. By these means we were able to reach isolated groups in locations quite distant from contact with trade or merchant ships. To reach these isolated groups often required going over rough and difficult trails since most of the islands being of volcanic formation are mountainous.

On reaching the isolated groups our greetings and the purpose of the mission were conveyed by our interpreters to the chiefs. Much time was often

94

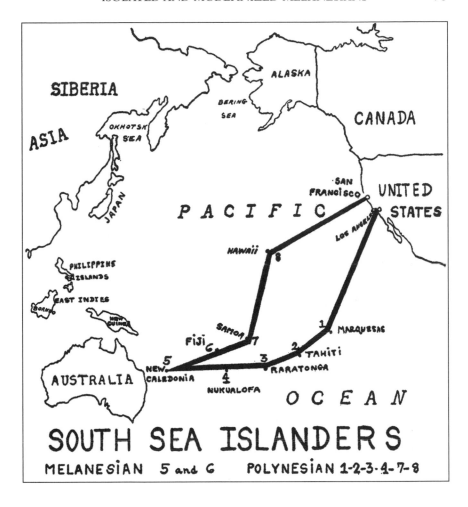

SOUTH SEA ISLANDERS
MELANESIAN 5 and 6   POLYNESIAN 1-2-3-4-7-8

lost in going through necessary ceremonials and feasting. In every instance we received a very cordial reception and excellent cooperation. In no instance was there antagonism. Through the underground telegraph they always seemed to know we were coming and had prepared for us. When these formalities were once over and our wishes made known, the chiefs instructed the members of their tribes to carry out our program for making examinations, recording personal data, making photographs, and collecting samples of foods for chemical analysis. The food samples were either dried or preserved in formalin.

The detailed records for every individual included data on the tribe, village and family, his age, previous residence, physical development, the kinds of foods eaten, the physical condition of every tooth, including presence or absence of cavities; the shape of the dental arches; the shape and development of the face; and detailed notes on divergencies from racial type. Special physical characteristics were photographed. A comparison was made of these factors for each of the more isolated members of the same tribe and those in the vicinity of the port or landing place of the island. Through the government officials detailed information was secured, usually in the form of the annual government statistical reports, showing the kind and quantity of the various ingredients and articles that were imported, and similarly those that were exported. Contact was made in each island group with the health officers, and the studies were usually made with their assistance. In many instances the only contact with civilization had consisted of the call of a small trading ship once or twice a year to gather up the copra or dried coconut, sea shells and such other products as the natives had accumulated for exchange. Payment for these products was usually made in trade goods and not in money. The following articles consisted nearly always of 90 percent of the total value: white flour and sugar. Ten percent consisted of wearing apparel or material for that apparel.

While the missionaries have encouraged the people to adopt habits of modern civilization, in the isolated districts the tribes were not able to depart much from their native foods because of the infrequency of the call of the trader ship. Effort had been made in almost all of the islands to induce the natives to cover their bodies, especially when in sight of strangers. In several islands regulatory measures had been adopted requiring the covering of the body. This regulation had greatly reduced the primitive practice of coating the surface of the body with coconut oil, which had the effect of absorbing the ultra-violet rays thus preventing injury from the tropical sun. This coating of oil enabled them to shed the rain which was frequently torrential though of short duration. The irradiation of the coconut oil was considered by the natives to provide, in addition, an important source of nutrition. Their newly acquired wet garments became a serious menace to the comfort and health of the wearers.

The early navigators who visited these South Sea Islands reported the people as being exceedingly strong, vigorously built, beautiful in body and kindly disposed. There were formerly dense populations on most of the inhabitable islands. In contrast with this, one now finds that on many of the islands the death rate has come to so far exceed the birth rate that the very existence of these racial groups is often seriously threatened.

The Island of New Caledonia is one of the largest of the Pacific. It is situated in the vicinity of 23 degrees south latitude and 165 degrees east longitude. The New Caledonians are pure Melanesian stock. They are broad shouldered, very muscular and in the past have been very warlike. These Islands are under French control. The foreign population is chiefly French, and limited mainly to the vicinity of the one port of Noumea. The subjugation of these people has been very difficult and as recently as 1917 a band from the interior in pro-

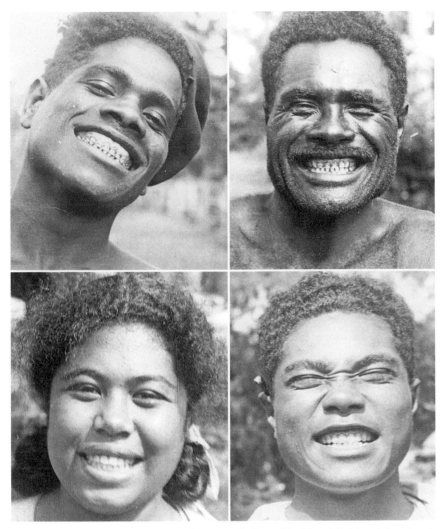

FIG. 28. These Melanesians are typical in general physical build and facial and dental arch form of their race which is spread over a wide area of Islands in the southeastern Pacific. The nutrition of all is adequate for them to develop and maintain their racial pattern.

test against efforts to establish a white colony and sugar plantation on a desirable section of coastal land swept down on the French colony in the night and massacred almost the entire population. Their contact with the required foods from the sea had been cut off. They believe they require sea foods to maintain life and physical efficiency. The physical development of the primitive people including their teeth and dental arches is of very high order. A comparison of the individuals living near the ports with those living in the

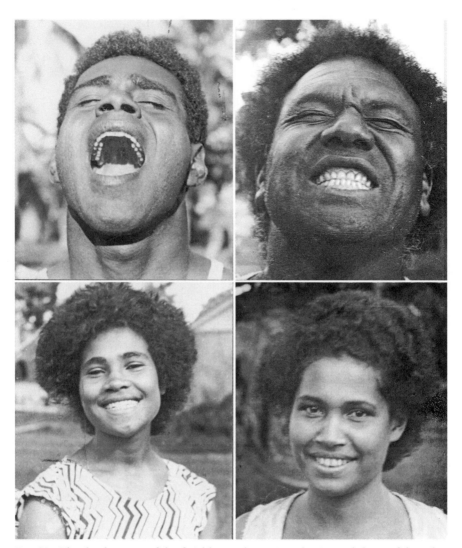

FIG. 29. The development of the facial bones determines the size and shape of the palate and the size of the nasal air passages. Note the strength of the neck of the men above and the well-proportioned faces of the girls below. Such faces are usually associated with properly proportioned bodies. Tooth decay is rare in these mouths so long as they use an adequate selection of the native foods.

isolated inland locations shows marked increase in the incidence of dental caries. For those living almost exclusively on the native foods the incidence of dental caries was only 0.14 percent; while for those using trade foods the incidence of dental caries was 26 percent. The splendid facial and dental arch development of these quite primitive Caledonians is shown in Fig. 28. Note also their kinky hair and strong neck and face muscles.

The Fiji Island group lies between 15 and 22 degrees south latitude and between 177 degrees west and 175 degrees east longitude, thus straddling the international date line. The Fiji Islanders are similar in physical development and appearance to the New Caledonians, and like them are largely, if not wholly, Melanesian in racial origin. The men have kinky hair and broad shoulders. In the past, they have been excellent warriors. They are not as tall as their hereditary enemies, the Tongans, to the east, and in order to make themselves look equally tall, they have adopted the practice of training their kinky hair straight out from the head to a height often reaching six or more inches. Typical facial and dental arch forms are shown in Fig. 29. They are British subjects, and where they have had supervision, in the districts near the ports and on those islands on which sugar plantations have been established, they have suffered very greatly from the degenerative diseases.

Since Viti Levu, one of the islands of this group, is one of the larger islands of the Pacific Ocean, I had hoped to find on it a district far enough from the sea to make it necessary for the natives to have lived entirely on land foods. Accordingly, with the assistance of the government officials and by using a recently opened government road I was able to get well into the interior of the island by motor vehicle, and from this point to proceed farther inland on foot with two guides. I was not able, however, to get beyond the piles of sea shells which had been carried into the interior. My guide told me that it had always been essential, as it is today, for the people of the interior to obtain some food from the sea, and that even during the times of most bitter warfare between the inland or hill tribes and the coast tribes, those of the interior would bring down during the night choice plant foods from the mountain areas and place them in caches and return the following night and obtain the sea foods that had been placed in those depositories by the shore tribes. The individuals who carried these foods were never molested, not even during active warfare. He told me further that they require food from the sea at least every three months, even to this day. This was a matter of keen interest, and at the same time disappointment since one of the purposes of the expedition to the South Seas was to find, if possible, plants or fruits which together, without the use of animal products, were capable of providing all of the requirements of the body for growth and for maintenance of good health and a high state of physical efficiency. Among the sources of animal foods was the wild pig from the bush.

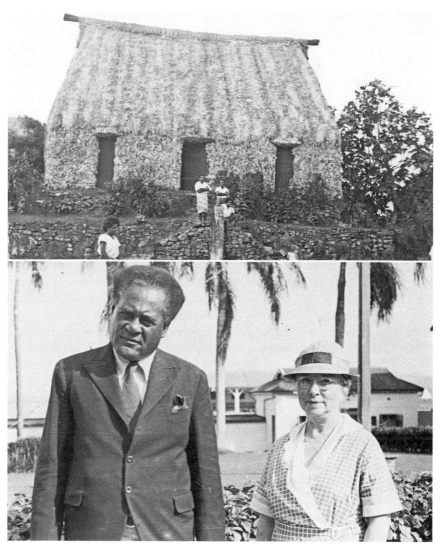

FIG. 30. The building above is the Fiji Council house and shows the typical form of native architecture; no nails or bolts are used. It is located on the King's Island Mbau. The hereditary monarch, Ratu Popi is seen with Mrs. Price. Note his splendid features. Beneath his coat he wears a native skirt and is barefooted.

These were not native, but imported into nearly all of the islands, and they have become wild where there is an abundance of food for them. Another animal food was that from coconut crabs which grow to a weight of several pounds. At certain seasons of the year the crabs migrate to the sea in great numbers from the mountains and interior country. They spend about three days in the sea for part of their reproductive program and return later to their mountain habitats. Their routes of travel are as nearly as possible in straight lines. At the season of migration, large numbers of the crabs are captured for food. These crabs rob the coconut trees of fruit. They climb the trees during the darkness and return to the ground before the dawn. They cut off the coconuts and allow them to drop to the ground. When the natives hear coconuts dropping in the night they put a girdle of grass around the tree fifteen or twenty feet from the ground, and when the crabs back down and touch the grass they think that they are down on the ground, let go their hold and are stunned by the fall. The natives then collect the crabs and put them in a pen where they are fed on shredded coconut. In two weeks' time the crabs are so fat that they burst their shells. They are then very delicious eating. Fresh water fish of various kinds are used where available from the mountain streams. Land animal foods, however, are not abundant in the mountainous interior, and no places were found where the native plant foods were not supplemented by sea foods.

Our first visit to the Fiji Islands was in 1934, and the second in 1936. On our first trip we had much personal assistance from Ratu Popi, hereditary king. His residence was on the royal island reserved exclusively for the king and his retinue. His picture is shown in Fig. 30 with that of Mrs. Price. He was very solicitous for the welfare of his people whom he recognized to be rapidly breaking down with modernization. The council house is also shown in Fig. 30. He gave us very important information regarding the origin of cannibalism, relating it to a recognition of special food values of special organs, particularly the livers.

There has been a very extensive development of sugar plantations on the larger islands of several of the Pacific archipelagos. The working of these plantations has required the importation of large numbers of indentured laborers. These have been brought chiefly from India and China. Since they are nearly all men, those who have married have obtained their wives from among the natives. This, the Chinese have done quite frequently. Since they are excellent workers they provide good homes and are good business men. They are, in many districts, rapidly becoming the landowners and are men of influence. This influx of Asiatics, together with that of Europeans, has had an important influence upon the purity of the native race around the ports and provided an opportunity to study the effect of intermingling of races upon the susceptibility to dental caries. No differences in extent of tooth decay due to ancestry were disclosed. The incidence of dental caries at the points of contact

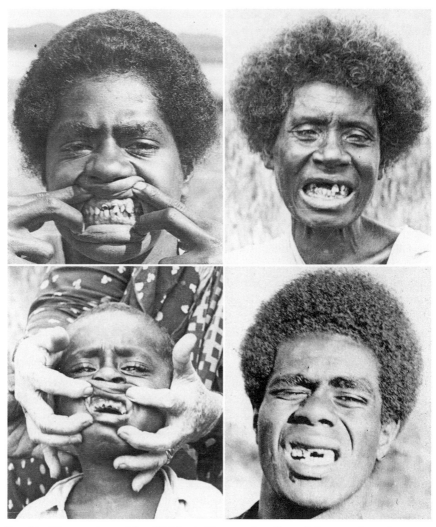

FIG. 31. These natives of the Fiji Islands illustrate the effect of changing from the native food to the imported foods of commerce. Tooth decay becomes rampant and with it is lost the ability to properly masticate the food. Growing children and child bearing mothers suffer most severely from dental caries.

with imported foods was 30.1 percent of teeth examined as compared with 0.42 for the more isolated groups living on the native foods of land and sea.

The physical changes which were found associated with the use of the imported foods included the loss of immunity to dental caries in practically all of the individuals who had displaced their native foods very largely with the modern foods. Dental caries was much worse, however, in the growing chil-

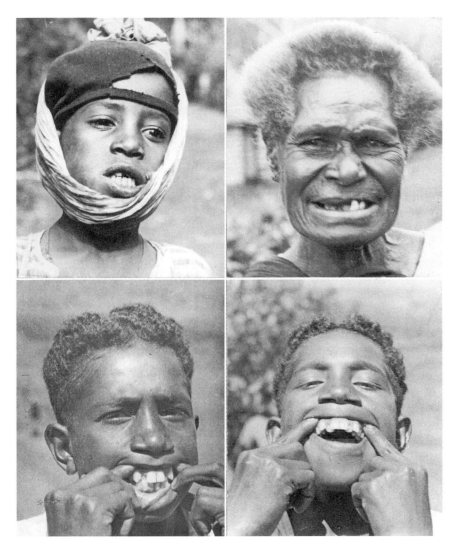

FIG. 32. No dentists or physicians are available on most of these islands. Toothache is the only cause of suicide. The new generation, born after the parents adopt the imported modern foods, often have a change in the shape of the face and dental arches. The teeth are crowded as shown above.

dren and motherhood group due to the special demands of these individuals. These conditions are illustrated in Figs. 31 and 32. The boy shown in Fig. 32 (upper, left) typifies the suffering brought by modernization. Abscessed teeth often cause suicide.

Another important phase of the studies included a critical examination of the facial form and shape of the dental arches which include very definite and typical changes represented by the narrowing of the features and the length-ening of the face with crowding of the teeth in the arch. These are illustrated in the lower half of Fig. 32.

The members of the Melanesian race living on the Fiji Islands of the Pacific, whether volcanic or coral in origin, have developed a very high im-munity to dental caries and well-formed faces and dental arches. Their native foods consisted of animal life from the sea eaten with plants and fruits from the land in accordance with a definite program of food selection. In their primitive state only 0.42 percent of their teeth were attacked by tooth decay. In the modernized groups this incidence increased to 30.1 percent. The change in the nutrition included a marked reduction in the native foods and their displacement with white-flour products, sugar and sweetened goods, canned foods and polished rice. In the succeeding generations after the parents had adopted the modern foods, there occurred distinct changes in facial form and shape of the dental arches.

Chapter 8

ISOLATED AND MODERNIZED POLYNESIANS

THE characteristics of the Polynesian race included straight hair, oval features, happy, buoyant dispositions and splendid physiques. When the Pacific Islands were discovered the Polynesians were found inhabiting the Hawaiian Islands, the Marquesas Islands, the Tuamotu group including Tahiti, the Cook Islands, the Tongan Islands and the Samoan group.

The first group studied was made up of the people of the Marquesas Islands which are situated 9 degrees south latitude and 140 degrees west longitude, about 4,000 miles due west of Peru. Few, if any, of the primitive racial stocks of the South Sea Islands were so enthusiastically extolled for their beauty and excellence of physical development by the early navigators. Much tooth decay prevails today. They reported the Marquesans as vivacious, happy people numbering over a hundred thousand on the seven principal islands of this group. Probably in few places in the world can so distressing a picture be seen today as is found there. A French government official told me that the native population had decreased to about two thousand, chiefly as a result of the ravages of tuberculosis. Serious epidemics of small-pox and measles have at times taken a heavy toll. In a group of approximately one hundred adults and children I counted ten who were emaciated and coughing with typical signs of tuberculosis. Many were waiting for treatment at a dispensary eight hours before the hour it opened. In the past some of the natives have had splendid physiques, fine countenances, and some of the women have had beautiful features. They are now a sick and dying primitive group. A trader ship was in port exchanging white flour and sugar for their copra. They have largely ceased to depend on the sea for food. Tooth decay was rampant. At the time of the examination, 36.9 percent of the teeth of the people using trade food in conjunction with the land plants and fruits had been attacked by tooth decay. The individuals living entirely on native foods were few. Some early navigators were so highly impressed with the beauty and health of these people that they reported the Marquesas Islands as the Garden of Eden.

Tahiti is the principal island of the Society group. It is situated 17 degrees south of the equator, 149 degrees west longitude. Fortunately, degeneration has not been so rapid nor so severe here. The Tahitian population, however, has reduced from over two hundred thousand, as early estimated, to a present

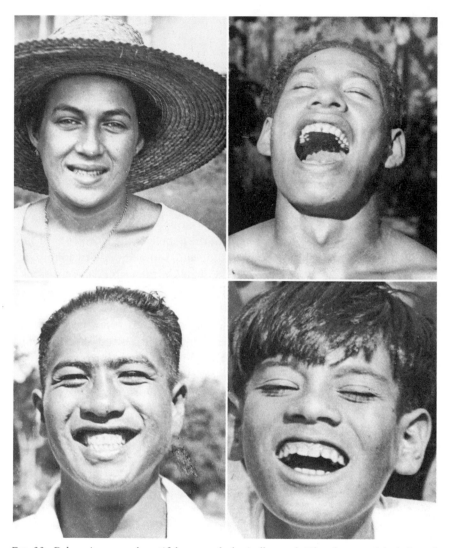

FIG. 33. Polynesians are a beautiful race and physically sturdy. They have straight hair and their color is often that of a sun tanned European. They have perfect dental arches.

native population estimated at about ten thousand. These islands are also a part of French Oceania. Many of the able bodied men were taken from these French Islands to France to fight in the World War. Only a small percentage, however, returned, and they were mostly crippled and maimed. The Tahitians are a buoyant, light-hearted race, fully conscious, however, of their rapid decline in numbers and health. Many of the more primitive are very fine looking and have excellent dental arches, as seen in Fig. 33.

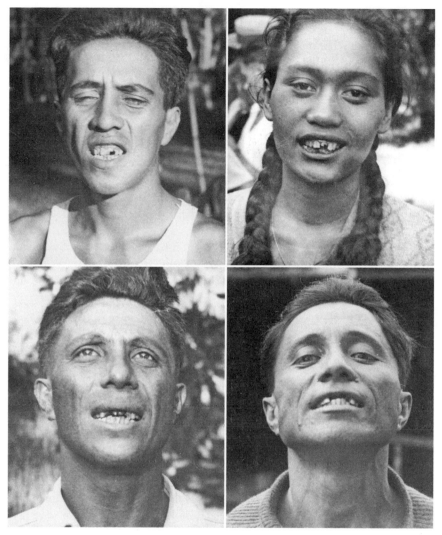

FIG. 34. Wherever the native foods have been displaced by the imported foods, dental caries become rampant. These are typical modernized Tahitians.

The capital of Tahiti, Papeete, is the administrative center for the French Pacific possessions. It has a large foreign population, and there is considerable commerce in and out of this port. Much imported food is used. Like on the Marquesas Islands, it was difficult to find large numbers of individuals living entirely on the native foods. Those that were found had complete immunity to dental caries. For the natives living in part on trade foods, chiefly white flour, sugar and canned goods, 31.9 percent of the teeth were found to be attacked by tooth decay. Typical extensive destruction of the teeth amongst the modernized Tahitians is shown in Fig. 34. There is a large colony of Chinese in Tahiti, brought there as indentured laborers. They have not returned. When the Tahitian men did not return from the war, their wives married the Chinese, who are good workers.

The Cook Islands are British and under the direct guidance of the New Zealand Government. Rarotonga is the principal island. It is situated in the Pacific Ocean in the vicinity of 21 degrees south latitude and 160 degrees west longitude. It has a delightful climate the year around. Racially according to legend, the Maori tribe, the native tribe of New Zealand, migrated there from the Cook Islands. In addition to being similar in physical development and appearance, their languages are sufficiently similar so that each can understand the other, even though their separation occurred probably over a thousand years ago.

It is a matter of great importance that the inhabitants of these South Sea Islands were skillful navigators and boat builders. It was a common occurrence for expeditions both peaceful and aggressive to make journeys of one and two thousand miles in crafts propelled by man power and wind and carrying in addition an adequate supply of water and food for their journey.

A large number were found in Rarotonga living almost entirely on native foods, and only 0.3 percent of the teeth of these individuals have been attacked by dental caries. In the vicinity of Avarua, the principal port, however, the natives were living largely on trade foods, and among these 29.5 percent of the teeth were found to have been attacked by dental caries. In Fig. 35 (top) are seen typically fine faces and teeth. However at the lower left is shown a child at the port whose parents were living on the imported food. This boy's upper lateral teeth are erupting inside the arch. In the lower right is a child with normal spacing of the deciduous teeth.

Under British guidance the Cook Islanders have much better health than the Marquesans or the Tahitians. Their population is not seriously decreasing, and is untroubled except for the progressive development of the degenerative diseases around the port. They are thrifty and happy, and are rapidly developing a local culture including a school system supported by natives.

The inhabitants of the Tongan Islands, the principal of which is Tongatabu, are Polynesian. This group, containing over 100 islands, is situated between 18 and 22 degrees south latitude and between 173 and 176 degrees west longitude, and has a native population of about 28,000. They have the distinction of being one of the last absolute monarchies of the world. While they are under the protection of Great Britain, they largely manage their own affairs. Their isolation is nearly complete except for a call from an infrequent trader. They seem to be credited by the inhabitants of the other islands as being the greatest warriors of the Pacific. The Tongans at least acknowledge that they

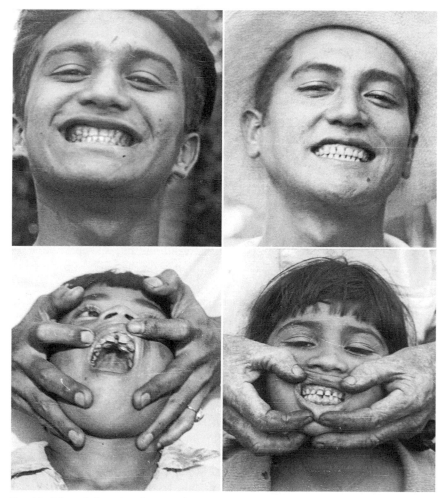

FIG. 35. These Polynesians live on the island of Rarotonga. At the top are two examples of typically fine faces and teeth. Below, at left, is seen a full-blood Polynesian child with the dental arch so small that the permanent laterals are developing inside the arch. His parents used imported food. At the right below is a mixed blood of white and Polynesian. Note the normal spacing of the temporary teeth before the permanent set appears. Parents used native foods.

are the greatest warriors, and indeed the greatest people of the world. They will not step aside to allow anyone to pass since they say that when the world was created and populated they were the first to be made, next was the pig, and last the white man. Ethnologically, they are said to be a mixture of the darker Melanesians with their kinky hair, and the fairer Polynesians of the eastern archipelagos with straight hair. It is said they have never been defeated in battle. For centuries they and the Fijian tribes 700 miles to the west have frequently been at war. The British government has very skillfully directed this racial rivalry into athletics. While we were in the Fiji Islands the British government provided a battle cruiser to carry the football team from Fiji to Nukualofa for the annual contest of strength.

These islanders have practiced eugenics by selecting tall strong mates. The queen of the islands was six feet three inches in height.

The limited importation of foods to the Tongan Islands due to the infrequent call of merchant or trading ships has required the people to remain largely on their native foods. Following the war, however, the price of copra went up from $40.00 per ton to $400.00, which brought trading ships with white flour and sugar to exchange for the copra. The effect of this is shown very clearly in the condition of the teeth. The incidence of dental caries among the isolated groups living on native foods was 0.6 percent, while for those around the port living in part on trade foods, it is 33.4 percent. The effect of the imported food was clearly to be seen on the teeth of the people who were in the growth stage at that time. Now the trader ships no longer call and this forced isolation is very clearly a blessing in disguise. Dental caries has largely ceased to be active since imported foods became scarce, for the price of copra fell to $4.00 a ton. The temporary rise in tooth decay was apparently directly associated with the calling of trader ships.

The Samoan Islands are located in the vicinity of 14 degrees south latitude and between 166 and 174 degrees west longitude. The native population of the Samoan Islands is Polynesian. The control of the Islands is divided between two governments. The eastern group is American. The western group is British since the World War, before which it was under German control. The western group is now under a mandate to New Zealand. Through the kindness of the Governor and Naval Officers of American Samoa transportation was provided on an auxiliary craft to the various islands of the American Samoan group. We were particularly indebted to Commander Stephenson, Director of Health, whose guests we were, for continued personal assistance in making favorable contacts in nearly all villages of the American Samoan group. In no islands of the Pacific did we find so excellent an organization for health service. Dispensaries have been established within reach of nearly all the villages besides hospital service at Pago Pago, the port of Tutuila. This is the finest port in the Pacific Ocean. Notwithstanding the regular monthly contact through merchant ships to and from America and Australia, many isolated groups were found living largely on the native foods. A dental survey had recently been made of this group by Lieutenant Commander Ferguson.[1]

The excellent facial and dental arch development of the Samoans is illustrated in the upper half of Fig. 36. The change in facial and dental arch form

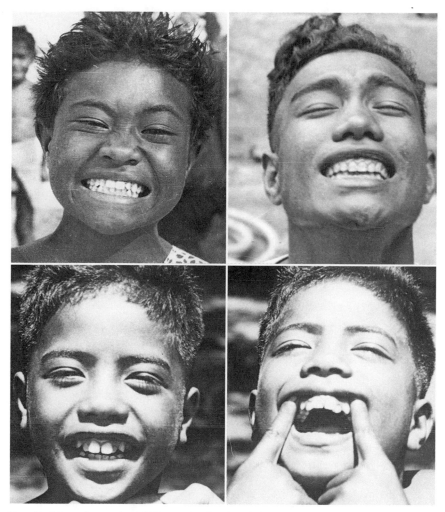

FIG. 36. Note the marked difference in facial and dental arch form of the two Samoan primitives above and the two modernized below. The face bones are underdeveloped below causing a marked constriction of the arches with crowding of the teeth. This is a typical expression of inadequate nutrition of the parents.

which follows the use of modern food by the parents is shown in the lower half of Fig. 36. Note the marked irregularity of the teeth. This is one of the few groups of islands in which the population is not rapidly decreasing, indeed there is some increase. The Navy personnel includes one dentist. Practically all his time is required for the personnel and families of the Navy at this station. Accordingly, he can do only a limited amount of emergency service such as extractions for the natives. About 90 percent of the inhabitants of

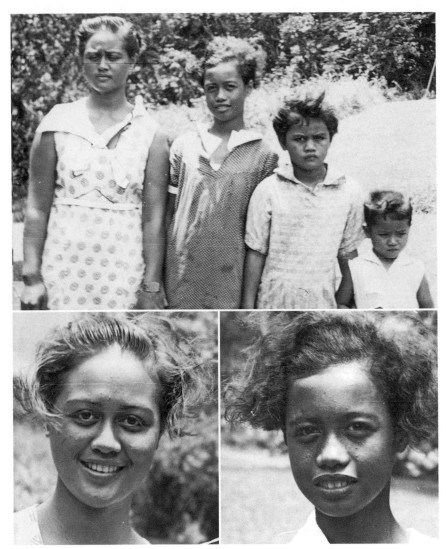

FIG. 37. Wherever the Polynesians are being modernized a change is occurring in facial form which is progressively more severe in the younger members of the family. These girls of an Hawaiian family demonstrate this. Note the change in facial form in the sister to the right. The face is longer and narrower, the nostrils pinched and the chin is receding. The tribal facial pattern is lost.

American Samoa are on the largest island, Tutuila, and due to the development of roads, a considerable number of the people have access to the main port, to which several of them come on ship days to sell their wares and to buy provisions to augment their native foods. The incidence of dental caries among those individuals living in part on imported foods at the port as compared with those in remote districts living on native foods was as follows: Those almost exclusively on native foods had 0.3 percent of the teeth attacked by dental caries, and for those on trade foods, 18.7 percent. Sea foods used here include many shell fish which are gathered and sold largely by the young people. The octopus, the sea crab and the beche-de-mere eaten raw were used.

The Hawaiian Islands lie between 18 and 22 degrees north latitude and between 154 and 160 degrees west longitude. These Islands are quite unlike any of the other Pacific Island groups previously discussed. Sugar and pineapple plantations cover vast areas and together constitute by far the most important industries of these Islands. In many districts the population is almost entirely foreign or of various blends, chiefly of Filipinos and Japanese with Hawaiians. There is a large American population and a considerable European. These different racial groups have largely brought their own customs which are rapidly submerging the native customs. Since the native population is so greatly reduced in comparison with the foreign population, and because intermarrying has been so general, it was difficult to find large groups of relatively pure-blooded Hawaiians either living almost entirely on native foods or on modernized foods. Though the number of the individuals in these groups is accordingly not large, important data were obtained for comparing the relative incidence of dental caries and other degenerative processes. While the preparation of foods on the various Pacific Islands has many common factors, all natives using the underground oven of hot stones for cooking, the Hawaiian Islands present one unique difference in the method of preparation of their taro. They cook the root as do all the other tribes, but having done so they dry the taro, powder it and mix it with water and allow it to ferment for several hours, usually twenty-four or more. This preparation called "poi" becomes slightly tart by the process of fermentation and has the consistency of heavy strap molasses or a very heavy cream. It is eaten by rolling it up on one or two fingers and sucking it from them. It accordingly offers no resistance to the process of mastication. In the districts where the natives are living on native foods the incidence of dental caries was only 2 percent of the teeth, whereas among those natives who are living in large part on the imported foods, chiefly white flour and sweetened goods, 37.3 percent of the teeth had been attacked by tooth decay. Typical Hawaiian faces are seen in Fig. 37. Typical modern tooth decay is shown in Fig. 38. This girl has tuberculosis also.

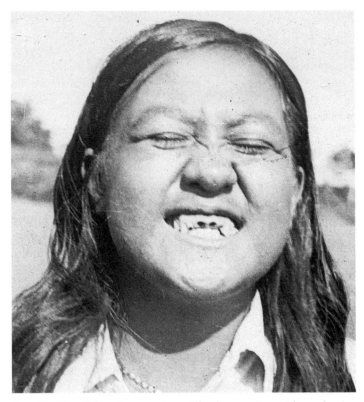

FIG. 38. The Polynesian race is rapidly disappearing with modernization. Tooth decay becomes extreme as shown in the girl above. This
girl has tuberculosis, one of the physical injuries which accompany
modernization. This is one of the bodily injuries as we will see later.

The study of the incidence of dental caries in these various South Sea
Island groups in its relation to diet was only one of several of the problems investigated. Since nutrition is the principal factor that has been found related
to the role of immunity and susceptibility to dental caries in my previous
field studies, the collection of foods for chemical analysis and the gathering
of detailed data regarding the articles of diet have been very important phases
of the activities of this group of studies.

Data were collected for relating the incidence of irregularities of the teeth
and dental arches to the types of nutrition. Similarly, studies were made of the
individuals who had been hospitalized, in the few places where hospitals existed, chiefly to obtain data regarding the classification of the individuals who
were suffering from tuberculosis. These were similar to the studies that I have

made among the Eskimos and Indians of Alaska and northern and central Canada.

If one will picture a community of several thousand people with an average of 30 percent of all the teeth attacked by dental caries and not a single dentist or dental instrument available for assistance of the entire group, a slight realization is had of the mass suffering that has to be endured. Commerce and trade for profit blaze the way in breaking down isolation's barriers, far in advance of the development of health agencies and emergency relief unwittingly made necessary by the trade contact.

While dental caries was most active in the periods of systematic overloads, such as growth, gestation and lactation, even the splendidly formed teeth of the adult men were wrecked by dental caries when the native foods were displaced with modern foods. In all of the groups living on native foods with a liberal intake of animal life of the sea, the health of the gums was generally excellent. When, however, the sea foods were quite limited in the dietary, heavy deposits formed and often were associated with a marked destruction of the supporting tissues with gingival infection. This condition was particularly prevalent among all groups near the ports, when the groups were displacing part of their native foods with imported foods.

In American Samoa through the cooperation of the educational authorities and the Director of the Department of Health, Commander Stephenson, and under the direct supervision of Lieutenant Commander Lowry, the dental surgeon, a group of four young men of the native teaching staff was selected and given instructions for the removal of the deposits. Equipment in the form of instruments has since been provided, in part through the kindness and generosity of some dental manufacturers. This probably constitutes the only native dental service that has ever been available in any of the Pacific Island groups. The intelligence and aptness with which these men were able to learn the fundamental principles, and their skill in carrying out a highly commendable prophylactic operation was indeed remarkable. I gave them pieces of soap and asked them to carve a reproduction of an extracted tooth which was given as a model and in which they were required to increase all diameters to a given amount. Their work would probably equal if not exceed in excellence that of the first effort of 90 percent of American dental students. Many of these natives are very dexterous with their fingers and are skilled artists in carving wood and other material.

A great service could be rendered to these people who are in the process of modernization, but who have no opportunity for dental assistance, by teaching some of the bright young men certain of the procedures for rendering first aid. They could be compensated by contributions of native foods and native wares much as our itinerant dentists were in earlier days. The people would not have money to pay an American or European dentist for his service until trade is carried on with currency.

Nearly all these racial stocks are magnificent singers for which Nature has well-equipped them physically. Their artistry can be judged by the fact that they sing very difficult music unaccompanied and undirected. A large native chorus at Nukualofa, in the Tongan Group, sang without accompaniment "The Hallelujah Chorus" from Handel's Messiah with all the parts and with phenomenal volume and modulation. Much of their work, such as rowing their largest boats, and many of their sports are carried out to the rhythm of hilarious music.

Many of the island groups recognize that their races are doomed since they are melting away with degenerative diseases, chiefly tuberculosis. Their one overwhelming desire is that their race shall not die out. They know that something serious has happened since they have been touched by civilization. Surely our civilization is on trial both at home and abroad.

The nutrition of the primitive Polynesians is continually reinforced with animal life from the sea which includes both soft- and hard-shell forms. The incidence of tooth decay varied from 0.6 percent for the most isolated groups to 33.4 percent for the modernized groups. Those individuals living in their native environment on their native foods have universally normal facial and dental arch form reproducing the characteristics of the race. Those living on the normal environment except for using the imported foods of white flour, sugar, sugar products, syrup, polished rice, and the like, have in the succeeding generations marked changes in facial and dental arch forms.

REFERENCE

[1] FERGUSON, R. A. A dental survey of the school children of American Samoa. *J. Am. Dent. Assoc.*, 21:534, 1934.

Chapter 9

ISOLATED AND MODERNIZED AFRICAN TRIBES

AFRICA has been the last of the large continents to be invaded and explored by our modern civilization. It has one of the largest native populations still living in accordance with inherited traditions. Accordingly, it provides a particularly favorable field for studying primitive racial stocks.

This study of primitive racial stocks, with the exception of some Indian groups, has been largely concerned with people living under physical conditions quite different from those found in the central area of a large continent.

Sea foods are within reach of the inhabitants of islands and coastal regions regardless of latitude. The inhabitants of the interior of a continent, however, have not access to liberal supplies of various forms of animal life of the sea. It was important, therefore, in the interest of the inhabitants of the United States, Canada, Europe, and other large continental interiors, to study primitive people living under environments similar to theirs. Africa is one of the few countries that can provide both primitive living conditions and the modern life of the plains and plateau country in the interior. The great plateau of eastern and central Africa has nurtured a score of tribes with superb physiques and much accumulated wisdom. We are concerned to know how they have accomplished this, and whether they or any other people can survive in that environment after adopting the formulas of our modern civilizations. Considering that the most universal scourge of modern civilization is dental caries, though it is only one of its many degenerative processes, it is important that we study these people to note how they have solved the major problems of living in so severe and disciplining an environment as provided in Africa.

This was done during the summer of 1935. Our route took us through the Red Sea and down the Indian Ocean to enter the African continent at Mombasa below the equator and then across Kenya and Uganda into Eastern Belgian Congo, and thence about 4,000 miles down the long stretch of the Nile through Sudan to the modernized civilization of Egypt. This journey covered most of the country around Ethiopia and gave us contact with several of the most primitive racial stocks of that country. These people are accordingly the neighbors of the Abyssinians or Ethiopians. Since the various tribes speak different languages and are under different governments, it was

117

necessary to organize our safari in connection with the local government officials in the different districts.

During these journeys in Africa which covered about 6,000 miles, we came in contact with about thirty different tribes. Special attention was given to the foods, samples of which were obtained for chemical analysis. Over 2,500 negatives were made and developed in the field. If any one impression of our experiences were to be selected as particularly vivid, it would be the contrast between the health and ruggedness of the primitives in general and that of the foreigners who have entered their country. That their superior ruggedness was not racial became evident when through contact with modern civilizations degenerative processes developed. Very few of the many Europeans with whom we came in contact had lived in central Africa for as much as two years without serious illness or distinct evidence of physical stress. That the cause was not the severity of the climate, but something related to the methods of living, was soon apparent. In all the districts it was recognized and expected that the foreigners must plan to spend a portion of every few years or every year outside that environment if they would keep well. Children born in that country to Europeans were generally expected to spend several of their growing years in Europe or America if they would build even relatively normal bodies.

One exacting condition of the environment that we encountered was the constant exposure to disease. Dysentery epidemics were so severe and frequent that we scarcely allowed ourselves to eat any food that had not been cooked or that we had not peeled ourselves. In general, it was necessary to boil all drinking water. We dared not allow our bare feet to touch a floor of the ground for fear of jiggers which burrow into the skin of the feet. Scarcely ever when below 6,000 feet were we safe after sundown to step from behind mosquito netting or to go out without thorough protection against the malaria pests. These malaria mosquitoes which include many varieties are largely night feeders. They were thought to come out soon after sundown. We were advised that the most dangerous places for becoming infected were the public eating houses, since the mosquitoes hide under the tables and attack the diner's ankles if they are not adequately protected. We rigidly followed the precaution of providing adequate protection against these pests. Disease-carrying ticks were so abundant in the grass and shrubbery that we had to be on guard constantly to remove them from our clothing before they buried themselves in our flesh. They were often carriers of very severe fevers. We had to be most careful not to touch the hides with which the natives protected their bodies from the cold at night and from the sun in the daytime without thorough sterilization following any contact. There was grave danger from the lice that infected the hair of the hides. We dared not enter several districts because of

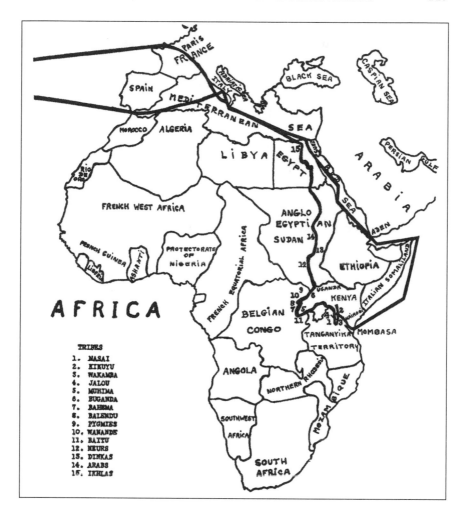

AFRICA

TRIBES
1. MASAI
2. KIKUYU
3. WAKAMBA
4. JALOU
5. MUHIMA
6. BUGANDA
7. BAHIMA
8. BALENDU
9. PYGMIES
10. WANANDE
11. BAITU
12. NEURS
13. DINKAS
14. ARABS
15. IKHLAS

the dreaded tsetse fly and the sleeping sickness it carries. One wonders at the apparent health of the natives until he learns of the unique immunity they have developed and which is largely transmitted to the offspring. In several districts we were told that practically every living native had had typhus fever and was immune, though the lice from their bodies could transmit the disease. One also wonders why people with such resistance to disease are not able to combat the degenerative diseases of modern civilization. When they adopt modern civilization they then become susceptible to several of our modern degenerative processes, including tooth decay.

Dr. Anderson who is in charge of a splendid government hospital in Kenya, assured me that in several years of service among the primitive people of that district he had observed that they did not suffer from appendicitis, gall bladder trouble, cystitis and duodenal ulcer. Malignancy was also very rare among the primitives.

It is of great significance that we studied six tribes in which there appeared to be not a single tooth attacked by dental caries nor a single malformed dental arch. Several other tribes were found with nearly complete immunity to dental caries. In thirteen tribes we did not meet a single individual with irregular teeth. Where the members of these same tribes had adopted modern civilization many cases of tooth decay were found. In the next generation following the adoption of the European dietaries dental arch deformities frequently developed.

We are concerned to know something of the origin of these people including the Ethiopians and to what extent racial ancestry has protected them. If we refer to an ethnographic map of African races we find there is evidence of a great movement northward from South Africa. These people had some things in common with the Melanesians and Polynesians of the South Pacific whom we studied the year previously. Their language carries some words of similar meaning. While there are many tribes existing today, it is of significance that they each possess some identifying characteristics of language, dress and food habits. Another great racial movement has apparently moved southward from Northern Africa. These tribes are of Hamitic origin and include Nilotic tribes and Abyssinians. The Nilotic tribes have a distinct physical pattern and mode of life. These great racial movements have met in the Upper Nile region of Eastern Africa near the equator, and have swayed back and forth with successive obliteration or absorption of those tribes that were least sturdy. The negro race occupied an area across Africa from the West to Central Africa. They were exposed to the aggression and oppression of these two great racial movements, resulting often in intermingling in various proportions of racial bloods. The Semitic race, chiefly Arabs, occupied Arabia and a great area in Northern Africa.

In this bird's-eye view we are observing changes that have been in progress during many hundreds or thousands of years. The Arabs have been the principal slave dealers working in from the east coast of Africa. They have maintained their individuality without much blending except on the coast. They have not become an important part of the native stock of the interior. These primitive native stocks can be largely identified on the basis of their habits and methods of living. The Nilotic tribes have been chiefly herders of cattle and goats and have lived primarily on dairy products, including milk and blood, with some meat, and with a varying percentage of vegetable foods. It was most interesting to observe that in every instance these cattle people dominated the surrounding tribes. They were characterized by superb physi-

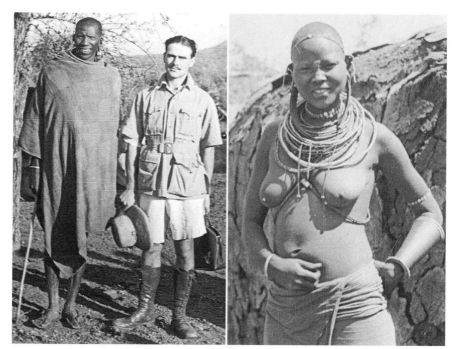

FIG. 39. These members of the Masai tribe illustrate the splendid nutrition provided by their diet of cattle products namely: meat, milk and blood. The chief beside our guide is well over six feet. This Masai belle wears the customary decorations of coils of copper wire bracelets and anklets which largely constitute the attire of the girls.

cal development, great bravery and a mental acumen that made it possible for them to dominate because of their superior intelligence. Among these Nilotic tribes the Masai forced their way farthest south and occupy a position between two of the great Bantu tribes, the Kikuyu and the Wakamba. Both of these latter tribes are primarily agricultural people.

Masai Tribe. The Masai are tall and strong. Fig. 39 shows a typical belle, also a Masai man who is much taller than our six-foot guide. It is interesting to study the methods of living and observe the accumulated wisdom of the Masai. They are reported to have known for over two hundred years that malaria was carried by mosquitoes, and further they have practiced exposing the members of their tribes who had been infected with syphilis by the Arabs to malaria to prevent the serious injuries resulting from the spirochetal infection. Yet modern medicine boasts of being the discoverer of this great principle of using malaria to prevent or relieve syphilitic infections of the spinal cord and brain.

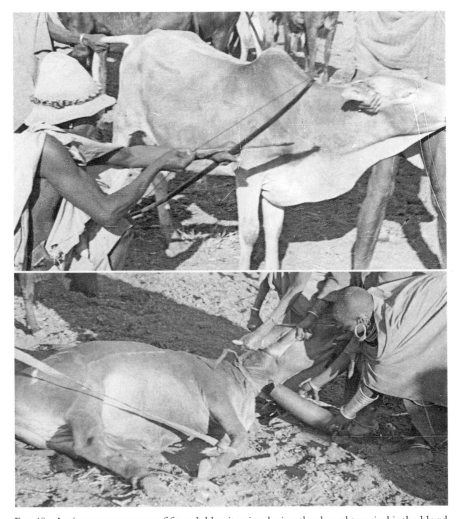

Fig. 40. An important source of fat-soluble vitamins during the drought period is the blood of the steers which is drawn about every thirty days. Above shows the lance tipped arrow being shot into the neck vein. If the animal is wild it is hobbled as shown below where the stream of blood is seen spurting into the gourd. The flow ceases when the compress is removed.

I saw the native Masai operating on their cattle with skill and knowledge. The Masai have no currency and all their transactions are made with cows or goats. A valuable cow was not eating properly, and I observed them taking a thorn out of the inside of her mouth. The surgical operation was done with a knife of their own making and tempered by pounding. The wound was treated by rubbing it with the ashes of a plant that acted as a very powerful styptic. Their knowledge of veterinary science is quite remarkable. I saw them treating a young cow that had failed to conceive. They apparently knew the cause and proceeded to treat her as modern veterinaries might do in order to overcome her difficulties. For their food throughout the centuries they have depended very largely on milk, meat and blood, reinforced with vegetables and fruits. They milk the cows daily and bleed the steers at regular intervals by a unique process. In Fig. 40 we see a native Masai with his bow and arrow, the latter tipped with a sharp knife which is guarded by a shoulder to determine the depth to which the arrow may enter the vein. If the animal is sufficiently tame, the blood is drawn while it is standing. If the animal is frightened it is quickly hobbled, as shown below. In this figure the stream of blood may be seen spurting from the jugular vein into a gourd which holds about a gallon. A torque is placed around the neck before the puncture is made. The animals did not even flinch when struck by the arrow, the operation is done so quickly and skillfully. When sufficient blood was drawn, the torque was removed and the blood immediately stopped flowing. A styptic made of ashes referred to above was used. This serves also to protect the wound from infection. The blood is defibrinated by whipping in the gourd. The fibrin is fried or cooked much as bacon or meat would be prepared. The defibrinated blood is used raw just as the milk is, except in smaller quantities. When available, each growing child receives a day's ration of blood as does each pregnant or lactating woman. Formerly, the warriors used this food exclusively. These three sources, milk, blood and meat provide them with liberal supplies of body-building minerals and the special vitamins, both fat-soluble and water soluble. Their estimate of a desirable dairy stock is based on quality not quantity. They judge the value of a cow for keeping in their herd by the length of time it takes her calf to stand on its feet and run after it is born, which is only a very few minutes. This is in striking contrast with the practice of our modern dairymen who are chiefly concerned with the quantity of milk and quantity of butter-fat rather than with its value as a source of special factors for nutrition. Many of the calves of the modern high-production cows of civilized countries are not able to stand for many hours after birth, frequently twenty-four. This ability to stand is very important in a country infested with predatory animals; such as lions, leopards, hyenas, jackals and vultures.

This reminded me of my experience in Alaska in studying the reindeer of the Eskimos. I was told that a reindeer calf could be dropped in a foot of snow and almost immediately it could run with such speed that the predatory animals, including wolves, could not catch it. And, moreover, that these fawns would go almost immediately after their birth with a herd on a stampede and never be knocked down.

The problem of combating the predatory animals, particularly the lions, calls for greater skill and bravery than is required by other tribes in Africa. The lions live on the large grazing animals, particularly the cattle, from which they select the strongest. In driving over the veldt we frequently saw one or two men or boys guarding an entire herd with only their spears. Their skill in killing a lion with a spear is one of the most superb of human achievements. I was interested to learn that they much prefer their locally made spears to those that are manufactured outside and brought in, because of their certainty that they will not break, will withstand straightening regardless of how much they are bent and because due to the process of manufacture will take a very sharp edge.

On one occasion, after we had been kept awake much of the night by the roaring of the lions and neighing of the zebras that were being attacked by the lions, we visited a Masai manyata nearby in the morning to learn that when they let their cattle and goats out of the corral of acacia thorns, three or four spearsmen went ahead in search of the lions that might be waiting to ambush the cattle. They apparently did not have the slightest fear. The lions evidently had made a kill nearby. This the natives determined by the number of jackals.

The heart and courage of these people has been largely broken by the action of the government in taking away their shields in order to prevent them pillaging the surrounding native tribes as formerly. They depended upon their shields to protect them from the arrows of the other tribes. The efforts to make agriculturists of these Masai people are not promising.

In a typical manyata the chief has several wives. Each one has a separate dwelling. Timber and shrubbery are so scarce in this vicinity that the dwellings are built of clay mixed with cow dung which is plastered over a framework of twigs. Many chiefs are over six feet in height.

The Masai live in a very extensive game preserve in which hundreds of thousands of grazing animals enjoy an existence protected from man since even the natives are not allowed to kill the animals as formerly. They seemed to be preserved for the numerous lions which occasionally become very bold since they have an abundance of food and no enemies. Recently the local government authorities found it necessary to shoot off eighty of the lions in a particular district because of their aggressiveness.

In the Masai tribe, a study of 2,516 teeth in eighty-eight individuals distributed through several widely separated manyatas showed only four individuals with caries. These had a total of ten carious teeth, or only 0.4 percent of the teeth attacked by tooth decay.

Kikuyu Tribe, Kiambu, Kenya. In contrast with the Masai, the Kikuyu tribe, which inhabits a district to the west and north of the Masai, are characterized by being primarily an agricultural people. Their chief articles of diet are sweet potatoes, corn, beans, and some bananas, millet, and Kafir corn, a variety of Indian millet. The women use special diets during gestation and lactation. The girls in this tribe, as in several others, are placed on a special diet for six months prior to marriage. They nurse their children for three harvests and precede each pregnancy with special feeding.

The Kikuyus are not as tall as the Masai and physically they are much less rugged. Like many of the central African tribes, they remove some lower incisors at the time these permanent teeth erupt. This custom is reported to have been established for the purpose of feeding the individuals in case of lockjaw. One of the striking tribal customs is the making of large perforations in the ears in which they carry many metal ornaments. A typical Kikuyu woman is shown in Fig. 41 (upper right). Typical Kikuyu men are also shown in Fig. 41. Note their fine teeth and dental arches.

A study of 1,041 teeth in thirty-three individuals showed fifty-seven teeth with caries, or 5.5 percent. These were 36.4 percent of the individuals affected.

Much of the territory occupied by the Kikuyu tribes was formerly forest. Their practice has been to burn down a section of forest in order to get new lands for planting. As soon as the virgin fertility is exhausted, which is usually in three to five years, they burn down another section of forest. By this process they have largely denuded their section of Kenya of its timber. This has resulted in a great waste of building material. There are few stands of native forest within easy reach of transportation.

Wakamba Tribe, Kenya. The Wakamba tribe point their teeth as shown in Fig. 41. They occupy the territory to the east of the Masai, who in past centuries have driven themselves as a wedge between the Kikuyu and the Wakamba tribes. The Masai until checked carried on a relentless warfare, consisting largely of raids, in which they slaughtered the men and carried off the women and children and drove away the cattle or goats. The Wakambas are intellectually superior to the Kikuyus and have distinct artistic skill in the carving of art objects. They are mechanical and like machinery. Many of them have important positions in the shops of the Kenya and Uganda railway.

An examination of 1,112 teeth of thirty-seven individuals showed sixty-nine teeth with caries, or 6.2 percent. Twenty-one and six-tenths percent of the individuals studied had dental caries.

Jalou Tribe, Kenya. This tribe occupies the territory along Lake Victoria and Kisumu Bay. They are one of the most intelligent and physically excellent native tribes. They were studied in two groups, one at Maseno, and the other at Ogado.

The group studied at the Maseno school were boys ranging from about ten years to twenty-two, totaling about 190 in all. The principal of the school presented the boys in military formation for inspection. Through him as interpreter I asked that all boys who had ever had toothache hold up their hands, and nineteen did so. Of the nineteen only one individual was found to have caries; two of his teeth were involved, which, out of 546 teeth for these individuals, gives 0.4 percent of the teeth with caries.

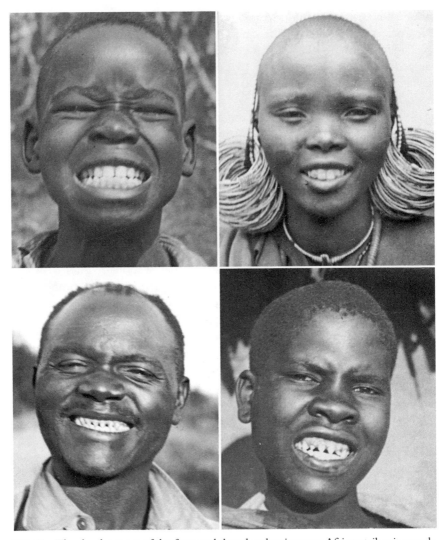

FIG. 41. The development of the faces and dental arches in many African tribes is superb. The girl at the upper right is wearing several earrings in the lobe of each ear. The Wakamba tribe shapes their teeth into points as shown below. This does not cause tooth decay while they live on their native food.

In the Ogado Mission a study of 258 teeth for ten individuals revealed no teeth affected with dental caries.

Jeannes School, Kenya. This school is located at Kabete. It is an institution where young married couples are trained in domestic science, agriculture, and similar subjects.

In 388 teeth of thirteen individuals, thirty-one teeth were found to have been attacked by dental caries, or 7.9 percent. These were in six individuals.

Pumwani Mission School, Kenya. This is a native suburb of Nairobi, and there the people have come under the influence of recent European contact.

In an examination of 588 teeth of twenty-one individuals twenty-six teeth had caries, or 4.4 percent.

C. M. S. School, Nukuru, Kenya. The children of this school belong to several tribes, chiefly Jalou. In a study of 312 teeth of eleven individuals, only one tooth was found to have been attacked by tooth decay, or 0.3 percent.

Chewya at Kisumu, Kenya. The natives of this district belong to the Maragoli tribe. They are very strong and physically well developed. They live within easy reach of Lake Victoria from which they obtain large quantities of fish which constitutes an important part of their diet, together with cereals and sweet potatoes.

A study of 552 teeth of nineteen individuals revealed only one tooth with dental caries, or 0.2 percent.

Muhima Tribe or Anchola, Uganda. This tribe resides in southern Uganda. They, like the Masai, are primarily a cattle raising people and live on milk, blood and meat. The district in which they live is to the east of Lake Edward and the Mountains of the Moon. They constitute one of the very primitive and undisturbed groups. While the Masai raise chiefly the hump-backed cattle, the herds of this Muhima or Anchola tribe are characterized by their large wide-spread horns. Like the Masai, they are tall and courageous. They defend their herds and their families from lions and leopards with their primitive spears. Like the other primitive cattle people, they dominate the adjoining tribes.

In a study of 1,040 teeth of thirty-seven individuals, not a single tooth was found with dental caries. This tribe makes their huts of grass and sticks.

Watusi Tribe. This is a very interesting tribe living on the east of Lake Kivu, one of the headwaters of the West Nile in Ruanda which is a Belgian Protectorate. They are tall and athletic. Their faces differ markedly from those of other tribes, and they boast a very noble inheritance. According to legend, a Roman military expedition penetrated into central Africa at the time of Anthony and Cleopatra. A phalanx remained, refusing to return with the expedition. They took wives from the native tribes and passed laws that thereafter no marriage could take place outside their group. They have magnificent physiques. Many stand over six feet without shoes.

Several of the tribes neighboring Ethiopia are agriculturists and grow corn, beans, millet, sweet potatoes, bananas, Kafir corn, and other grains, as their chief articles of food. Physically they are not as well built as either the tribes using dairy products liberally or those using fish from the fresh water lakes and streams. They have been dominated because they possess less courage and resourcefulness.

The Government of Kenya has for several years sponsored an athletic contest among the various tribes, the test being one of strength for which they use a tug-of-war. One particular tribe has carried off the trophy repeatedly. This tribe resides on the east coast of Lake Victoria and lives very largely on fish. The members are powerful athletes and wonderful swimmers. They are said not to have been conquered in warfare when they could take the warfare to the water. One of their methods is to swim under water to the enemy's fleet and scuttle their boats. They fight with spears under water with marvelous skill. Their physiques are magnificent. In a group of 190 boys who had been gathered into a government school near the east coast of Lake Victoria only one boy was found with dental caries, and two of his teeth had been affected. The people dry the fish which are carried far inland.

Uganda which lies to the north and west of Lake Victoria and west of Kenya, is high and although on the equator, has an equitable climate with an abundance of native foods. Two crops per year are produced, and many varieties of bananas grow wild. The Buganda Tribe, Uganda, is the chief tribe of this region. Uganda has been called the Garden of Eden of Africa because of its abundance of plant foods, chiefly bananas and sweet potatoes, and because of its abundance of fresh water fish and animal life. The natives are thrifty and mentally superior to those of most other districts. They have a king and a native parliament which the British Government recognizes and entrusts with local administrative affairs. A typical group was studied in a mission at Masaka. An examination of 664 teeth of twenty-one individuals revealed only three teeth with caries, or 0.4 percent.

West Nile Laborers from the Belgian Congo. The West Nile Laborers studied at Masaka represent a very strong and dependable group. They come from districts north of Lake Albert in Belgian Congo. They are much sought for in industrial enterprises and are often moved in groups for a considerable distance.

A study of 984 teeth of thirty-one individuals revealed that only three teeth had ever been attacked by tooth decay, or 0.3 percent. Only one individual had dental caries.

As one travels down the West Nile and later along the western border of Ethiopia many unique tribes are met. A typical negroid type of the upper Nile region is shown in Fig. 42. Members of these tribes wear little or no clothing. They have splendid physiques and high immunity to dental caries.

After the confluence of the White Nile and West Nile, the former draining Lake Victoria and the Uganda lakes through Uganda, and the latter, Lakes Kivu, Edwards and Albert and eastern Belgian Congo, the volume of water moving northward is very large. A unique obstruction to navigation has developed due to the fact that the Nile runs underground for a considerable distance. In this district vegetation is rank and prolific, including large quantities of water plants which form islands that are often attached temporarily

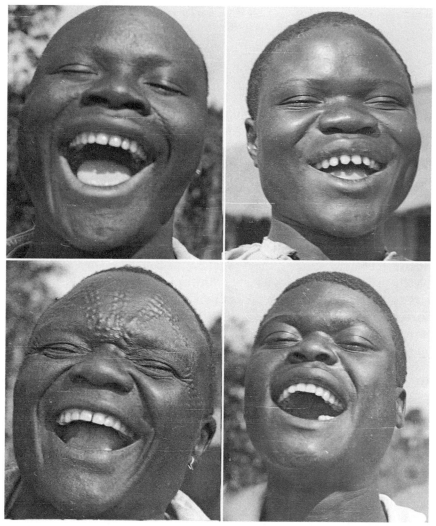

FIG. 42. The reward of obeying nature's laws of nutrition is illustrated in this west Nile tribe in Belgian Congo. Note the breadth of the dental arches and the finely proportioned features. Their bodies are as well built as their heads. Exceedingly few teeth have been attacked by dental caries while on their native foods.

to the shore. The water carries large quantities of alluvia which furnish an abundance of nutriment to the floating plant life. Accordingly, in many of these floating islands a large quantity of soil is enmeshed in the plant roots. At some period in the past the river became bridged across in upper Sudan near its southern border. With the progressive addition of new material a large natural bridge has been raised on which trees are now growing, and across which are elephant trails. This and a series of rapids require a detour of over a hundred miles.

The elephants are so plentiful in this district that both in Uganda and Sudan the governments have been required to send in special hunters to reduce the herds. In one district in Uganda two hundred were said to have been slaughtered. They are very destructive to banana plantations. They break the banana trees over or pull them up by the roots and eat the succulent heart as well as the fruits. In a night a herd may destroy an entire plantation. The only people in the districts who are permitted to kill the elephants without license are the pygmies. They are also the only ones not required to pay a head tax. There are many tribes of them in the great forest area in Belgian Congo and Uganda. Their skill with spears is remarkable and they are able to kill an elephant while the animal remains unaware of his danger. It takes them one to two days to hamstring an elephant by working stealthily from behind, always keeping out of the elephant's sight. Although an elephant can scent a human for a long distance, these pygmies can disguise themselves so completely that the elephant is unaware of their presence. After disabling him by cutting the tendons of both hind legs, they attack him openly and, while one attracts his attention, the other slowly but progressively hacks off his trunk. In this manner he bleeds to death. They are particularly fond of elephant meat and a slaughter means a great feast. While we were in one of the pygmy colonies two of them brought in the tusks of an elephant they had just killed. We had the rare opportunity of witnessing the celebration in the colony, which included the special reproduction in pantomime of the attack and method of killing the elephant. The pygmy mother of these two men is shown in Fig. 43 (lower half). It will be noticed that she is a full head shorter than Mrs. Price, who is five feet three inches tall. This rugged, though small, woman is the mother of five grown men, two of whom are shown in Fig. 43 with the tusks of the elephant. Note their homemade spears. As marksmen with bows and arrows and as trappers, these pygmies have wonderful skill. Their arrows are tipped with iron of their own manufacture and have receptacles for carrying drugs which they extract from plants. These drugs temporarily paralyze the animals. For animals which they wish to destroy the arrows carry a poison which rapidly produces death. The home life of the pygmies in the forest is often filled with danger. Just before our arrival two babies had been carried off by a leopard. This stealthy night prowler is one of the most difficult animals to combat and probably has been one of the reasons the pygmies build cabins in the trees. Ordinarily their homes are built on the ground in a little clearing in the big forest. They consist of low shelters covered with banana leaves and other plants, built over a frame work. The native missionary dispensed our gift of salt which is one of their most prized gifts. They put on a dance for us.

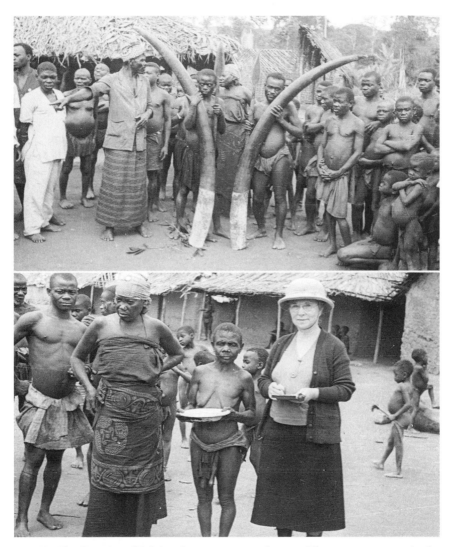

FIG. 43. The Pygmies of Belgian Congo are expert hunters. The two young men in the center above have slain single handed the large bull elephant whose tusks they are holding. The spears used are shown. They are two of five grown sons of the pygmy mother standing next to Mrs. Price in the lower picture. Their teeth are excellent and their knowledge of foods unique.

Pygmies, Ituru Forest, Belgian Congo. These people are said to have originally lived in the trees and they were exceedingly shy and difficult to contact. We were taken to several of their villages in the heart of the dense Ituru forest. We found them very well disposed through the confidence that has been established by the mission workers. Their shyness, however, together with the difficulty of making them understand through two transfers of languages, made an examination of their teeth very difficult.

A study of 352 teeth of twelve individuals revealed eight teeth had been attacked by tooth decay, or 2.2 percent.

The native tribes of Africa have depended to a great extent on fresh water fish from the numerous lakes and rivers for certain of their essential food factors. After being dried in the sun these fish are carried long distances into the interior. The Nile perch grows frequently to a weight of 150 pounds. The natives of Africa know that certain insects are very rich in special food values at certain seasons, also that their eggs are valuable foods. A fly that hatches in enormous quantities in Lake Victoria is gathered and used fresh and dried for storage. They also use ant eggs and ants.

Nyankunde Mission, Irumu, Belgian Congo. This group is made up of members of the Bahema, Babira, Alur and Balendu tribes. We will consider the representatives of these different tribes collectively since they live largely on a common dietary consisting chiefly of cereals. Only the Bahemas of this group have small herds of cattle. Some of the others have a few goats. This district is located southwest of Lake Albert.

A study of 6,461 teeth of 217 individuals revealed 390 teeth with dental caries, or 6 percent. Thirty-eight and seven-tenths percent of the individuals suffered from dental caries.

Bogora Mission, Belgian Congo. This mission is located west of Lake Albert and includes members of the Bahema and Balendu tribes. While the Bahema tribe originally lived very largely on cattle products, milk, blood and meat, in this district, the herds were small and they were using a considerable quantity of cereals, chiefly corn and beans, some sweet potatoes and bananas. These latter were the chief foods of the other tribes, in addition to goats' milk.

An examination of 2,196 teeth of seventy-seven individuals revealed 160 teeth with caries, or 7.2 percent. Fifty-three percent of the individuals had caries.

Kasenyi Port, Lake Albert, Belgian Congo. These natives were members of several tribes surrounding this district who were for the most part temporary residents as laborers. The people had been living largely on a cereal diet and now during their temporary residence at the port had had fish.

An examination of 1,940 teeth of sixty-three individuals revealed 120 teeth with dental caries, or 6.1 percent of the teeth. Fifty and eight-tenths percent of the individuals had dental caries.

Wanande Tribe, Belgian Congo. This tribe is located at Lubero in Belgian Congo. Their diet consists largely of bananas, sweet potatoes, cereals and goats' milk.

In an examination of 368 teeth of thirteen individuals, there were eight teeth with caries, or 2.2 percent. Fifteen and four-tenths percent of the individuals were affected.

Baitu Tribe, Nyunge, Ruanda, Belgian Protectorate. This district lies south of Uganda and east of Belgian Congo proper, northwest of Tanganyika. It lies just east of Lake Kivu. When we learn that Lake Kivu was only discovered in 1894, even though it is one of the important sources of the Nile waters, we realize the primitiveness of the people of this and adjoining districts. This group lives largely on dairy products from cattle and goats, together with sweet potatoes, cereals and bananas.

In a study of 364 teeth of thirteen individuals, not a single tooth was found to have been attacked by dental caries.

Native Hotel Staff at Goma, Belgian Congo. This group consisted of the inside and outside servants of a tourist hotel on Lake Kivu.

An examination of 320 teeth of ten individuals revealed twenty teeth with caries, or 6.3 percent. It is significant that all of these carious teeth were in the mouth of one individual, the cook. The others all boarded themselves and lived on native diets. The cook used European foods.

Where the members of the African tribes had attached themselves to coffee plantations and were provided with the imported foods of white flour, sugar, polished rice and canned goods, tooth decay became rampant. This is typically illustrated in Fig. 44.

Anglo-Egyptian Sudan has an area approximately one-third that of the United States. It is traversed throughout its length from south to north by the Nile. There are several tribes living along this great waterway, which are of special interest now owing to their close proximity to Ethiopia. There are wonderful hunters and warriors among them. In hunting they use their long-bladed spears almost entirely. The shores of the Nile for nearly a thousand miles in this district are lined with papyrus and other water plants to a depth of from several hundred yards to a few miles. Back of this area the land rises and provides excellent pasturage for the grazing cattle. These tribes, therefore, use milk, blood and meat from cattle and large quantities of animal life from the Nile River. Some of the tribes are very tall, particularly the Neurs. The women are often six feet or over, and the men seven feet, some of them reaching seven and a half feet in height. I was particularly interested in their food habits both because of their high immunity to dental caries which approximated one hundred percent, and because of their physical development. I learned that they have a belief which to them is their religion, namely, that every man and woman has a soul which resides in the liver and that a man's character and physical growth depend upon how well he feeds that soul by eating the livers of animals. The liver is so sacred that it may not be touched by human hands. It is accordingly always handled with their spear or saber, or with specially prepared forked sticks. It is eaten both raw and cooked.

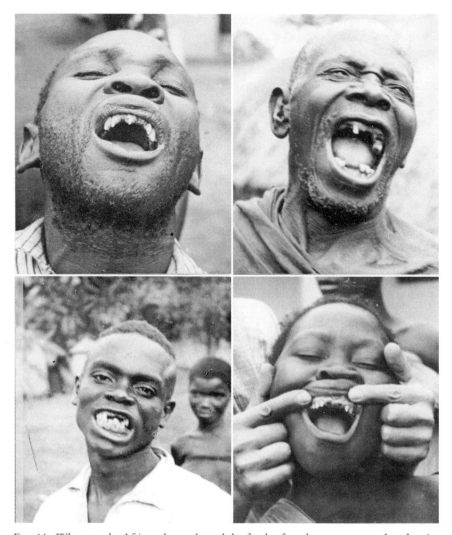

FIG. 44. Wherever the Africans have adopted the foods of modern commerce, dental caries was active, thus destroying large numbers of the teeth and causing great suffering. The cases shown here are typical of workers on plantations which largely use imported foods.

Many of these tribes, like the Neurs, wear no clothing and decorate their bodies with various designs, some of them representing strings of beads produced by putting foreign substances under the skin in definite order. They have maintained a particularly bitter warfare against the Arab slave dealers who have come across from the Red Sea coast to carry off the women and children. In isolated districts even to this day they are suspicious of foreigners. We were told that in one district adjoining Ethiopia all light skinned people are in danger and cannot safely enter that territory without a military escort.

Terrakeka, Upper Nile, Sudan. These people are tall and live largely on fish and other animal life. This part of Sudan consists of many districts of great marshland called the sudd. It is covered with rank papyrus to the height of fifteen to thirty feet. This jungle of rank marsh growth swarms with a wide variety of animal life, large and small.

An examination of 548 teeth of eighteen individuals revealed that not a single tooth had been attacked by dental caries, or 100 percent immunity.

Neurs, Malakal, Sudan. The Neurs at Malakal on the Nile River are a unique tribe because of their remarkable stature. Many of the women are six feet tall and the men range from six feet to seven and a half feet in height. Their food consists very largely of animal life of the Nile, dairy products, milk and blood from the herds.

A study of 1,268 teeth of thirty-nine individuals revealed only six teeth with dental caries, or 0.5 percent. Only three individuals had caries, or 7.7 percent.

Dinkas, Jebelein, Sudan. This tribe lives on the Nile. Its members are not as tall as the Neurs. They are physically better proportioned and have greater strength. They use fish from the Nile and cereals for their diet. They decorate their bodies profusely with scars.

An examination of 592 teeth of twenty-two individuals revealed only one tooth with caries, or 0.2 percent.

Arab Schools at Khartoum and Omdurman, Sudan. The Arabs are the chief occupants of the territory of Northern Sudan. Omdurman on the west bank of the White Nile opposite Khartoum is the largest purely Arab city in the world. It has been but slightly influenced by modern civilization. Khartoum, on the contrary, just across the river from Omdurman and the capital of Anglo-Egyptian Sudan, has districts which are typically modern. These include the government offices and administration organization. The Arab section of Khartoum has been definitely influenced by contact with the Europeans. This makes possible a comparative study of similar groups in the two cities-modernized Khartoum and primitive Omdurman.

A study of 1,284 teeth of fifty-two individuals in an Arab school at Khartoum revealed that 59 teeth or 4.7 percent had been attacked by dental caries, or 44.2 percent of the individuals studied.

In Omdurman a study of 744 teeth in thirty-one individuals, revealed only nine teeth that had been attacked by tooth decay, or 1.2 percent. In this group only two or 6.4 percent of the individuals had dental caries.

The groups examined were selected with the assistance of the government officials and consisted of the higher grade pupils in two advanced native schools, one in Khartoum and one in Omdurman.

It is of interest that of the two boys in the Arab school at Omdurman with dental caries one was the son of a rich merchant and used liberally sweets and European foods.

Native Hospital, Khartoum, Sudan. The individuals studied in this institution were from quite remote areas distributed through Sudan. Some had traveled many days on camels to obtain the help that the hospital provided.

A study of 288 teeth of ten individuals revealed that thirteen had been attacked by tooth decay, or 4.5 percent.

Ikhlas School, Cairo, Egypt. This is a native school in which the individuals are comparable in many respects to those in the native schools at Khartoum and Omdurman. Their nutrition is highly modernized by living in a modern city.

A study of 2,092 teeth of eighty-five individuals revealed that 353 teeth or 12.1 percent had been attacked by tooth decay. Seventy-five percent of the individuals of this group had dental caries.

The total number of teeth examined in the preceding groups was 28,438. Of this number, 1,346 were found with dental caries or 4.7 percent. This represents a total of 1,002 individuals examined, of whom 300 had one or more carious teeth, or had lost teeth by caries, making 29.9 percent of the individuals with dental caries. Of this total number of individuals studied in twenty-seven groups, there were several groups with practically complete immunity to dental caries, while other groups had relatively high incidence of that disease.

Facial and Dental Arch Deformities. The purpose of these studies has included the obtaining of data which will throw light also on the etiology of deformities of the dental arches and face, including irregularity of position of the teeth.

A marked variation of the incidence of irregularities was found in the different tribes. This variation could be directly associated with the nutrition rather than with the tribal pattern. The lowest percentage of irregularity occurred in the tribes living very largely on dairy products and marine life. For example, among the Masai living on milk, blood and meat, only 3.4 percent had irregularities. Among the Kikuyu and Wakamba, 18.2 and 18.9 percent respectively had irregularities. These people were largely agriculturists living primarily on vegetable foods. In the native Arab school at Omdurman, among the pupils living almost entirely according to the native customs of selection and preparation of foods, 6.4 percent had irregularities, while in the native school at modernized Khartoum 17 percent had irregularities. In the Ikhlas school at Cairo, under modern influence, 16.5 percent had irregularities. In the native hospital at Khartoum, 70 percent had irregularities. In the Pygmy group 33.3 percent had irregularities, and among the grain eaters of the west Nile, 25.5 percent had irregularities. The Jeannes School had 46.1 percent and the Ogado mission 30 percent.

While the primitive racial stocks of Africa developed normal facial and dental arch forms when on their native foods, several characteristic types of

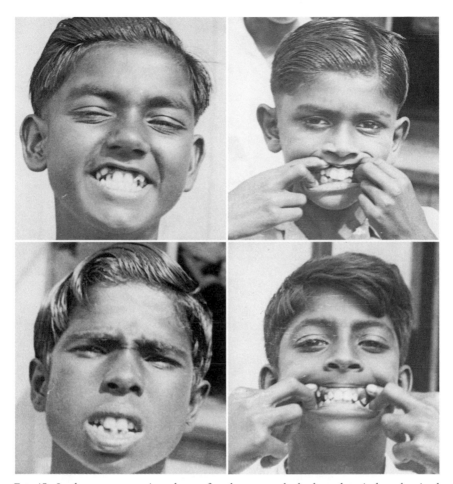

Fig. 45. In the new generations, born after the parents had adopted typical modernized diets of Europeans, there was a marked change in the facial and dental arch forms of the adolescent children. Note the narrowing of the nostrils and dental arches and the crowding of the teeth in these four typical young men.

deformity frequently developed in the children of the modernized groups. One of the simplest forms, and one which corresponds with a very common deformity pattern in the United States, involves the dropping inward of the laterals with narrowing of the upper arch making the incisors appear abnormally prominent and crowding the cuspids outside the line of the arch. Typical illustrations of this are shown in Fig. 45. Where the nutritional deficiency is very severe, as at Mombasa on the coast, more severe changes in facial form are found.

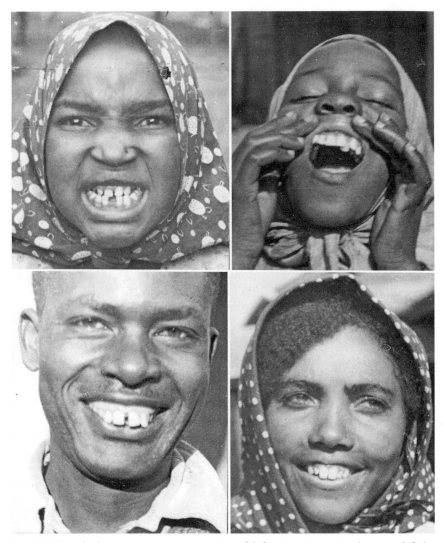

FIG. 46. Disturbed nature may present a variety of deformity patterns. In the upper left the upper arch is much too small for the lower and nearly goes inside it. The upper right is narrowed with crowding of the teeth. Both lower cases demonstrate an underdevelopment of the mandible of the lower jaw.

Among the deformity patterns a lack of development forward of the middle third of the face or of the lower third of the face often appeared in the more highly modernized groups. An illustration of the former is seen in Fig. 46 (upper left), and of the latter in Fig. 46 (lower left and right). In the girl at the upper left, the upper arch tends to go inside the lower arch all

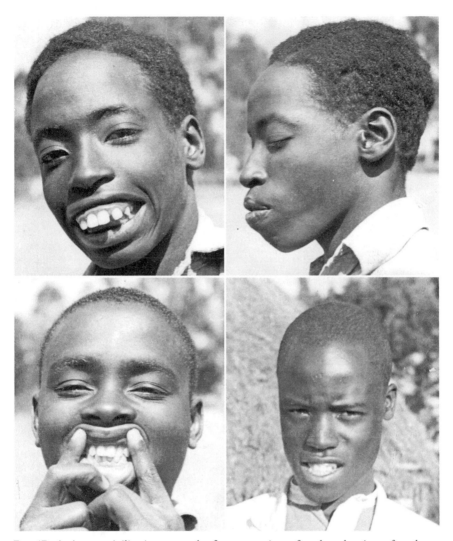

FIG. 47. As in our civilization, even the first generation, after the adoption of modernized foods may show gross deformities. Note the extreme protrusion of the upper teeth with shortening of the lower jaw in the upper pictures and the marked narrowing with lengthening of the face in the lower views. The injury is not limited to the visible structures.

around. This girl is of the first generation, in a mission in Nairobi, following the adoption of the modernized foods by the parents.

A more extreme and severe type of facial change involves an abnormal narrowing with marked distortion of both upper and lower arches. This is shown typically in Fig. 47.

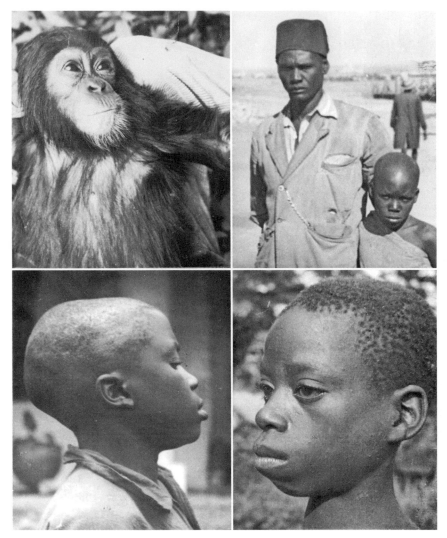

FIG. 48. A very frequent injury appearing in the offspring after the adoption of less efficient foods often involves a marked depression of the middle third of the face as illustrated
in the three boys in this view. Note the comparison with the chimpanzee face.

These extreme deformities often produce facial expressions that are sug-
gestive of the faces of some of the monkeys. This is illustrated by the three
boys shown with the monkey in Fig. 48.

The Arabs in several districts use camels' milk extensively. It is nutritious,
and in much of the desert country constitutes the mainstay of the nomads for
months at a time. The primitive Arabs studied had fine dental arches with very

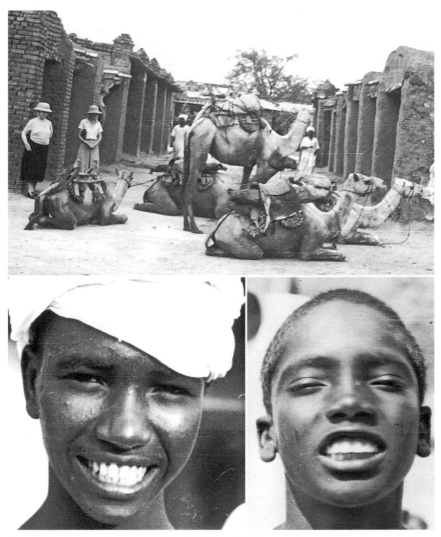

FIG. 49. In the hot desert countries of Asia and Africa, camel's milk is an important item of human nutrition. The teeth of the Arabs, as illustrated below, are excellent. Large areas could not maintain human life without the camel and its milk.

little deformity. Even the horses ridden by the Arab chiefs in moving their camel herds across the desert are often dependent, sometimes for as long as three months, upon the milk of the camels for their nutrition. Typical Arab faces and a camel caravan at rest are shown in Fig. 49. The primitive Arab girls have splendidly developed faces and fine dental arches. Their natural beauty, however, is rapidly lost with modernization, as illustrated in Fig. 50.

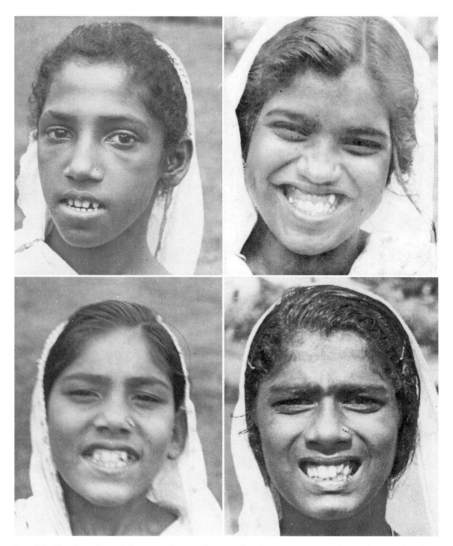

FIG. 50. Both girls and boys in the modernized colonies in Cairo showed typical deformity patterns in faces and dental arches. The health of these groups is not comparable to that of those living on the native dietaries. Reproductive efficiency in these generations is greatly reduced.

Dr. Hrdlička has called attention to the occasional development in several racial stocks of individuals who travel on all fours instead of upright. I saw several individuals of this type in Africa scooting around about as rapidly as the dogs. They were, accordingly, difficult to photograph. Two are shown in Fig. 51.

While slavery of the old form no longer exists in the so-called civilized countries, in its new form it is a most tragic reality for many of the people.

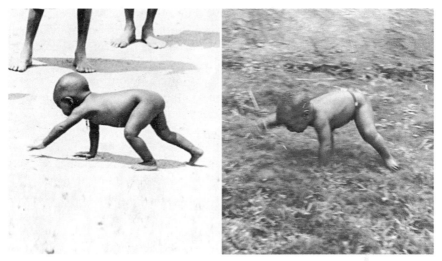

FIG. 51. These two native African children scooted around on all fours so swiftly that it was difficult to take their pictures. We did not see them stand up. They behaved very much like tame chimpanzees.

Taxes and the new order of living make many demands. For many of these primitive tribes a new suit of clothes could formerly be had every day with no more trouble than cutting a new banana leaf. With the new order they are requested to cover their bodies with clothing. Cloth of all kinds including the poorest cotton has to be imported. They must pay an excessive charge due to the long transportation cost for the imported goods, a charge which often exceeds the original cost in the European or American markets by several fold. In order to pay their head tax they are frequently required to carry such products as can be used by the government officials, chiefly foods, over long distances and for part of each year. These foods are often those which not only the adults, but particularly the growing children sorely need for providing body growth and repair. This naturally has produced a current of acute unrest and a chafing under the foreign domination.

As we encircled Ethiopia we found the natives not only aware of what was going on in that border country, but deeply concerned regarding the outcome. From their temper and sympathetic attitude for the oppressed Ethiopians, it would not be surprising if sympathizers pass over the border into that country to support their crushed neighbors. The problem is accordingly very much larger than the interest of some particular foreign power. It deals directly with the future course of events and the attitude of the African natives in general toward foreign domination. The native African is not only chafing under the taxation by foreign overlords, but is conscious that his race becomes blighted when met by our modern civilization. I found them well aware of the fact that those of their tribes who had adopted European methods of living and foods not only developed rampant tooth decay, but other degenerative processes.

In one of the most efficiently organized mission schools that we found in Africa, the principal asked me to help them solve a serious problem. He said there was no single question asked them so often by the native boys in their school as why it is that those families that have grown up in the mission or government schools were physically not so strong as those families who had never been in contact with the mission or government schools. These young men were thinking. I was even asked several times by them whether or not I thought that the native Africans must go the way of the Red Indians of America.

The happiness of the people in their homes and community life is everywhere very striking. A mining prospector who had spent two decades studying the mineral deposits of Uganda was quoted to me as stating that if he could have the heaven of his choice in which to spend all eternity it would be to live in Uganda as the natives of Uganda had lived before modern civilization came to it.

While inter-tribal warfare has largely ceased, a new scourge is upon them, namely the scourge which comes with modern civilization. As in the primitive racial stocks previously studied and reported, we found that modernizing forces were often associated with a very marked increase of the death rate over the birth rate. In some districts in Africa a marked degeneration is taking place. Geoffrey Gorer in his book, *Africa Dances*,[1] which was written after making studies in West Africa, discusses this problem at length.

He quotes figures given by Marcel Sauvage[2] in his article on French Equatorial Africa: "In 1911 French Equatorial Africa had twenty million negro inhabitants; in 1921 there were seven and a half million; in 1931 there were two and a half million."

He states regarding the quotation: "These figures were given in a responsible French conservative paper and have not been denied." Major Browne, a high official of the British Government Administrative Department of Kenya, with long experience, states in the closing paragraph of his book entitled, *The Vanishing Tribes of Kenya*,[3] the following:

> It must also be remembered that the "blessings of civilization" are not in practice by any means as obvious as some simple-minded folk would like to believe. It can be said with fair accuracy that among the tribes with which we have been dealing there is, in their uncontaminated society, no pauperism, no paid prostitution, very little serious drunkenness, and on the whole astonishingly little crime; while practically everyone has enough to eat, sufficient clothing, and an adequate dwelling, according to the primitive native standard. Of what civilized community can as much be said?

Civilizations have been rising and falling not only through all the period of recorded history, but long before as evidenced by archeological findings. If we think of Nature's calendar as one in which centuries are days and civilizations are years, the part current events are playing in the history of a great continent like Africa may be mere incidents.

This much we do know that throughout the world some remnants of several primitive racial stocks have persisted to this day even in very exacting environments and only by such could they have been protected.

In my studies of these several racial stocks I find that it is not accident but accumulated wisdom regarding foods that lies behind their physical excellence and freedom from our modern degenerative processes, and, further, that on various sides of our world the primitive people know many of the things that are essential for life—things that our modern civilizations apparently do not know. These are the fundamental truths of life that have put them in harmony with Nature through obeying her nutritional laws. Whence this wisdom? Was there in the distant past a world civilization that was better attuned to Nature's laws and have these remnants retained that knowledge? If this is not the explanation, it must be that these various primitive racial stocks have been able through a superior skill in interpreting cause and effect, to determine for themselves what foods in their environment are best for producing human bodies with a maximum of physical fitness and resistance to degeneration.

Primitive native races of eastern and central Africa have in their native state a very high immunity to dental caries, ranging from 0 to less than 1 percent of the teeth affected for many of the tribes. Where modernized, however, the incidence increased to 12.1 percent.

In the matter of facial deformity thirteen tribes out of twenty-seven studied presented so high a standard of excellence that not a single individual in the group was found with deformed dental arches.

Their nutrition varied according to their location, but always provided an adequate quantity of body-building and repairing material, even though much effort was required to obtain some of the essential food factors. Many tribes practiced feeding girls special foods for an extended period before marriage. Spacing of children was provided by a system of plural wives.

REFERENCES

[1] GORER, G. *Africa Dances*. N.Y., Knopf, 1935.
[2] SAUVAGE, M. Les secrets de l'Afrique Noire. *Intransigeant*, July–Aug., 1934.
[3] BROWNE, G. *The Vanishing Tribes of Kenya*. London, Seeley Service, 1925.

Chapter 10

ISOLATED AND MODERNIZED
AUSTRALIAN ABORIGINES

OUR problem of throwing light upon the cause of the physical break-down of our modern civilization, with special consideration of tooth decay and facial deformity, requires a critical examination of individuals living in as wide a range of physical conditions as may be possible. This requires that the Aborigines of Australia be included in this examination of human reactions to physical environments. These were studied in 1936.

In selecting the individuals in the various groups special effort was made to include children between the ages of ten and sixteen years in order to have an opportunity to observe and record the condition of the dental arches after the permanent teeth had erupted. This was necessary because the deciduous dentition or first set of teeth may be in normal position in the arches with a correct relationship between the arches, and the permanent dentition show marked irregularity. The shape of the dental arches of the infant at birth and the teeth that are to take their place in the arches have a considerable degree of their calcification at birth. The development of the adult face, however, does not occur until the permanent teeth have erupted. The general shape or pattern is largely influenced by the position and direction of the eruption of the permanent teeth. These studies, accordingly, have included a careful, detailed record of the shape of the dental arch of each individual.

The Australian Aborigines constitute one of the most unique primitive races that have come out of the past into our modern times and they are probably the oldest living race. We are particularly concerned with those qualities that have made possible their survival and cultural development.

The Aborigines are of special interest because they have come out of a very distant past and are associated with animal life which is unique in being characterized as a living museum preserved from the dawn of animal life on the earth. Many of the animal species that are abundant in Australia are found only in fossil form on other continents. The evidence indicates that they crossed on a land bridge which connected Australia with Asia. After the bridge was submerged the animals persisted in that protected island continent which never has known any of the animal species of later development. Among these animals the marsupials play an important role and constitute a large variety. The

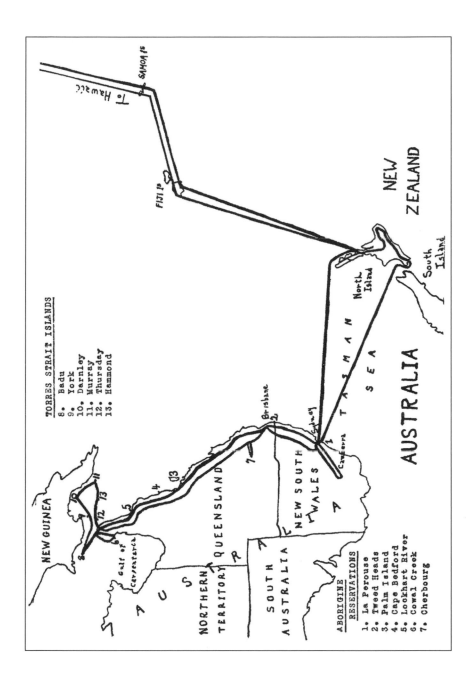

American continent has only one or two of the many forms found in Australia. These are the opossum of the marsupial family and the sloth. One of the most curious animals living on the earth today, or that has left its remains in the petrified skeletons of early periods of the earth's history, is the duckbill platypus. It has the unique distinction of having the characteristics of several animal species. It lays eggs like a bird and hatches them with the heat of its body in its pouch. It has webbed, five-toed feet, like the water birds, a bill like a duck and hair and tail like a beaver. The typical marsupial pouch for carrying its young, is another characteristic of this strange animal. Like other mammals it provides milk for its young. Its milk is similar in chemical constituents to that of other mammals. Most rudimentary in form are the mammary glands of the platypus. The young, when hatched in the pouch, nuzzle the lining membrane of the pouch and the milk exudes through minute openings. There is no nipple. The animal lives chiefly in the water. Its home is built above the water level on the bank, but the entrance to it is underneath the water. They are exceedingly playful creatures, apparently more at home in the water than on land. They live on both animal life and plant food found under the water. They seem to be related to an early era of differentiation of animal species.

The Aborigines are credited with having the most primitive type of skeletal development of any race living today. The eyes are very deep set, the brows very prominent giving them an expression that identifies them as a distinct racial type. See Fig. 52. Professor Weidenreich has shown that they resemble in this regard the recently discovered ancient Peking man. While they are still in the Stone Age stage in their arts and crafts, they have developed further in some respects than has any other ancient race. Their skill in tracking and outwitting the fleet and very cunning animal life of their land is so remarkable that they have been accredited with a sixth sense. They have been able to build good bodies and maintain them in excellent condition in a country in which the plant life, and consequently the lower animal life can be maintained at only a very low level because of the absence of rain. Over half of Australia has less than ten inches of rain a year. It is significant that the natives have maintained a vigorous existence in districts in which the white population which expelled them is unable to continue to live. Among the white race there, the death rate approaches or exceeds the birth rate.

They have developed a device for throwing spears, which makes them more deadly than any in the world. I witnessed a group of the present-day natives throwing their spears at a target which consisted of a banana stalk much smaller than a man's body. They threw the spears from a distance which I estimated to be seventy-five yards. About thirty spears were thrown and several pierced the banana stalk and the others were stuck in the ground close around it. This was accomplished by means of a wamara or throwing stick approximately as long as the arm, with a strong hand grip at one end and a device on the other end for engaging in a depression in the butt of the spear. This was thrown by poising

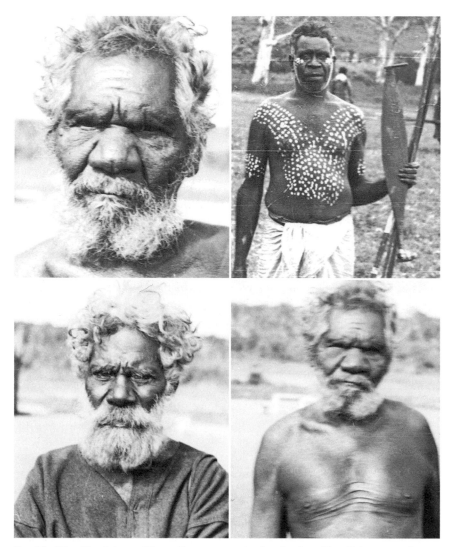

FIG. 52. The Aborigines of Australia are recognized to be the oldest living race of man-kind. Note the prominent eyebrows and deep set eyes. The man at the upper right is hold-ing his spears and wamara, or spear thrower. They are very fond of decorations on their bodies. Little baldness was seen even in the very old.

the spear about the level of the shoulder, the spear supported by the fingers of the hand which swung the throwing stick. The latter extended back over the shoulder. The impact of their spears has often been demonstrated to be sufficient to completely penetrate a man's body. Their method of tempering wood for the points of the spears was such that the spearheads offered great resistance. A throwing stick is shown in Fig. 52 (upper right).

These natives decorate their bodies with paints for dances and sports. They know the habits of all of the animals and insects so well that they are able to reproduce the calls of the animals and thus decoy them into traps. Some of the water birds maintain sentinels at lookout points to guard those in the water. The Aborigines are able to decoy these birds by most ingenious methods. They travel with their bodies disguised by grass and shrubbery and enter the water with a headgear made from feathers of one of the birds. Once in the water, they then maneuver in a manner similar to that of the birds and go among the flock of wild ducks or swans. Working entirely under water, they draw the birds under one by one and take load after load to shore without raising the suspicion of the flock. When working among the kangaroos they are so skilled in preparing movable blinds that they can kill many in a grazing wild pack without alarming the rest, always striking when the animal is grazing. Their skill at fishing probably exceeds that of any other race. They are so highly trained in the knowledge of the habits of the fish and the type of movement that the fish transmits to the water and to the reeds in the water, that one of their important contests between tribes is to see how many fish can be struck in succession with a spear, the fish never being seen, their only information as to its whereabouts being the change in the surface of the water and movement of grasses that are growing in the water as the fish moves. The fish are startled by the umpire's striking the water. The experts bring up a fish six times out of eight. These fishing contests are held along the banks of lakes and rivers where the water is deep enough for some of the reeds and grasses to come to the surface. The contestants travel in canoes.

The native canoe is cut in one piece from the side of a tree, the cutting being done with stone axes. The canoe offers an exceedingly treacherous platform from which a standing man must throw his spear. For some of the contests the canoe carries a paddler, but in the most exacting contests the spear man must manage his own flat-bottomed canoe.

The skill of the Aborigines in tracking is so phenomenal that practically every large modern town or city in Australia has one or more of these men on its police staff today to track criminals. For weeks, they carry the detailed information about the characteristics of the prisoner's foot across the desert, and when they come across the man's foot print they recognize it among all others in the same path. Every leaf that is turned over or grain of sand on bare rocks has meaning for them.

Their social organization is such that almost every person who had been in intimate contact with them, testified that they had never known any of the Aborigines to be guilty of the theft of anything. Even where partly modernized, as they are in the large government reservations they are trustworthy. A nurse in an emergency hospital told me that she continually left her money, jewelry and other objects of personal property freely exposed and available where many of the hundreds of primitives passing could pick them up, and that she had never known them to take anything. The other nurses had had the same experience.

Every boy and girl among these Aborigines must pass many examinations. Their early schooling includes the tracking of small animals and insects. The small boys begin throwing spears almost as soon as they can stand up straight. No young man can even witness a meeting of the council, let alone become a member of it, until he has passed three supreme tests of manhood. First, he is tested for his ability to withstand hunger without complaint. The test for this is to go on a march for two or three days over the hot desert and assist in preparing the meals of roast kangaroo and other choice foods and not partake of any himself. He must not complain. If he becomes too weak, he is given a small portion. There are tests for fear in which he is placed under the most trying ordeals without knowing that it is part of his examination, and he must demonstrate that he will accept death rather than flee. No member of their society would be allowed to continue to live with the tribe if he had defied the ideals of the group. Immorality is cause for immediate death.

The growing boys among the Aborigines are taught deference and esteem for their elders in many impressive ways. A boy may not kill or capture a slow moving animal. That is left for the older men, whom he must call. He must limit his hunting primarily to the fast fleeing and canny kangaroos and wallabies, whom even a man on horseback cannot outdistance. Racketeers and such unsocial beings could not exist in this type of civilization.

Marriages are arranged according to very distinct tribal patterns and every girl is provided with a husband at a time decided by the council. Their code of ethics is built around the conception of a powerful Supreme Force that is related to the sun. They believe that there is an after-existence in which the myriads of stars represent the spirits of the Aborigines that lived before. The boys and girls are taught the names of the great characters that make up the different constellations. These were individuals who had conquered all of the temptations of life and had lived so completely in the interest of others that they had fulfilled the great motivating principle of their religion, which is that life consists in serving others as one would wish to be served. The seven stars of Pleiades were seven beautiful maidens that had surpassed most other girls in their devotion and service in the interest of their tribe. It is most remarkable how closely this concept is related to the classical myth regarding the seven daughters of Atlas and the nymph, Pleione.

A part of a young man's examination to determine his ability to withstand pain and his power of self-control consists in performing an operation at the time of his graduation. This operation is at the same time calculated to provide him with his badge of attainment. It consists of the boy's lying on his back and allowing the appointed operator to knock out one of his front upper teeth. This is done by putting a peg against the tooth and hitting it a series of sharp blows with a stone. He must endure this without flinching. We saw scores that carried this diploma. Prior to this, other very severe tests of physical endurance had been successfully completed.

The marvelous vision of these primitive people is illustrated by the fact that they can see many stars that our race cannot see. In this connection it is authoritatively recorded regarding the Maori of New Zealand that they can see the satellites of Jupiter which are only visible to the white man's eye with the aid of telescopes. These people prove that they can see the satellites by telling the man at the telescope when the eclipse of one of the stars occurs. It is said of these primitive Aborigines of Australia that they can see animals moving at a distance of a mile which ordinary white people can not see at all.

While these evidences of superior physical development command our most profound admiration, their ability to build superb bodies and maintain them in excellent condition in so difficult an environment commands our genuine respect. It is a supreme test of human efficiency. It is doubtful if many places in the world can demonstrate so great a contrast in physical development and perfection of body as that which exists between the primitive Aborigines of Australia who have been the sole arbiters of their fate, and those Aborigines who have been under the influence of the white man. The white man has deprived them of their original habitats and is now feeding them in reservations while using them as laborers in modern industrial pursuits. This contrast between the primitive Aborigines as they still exist in isolated communities in Australia and the modern members of the clans is not, however, much greater than that between these excellent primitives and the whites, near whom they are living.

In my comparative study of primitive races in different parts of the world, of modernized members of their groups and of whites who have displaced them, as well as in my study of our typical modern social organization, I have seldom, if ever, found whites suffering so tragically from evidence of physical degeneration, as expressed in tooth decay and change in facial form, as are the whites of eastern Australia. This has occurred on the very best of the land that these primitives formerly occupied and becomes at once a monument to the wisdom of the primitive Aborigines and a signboard of warning to the modern civilization that has supplanted them. Their superb physical excellence is demonstrated in every isolated group in the primitive stocks with which we came in contact. For tribes that have lived along the coast and had access to the sea foods, their stature was large and well formed.

When living in the Bush they are largely without clothing. Where they are congregated in the reservations they are required to wear clothing. It is important to note in these people the splendid proportions of the faces, all of which are broad, with the dental arches wide and well contoured. This is

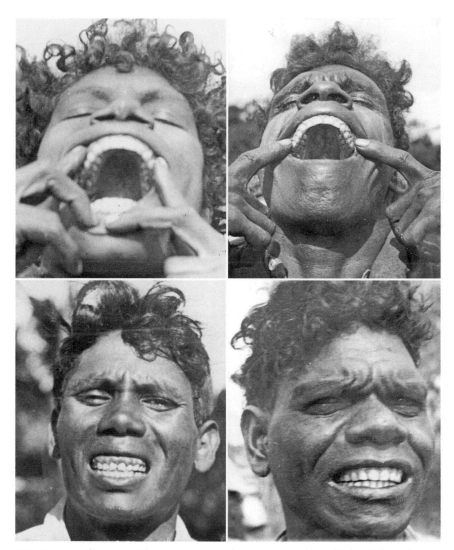

FIG. 53. No other primitive race seems to deserve so much credit for skill in obeying nature's laws as these primitive Aborigines because of the perpetual drought hazards of much of the land they live in. Half of Australia has less than ten inches of rain per year. Note the magnificent dental arches and beautiful teeth of these primitives. Tooth decay was almost unknown in many districts.

Nature's normal form for all humans and is shown in Figs. 53 and 54 (upper right). The person in Fig. 53 (upper left) is a woman.

Various factors in the changed environment were studied critically. Samples of foods were gathered for chemical analysis; and the changes in the modern diet from that which was characteristic of the primitives were studied.

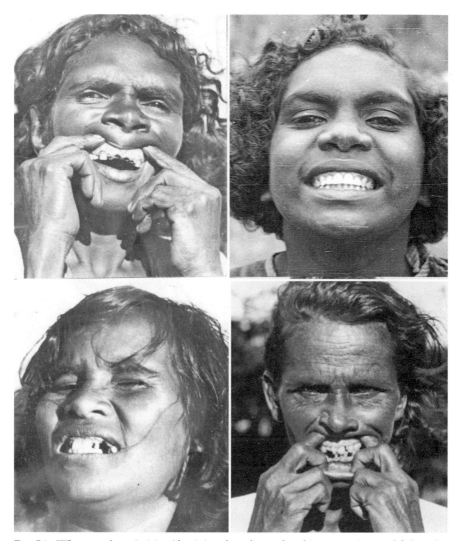

FIG. 54. Wherever the primitive Aborigines have been placed in reservations and fed on the white man's foods of commerce, dental caries has become rampant. This destroys their beauty, prevents mastication, and provides infection for seriously injuring their bodies. Note the contrast between the primitive woman in the upper right and the three modernized women.

When the teeth of the primitives and the teeth found in the skulls that had been assembled in the museums were examined, it was found that dental caries or tooth decay was exceedingly rare among the isolated groups. Those individuals, however, who had adopted the foods of the white man suffered extremely from tooth decay as did the whites. Where they had no opportunity to get native food to combine with the white man's food their condition was desperate and extreme. This is readily disclosed in Fig. 54. Note contrast with upper right. It is quite impossible to imagine the suffering that these people were compelled to endure due to abscessing teeth resulting from rampant tooth decay. As we had found in some of the modernized islands of the Pacific, we discovered that here, too, discouragement and a longing for death had taken the place of a joy in living in many. Few souls in the world have experienced this discouragement and this longing to a greater degree.

One of the most important phases of our special quest was to get information that would throw light on the degeneration of the facial pattern that occurs so often in our modern civilization. This has its expression in the narrowing and lengthening of the face and the development of crooked teeth. It is most remarkable and should be one of the most challenging facts that can come to our modern civilization that such primitive races as the Aborigines of Australia, have reproduced for generation after generation through many centuries—no one knows for how many thousands of years—without the development of a conspicuous number of irregularities of the dental arches. Yet, in the next generation after these people adopt the foods of the white man, a large percentage of the children developed irregularities of the dental arches with conspicuous facial deformities. The deformity patterns are similar to those seen in white civilizations. Typical illustrations of this will be seen in Figs. 55 and 56. Severe deformities of the face were frequently seen in the modernized groups, as evidenced in Fig. 57.

The data obtained from a study of the native Australians who are located in a reservation near Sydney, at La Perouse, revealed that among the Aborigines 47.5 percent of the teeth had been attacked by dental caries, and 40 percent of the individuals had abnormal dental arches. For the women of this group, 81.3 percent of all the teeth had been attacked by dental caries, and for the men, 60.4 percent, and for the children, 16.5 percent. In this group 100 percent of the individuals were affected by dental caries.

Palm Island is a government reservation situated in the ocean about fifty miles from the mainland, off the east coast of Australia, about two-thirds of the way up the coast. It was reached by a government launch. Included in the population of this reservation are a large number of adults who have been moved from various districts on the mainland of Central and Eastern Australia and many children who were born either before or after their parents were moved to this reservation. The food available on the Island is almost entirely that provided by the government. Of ninety-eight individuals examined and measured, 53.1 percent of them had dental caries. For the group as a whole, 8.9 percent of all of the teeth were affected; for the women, 21.2 percent; for the men, 14.2 percent; and for the children, 5.8 percent. Fifty percent of the children had deformed dental arches, which occurred in only 11 percent of the adults.

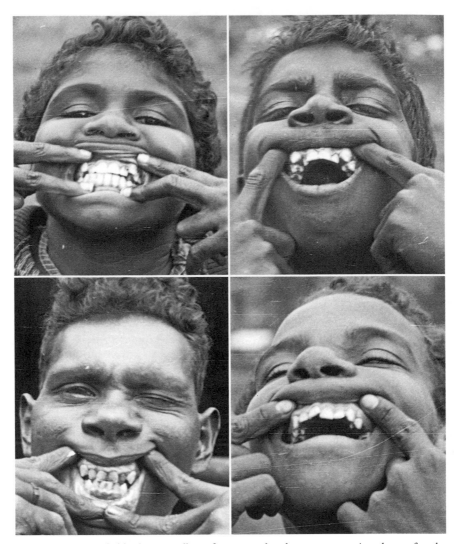

FIG. 55. It is remarkable that regardless of race or color the new generations born after the adoption by primitives of deficient foods develop in general the same facial and dental arch deformities and skeletal defects. Note the characteristic narrowing of the dental arches and crowding of the teeth of this modernized generation of Aborigines and their similarity to the facial patterns of modern whites.

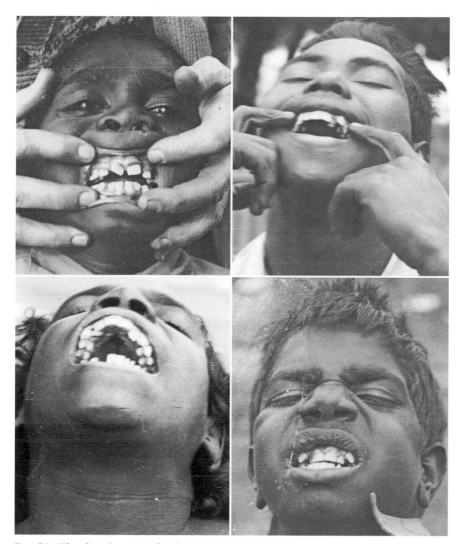

FIG. 56. The disturbance in facial growth is often so serious as to make normal breathing through the nose very difficult. This is primarily due to faulty development of the maxillary bones.

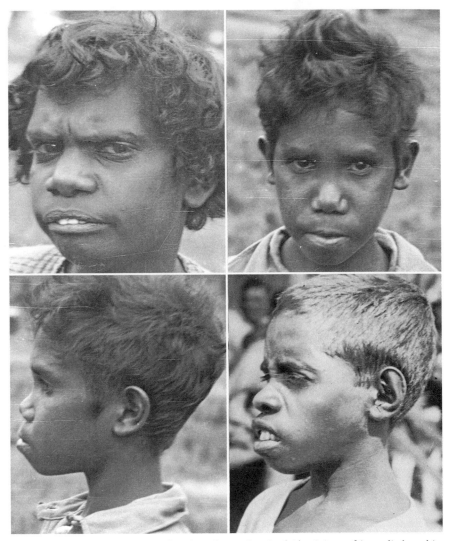

FIG. 57. Deformity patterns produced in the modernized Aborigines of Australia by white men's food. Note the undershot mandible, upper left, the pinched nostrils and facial deformity of all four.

Cape Bedford is situated about three-fourths of the way up the east coast and is so isolated that it was necessary for us to use a special aeroplane to reach it. Landing was made on the beach. This group of people is under the management of a German Lutheran missionary. They are dependent almost entirely on the food provided by the mission and the government. The official in charge had spent fifty years in devoted service to these native people. We found him exceedingly sad because of the very rapid breakdown that was in progress among the natives in his care. The dental caries for the group of eighty-three individuals studied was 12.4 percent of their 2,176 teeth examined. For the women, this amounted to 37.2 percent of the teeth; for the men, 8.4 percent; and for the children, 6.1 percent. Of the eighty-three individuals, 48.1 percent had been affected by dental caries. Many of the adults in this group had been born on plantations under the influence of the modern nutrition, and many of the children had been born in the mission. For the adults, 46 percent had abnormally formed dental arches, and for the children, 41.6 percent. We were advised that deaths occurred very frequently from tuberculosis. This reservation does not provide the natives with natural hunting grounds capable of providing the people with animal life for food. The coast for some distance inland is a series of sand dunes which are slowly being transferred over the vegetation by wind, completely smothering it. While the coast is well supplied with a variety of deep-water fish the natives have practically no equipment for obtaining them, a condition which restricts them very largely to the use of the imported foods supplied by the officials.

Our next stop, using the special aeroplane, was at Lockhart River, which is about four-fifths of the way up the east coast of Australia. Here again we were able to land on the beach near a large group of primitive Aborigines. The isolation here is so nearly complete that they are dependent upon the sea and the land for their foods. This part of Australia, namely, the York Peninsula, is still so primitive that there has been very little encroachment by the white population. It will be remembered that in this area there are no roads, the country being a primitive wilderness. Of fifty-eight individuals examined, their 1,784 teeth revealed that only 4.3 percent had been attacked by dental caries. For the women, this amounted to 3.4 percent; for the men, 6.1 percent; and for the children, 3.2 percent. Some of these men had at some time worked on cattle ranches for the white men. Of the children, only 6.3 percent had abnormal dental arches, and of the adults, 8.7 percent. In this group, therefore, 91.4 percent of all ages had reproduced the typical racial pattern as compared with 56 percent of the group at Cape Bedford, 62 percent of the group at Palm Island, and 60 percent at La Perouse. At Lockhart River, 32.7 percent of the individuals had dental caries.

A reservation called Cowall Creek on the west side of York Peninsula situated on the Gulf of Carpenteria, was reached by flying our special plane to Horn Island in the Torres Strait north of Australia and proceeding from there by boat to Thursday Island, and on, by boat, to Cowall Creek. In this reservation thirty-five individuals were studied and found to be in a very pathetic condition. We were told that deaths occurred frequently. Of the 976 teeth examined, 24.6 percent had been attacked by tooth decay. For the women, this amounted to 60.7 percent; for the men, 30.4 percent; and for the children,

8.9 percent. Forty-nine and six-tenths percent of the individuals studied had abnormal dental arches. Of the children 66.6 percent had deformed dental arches, and 9 percent of the adults. Many of these adults had been raised in the bush. Of the individuals studied, 68.6 percent had had dental caries. One can scarcely visualize, without observing it, the distress of a group of primitive people situated as these people are, compelled to live in a very restricted area, forced to live on food provided by the government, while they are conscious that if they could return to their normal habits of life they would regain their health and again enjoy life. Many individuals were seen with abscessing teeth. One girl with a fistula exuding pus on the outside of her face is shown in Fig. 58 (upper right). In their native life where they could get the foods that keep them well and preserve their teeth, they had no need for dentists. Now they have need, but have no dentists. It is easy to chide and blame the officials who provide them with the modernized foods under which they are breaking, but it must be remembered that practically all modern civilizations are more or less in the same plight themselves.

An opportunity was provided for examining a group of the native Aborigines of Australia who made up the crew of eighteen for a pearl-fishing boat. Of this group, 5.7 percent of their 554 teeth had been attacked by tooth decay. These individuals could be readily divided into two groups; namely, those who had been raised in the Bush and those who had been raised in missions. For the thirteen raised in the Bush, not a single tooth of their 364 teeth had ever been attacked by tooth decay and not a single individual had deformed dental arches. In contrast with this, of the five raised in the mission, 19.3 percent of their 140 teeth had been attacked by tooth decay and 40 percent of these individuals had abnormal dental arches.

The cook on the government boat was an aboriginal Australian from Northern Australia. He had been trained on a military craft as a dietitian. Nearly all his teeth were lost. It is of interest that while the native Aborigines had relatively perfect teeth, this man who was a trained dietitian for the whites had lost nearly all his teeth from tooth decay and pyorrhea.

In the group of Aborigines so far reported, there were many who had come from the interior districts of Australia and many who had always lived near the coast. These two types of districts provided quite different types of foods. Those near the coast were able to obtain animal life from the sea, including fish, dugong or sea cow, a great variety of shell fish, and some sea plants. Those from the interior districts could not obtain animal life of the sea, but did obtain animal life of the land which was eaten with their plant foods in each case. It was quite important to reach a group of Aborigines who had always lived inland and who were on a reservation inland. This contact was made with the group at a government reservation called Cherbourg. A typical group of individuals was examined. Of forty-five individuals with 1,236

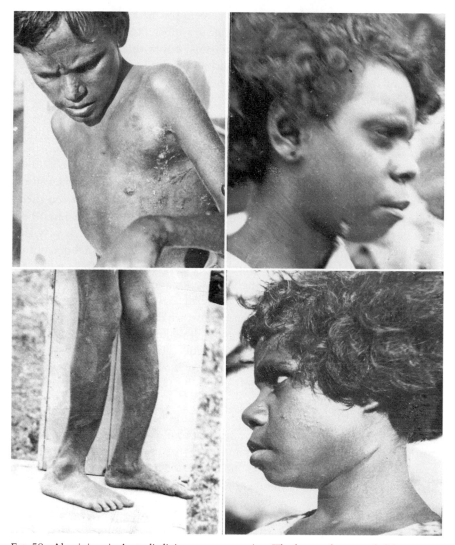

FIG. 58. Aborigines in Australia living on a reservation. The boy at the upper left has suppurating tubercular axillary glands. The girl at the upper right has pus running to the outside of her face from an abscessed tooth. The boy whose legs are shown at the lower left has a badly deformed body from malnutrition. The girl at the lower right has tubercular glands of the neck.

teeth, 42.5 percent of the teeth had been attacked by tooth decay. For the women, this constituted 43.7 percent; for the men, 64.6 percent; and for the children, 5.6 percent. Of all of the individuals here examined 64.5 percent had dental caries. It is of interest that many of these men had worked on white men's cattle ranches. While the adults showed 11.7 percent to have deformed dental arches, this rose to 50 percent for the children of the group. We were informed that in all of these groups tuberculosis was taking a very heavy toll. In Fig. 58, upper left, will be seen a boy with a supperating tubercular gland of the axilla; at the right, a girl with a fistula draining pus onto the outside of the face from an abscessed tooth; below, deformed legs and a girl with tubercular glands of the neck.

A reservation situated on the coast where sea foods were available might be expected to make available a particular type of nutrition through sea foods. The individuals in a reservation for the Aborigines at Tweed Heads, which is so situated, were studied. Of the twenty-seven individuals examined, 89 percent had dental caries. Of their 774 teeth, 39.7 percent had been attacked by dental caries. For the women, this amounted to 62.5 percent; for the men, 70.9 percent; and for the children, 20.8 percent. Most of these children had been born in this environment while their parents were being fed, largely, the foods provided by the government and mission. In this group, 83.4 percent of the children had deformed dental arches, and 33.3 percent of the adults.

An interesting incident was brought to my attention in one of the Australian reservations where the food was practically all supplied by the government. I was told by the director in charge, and in further detail by the other officials, that a number of native babies had become ill while nursing from their mothers. Some had died. By changing the nutrition to a condensed whole milk product, the babies recovered. When placed back on their mother's breast food they again became ill. The problem was: Why was not their mothers' milk adequate?

I was later told by the director of a condition that had developed in the pen of the reservation's hogs which were kept to use up the scraps and garbage from the reservation's kitchens. He reported that one after another the hogs went down with a type of paralysis and could not get up. The symptoms were suggestively like vitamin A deficiency in both the babies and the hogs, and indicated the treatment.

The rapid degeneration of the Australian Aborigines after the adoption of the government's modern foods provides a demonstration that should be infinitely more convincing than animal experimentation. It should be a matter not only of concern but deep alarm that human beings can degenerate physically so rapidly by the use of a certain type of nutrition, particularly the dietary products used so generally by modern civilization.

The child life among the Aborigines of Australia proved to be exceedingly interesting. Children develop independence very young and learn very early to take care of themselves. Mothers are very affectionate and show great concern when their children are not thriving. Two typical mothers with their children are shown in Fig. 59. These children, as suggested in the picture, were keenly interested in everything that I did, but were not alarmed or frightened.

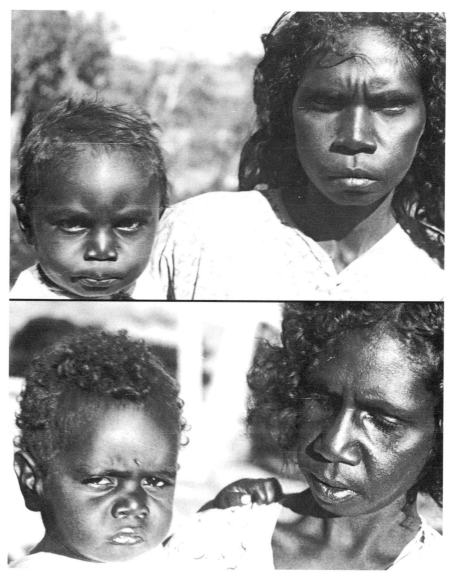

Fig. 59. Typical Aborigine mothers with their children.

The wonderful wisdom of these primitive people was attested by the principal of the public school at Palm Island. A mother died and her nursing infant was taken care of by its maternal grandmother, who had not recently given birth to a child. She proceeded to carry out the primitive formula for providing breast food by artificial means. Her method was to make an ointment of the fresh bodies of an insect which made its nest in the leaves of a certain tree. This she rubbed on her breast and in a short time produced milk liberally for this foster child. I was shown the type of insect, photographed its nest and the colony inside when the nest was opened. The people who vouched for this circumstance declared that they had seen the entire procedure and knew the facts to be as stated. They further stated that this was common knowledge among the Aborigines.

Another important source of information regarding the Aborigines of Australia was provided by a study of the skeletal material and skulls in the museums at Sydney and Canberra, particularly the former. I do not know the number of skulls that are available there for study, but it is very large. I examined many and found them remarkably uniform in design and quality. The dental arches were splendidly formed. The teeth were in excellent condition with exceedingly little dental caries. A characteristic of these skulls was the evidence of a shortage of material for those that had been transferred to a museum from the interior arid plains country. Those skulls, however, that had come from coastal areas where sea foods were available, show much more massive dimensions of the general pattern. In Fig. 60 will be seen typical skulls showing the normal dental arches and general design of the head. It is of interest to note the very heavy orbital ridges which characterize this race.

I have previously referred to a report by Professor Weidenreich regarding the resemblance of the Australian natives' skulls to those of the recently discovered Peking man in the caves of China. In Fig. 60 are two views for comparison. The skull at the left is that of an Australian primitive photographed in a museum in Sydney, and an outline of the Peking skull is shown at the right. Professor Weidenreich has emphasized the observations that when three skulls are put in series, namely, the Australian primitive, the Peking skull and a chimpanzee skull, the Peking skull appears to be about half way between the two in design and developmental order. The Australian primitive's skull is higher in the crown, showing much greater brain capacity. The supra-orbital depressions are less deep in the Peking than in the chimpanzee, and still less deep in the Australian primitive. The supra-orbital ridges which produce the prominent eyebrows are less pronounced in the Australian primitive than in the Peking man, and still more prominent in the chimpanzee. The prominent supra-orbital ridges of the chimpanzee face are shown in Fig. 48.

The age of the Peking skulls has been variously placed from several hundred thousand to a million years. A distinguished anthropologist has stated that the Australian primitives are the only people living on the earth today that could be part of the first race of mankind. It is a matter of concern that if a scale were extended a mile long and the decades represented by inches, there would apparently be more degeneration in the last few inches than

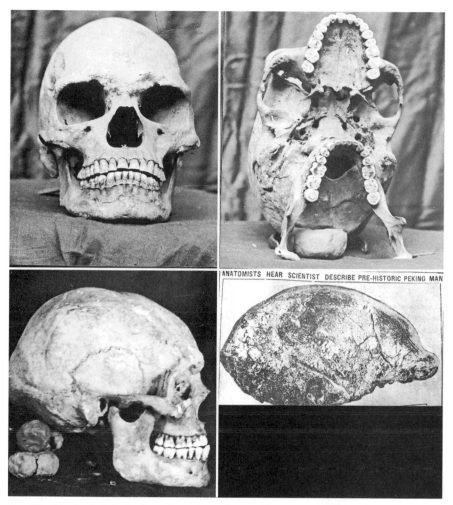

FIG. 60. The buried skulls throughout Australia provide a dependable record of their physical excellence and splendid facial and dental arch forms. In the lower pictures are shown the skull dome of a typical Australian Aborigine for comparison with that of the recently discovered Peking man who possibly lived a million years ago.

in the preceding mile. This gives some idea of the virulence of the blight contributed by our modern civilization.

The foods available for these people are exceedingly limited in variety and quantity, due to the absence of rains, and unfertility of the soil. For plant foods they used roots, stems, leaves, berries and seeds of grasses and a native pea eaten with tissues of large and small animals. The large animals available are the kangaroo and wallaby. Among the small animals they have a variety of rodents, insects, beetles and grubs, and wherever available various forms of animal life from the rivers and oceans. Birds and birds' eggs are used where available. They are able to balance their rations to provide the requisites for splendid body building and body repair. In several parts of Australia, which originally supported a large population of the primitives, none are left except a few score in reservations. These also are rapidly disappearing. Their fertility has been so greatly reduced that the death rate far exceeds the birth rate.

This group provides evidence of exceptional efficiency in obeying the laws of Nature through thousands of years, even in a parched land that is exceedingly inhospitable because of the scant plant foods for either men or animals. While the Aborigines are credited with being the oldest race on the face of the earth today, they are dying out with great rapidity wherever they have changed their native nutrition to that of the modern white civilization. For them this is not a matter of choice, but rather of necessity, since in a large part of Australia the few that are left are crowded into reservations where they have little or no access to native foods and are compelled to live on the foods provided for them by our white civilization. They demonstrate in a tragic way the inadequacy of the white man's dietary programs.

Chapter 11

ISOLATED AND MODERNIZED
TORRES STRAIT ISLANDERS

IN STUDYING the relationship between nutrition and physical characteristics, it is important to make observations at the point of contact with civilization where as few factors as possible in the environment have been modified by that contact. My previous studies have shown that wherever groups of people were utilizing sea foods abundantly in connection with land plants including roots, greens and fruits, they enjoyed fine physical development with uniform reproduction of the racial pattern and a very high immunity to dental caries. For this particular study we wished to select a racial group living on islands in tropical or subtropical climate, whose ancestral stocks differed from those previously observed, and which was located at points of contact with modern civilization. A high level of excellence might be expected among the groups who were in process of being modernized but were still utilizing the native foods.

For this study the inhabitants of islands north of Australia were chosen in order to record the effect on the Asiatic and Malay stocks at the points of contact of the north with the south and of the east with the west. In the Torres Strait there are a number of fertile islands supporting populations of from several hundred to a few thousand individuals each. These groups are in an area of the sea that is well stocked with sea animal life, and during the past they have been sufficiently isolated to provide protection. The racial stocks have retained their identities and include Papuans, New Guineans, Mobuiags, Arakuns, Kendals and Yonkas. The splendid dental arches of these groups will be seen in the various illustrations. Many of the girls are quite prepossessing, as may be seen in Fig. 61.

With the valuable assistance of the officials of the Australian Government we were able to make investigations on several islands in the Torres Strait. The local administrator provided us with a government boat and personal introductions to the local chief and local representatives of the government. We were accompanied by the administrator and by the general manager of the government stores. These stores have been located on the various islands, and the profit derived from them is used for administrative expenses of the government. They provide modern clothing in addition to foods, chiefly white flour, polished rice, canned goods, and sugar. Studies were made on the various

167

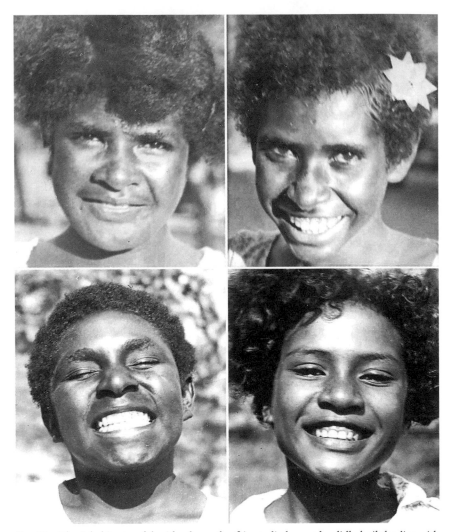

FIG. 61. The inhabitants of the islands north of Australia have splendidly built bodies with fine facial and dental arch form.

islands in the order in which the stores had been installed on them. It is important to have in mind the nature of these islands. Some are of volcanic origin and have rugged interiors with deep bays; others are of coral origin. All are in a zone that is abundantly supplied with sea animal life, this being the scene of the richest pearl fishing industry in the world.

Badu Island had had the store for the longest period, namely twenty-three years. Of the 586 teeth of twenty individuals examined, 20.6 percent had been attacked by tooth decay. Of the individuals examined 95 percent had dental caries. Unfortunately, our stay at this island was accompanied by a torrential downpour which made it very difficult for us to carry forward our investigations. Had we been able to examine the mothers the figures doubtless would have been much higher. The children were examined at the school and showed 18.8 percent of the teeth to have been attacked by tooth decay. The men examined showed 21.9 percent. Figures given me by Dr. Gibson, who had been taken by the government to the island to make extractions, showed that he found as high as 60 percent of the teeth had been attacked by tooth decay. For the children of this group, 33.3 percent had abnormal dental arches, whereas only 9.1 percent of the adults' arches were abnormally formed.

On York Island, 1,876 teeth of sixty-five individuals showed that 12.7 percent had been attacked by tooth decay. For the women, this was 20.2 percent; for the men, 12.1 percent; and for the children, 7 percent. For the children, 47.1 percent had abnormal dental arches; for the adults, 27 percent were affected. The individuals on this island had been in contact with the pearl fisheries industry for several years. Several of the men had been working on the fishing boat. Of the sixty-five individuals examined, 67.6 percent had dental caries.

On Darnley Island, thirty-three individuals showed that of their 900 teeth 5.7 percent had been attacked by tooth decay. The store had been established on this island recently. For the women, 16.6 percent of the teeth had been attacked; for the men, 6.3 percent; and for the children, 4.1 percent. On this island, 29.6 percent of the children showed abnormal dental arches, and 14.3 percent of the adults. Of the whole group, 46.1 percent had been attacked by dental caries.

On Murray Island where a store had recently been established, of the 1,074 teeth examined for 39 individuals, only 0.7 percent of the teeth had been attacked by tooth decay. For the women, this amounted to 2 percent; for the men, 1.7 percent; and for the children, 0.26 percent. Only 12.8 percent of the group had dental caries. It is significant that the natives were conscious of a danger from the presence on the island of a store providing imported foods. This had been so serious a problem that there was a question whether it would be safe for us to land, since on the last visit of the government officials, blood was almost shed because of the opposition of the natives to the government's program. The result of our examination indicates that dental caries on these islands shows an incidence which has an apparent direct relationship to the length of time government stores have been established there. The immunity to dental caries on this island is nearly 100 percent. Of the adults, 14.3 percent had abnormal dental arches, and of the children, 34.4 percent.

Thursday Island is the location of the administrative center for the group. Although it is the best sheltered harbor and affords protection for small boats in the Torres Strait, it was not originally inhabited by the natives. They considered it unfit for habitation because the soil was so poor that it could not provide the proper plant foods to be eaten with the sea foods which are abundant about all of the islands. Nearly all of the whites inhabiting the islands of this district live on this island. They are the families of the administrative officers and of merchants who are engaged in the pearl industry. Owing to the infertility of the soil, practically all of the food has to be shipped in except the little that the whites obtain from the sea. On the island there were many native families, with children attending the native school, while their fathers worked in the pearling fleets. Thirty individuals in three fleets were examined, and of their 960 teeth only thirty-five had been attacked by dental caries, or 3.6 percent. Of these thirty individuals, five, or 16.3 percent had abnormal dental arches. The men who had teeth attacked by dental caries informed me that this had happened after they had engaged on the pearling vessels and began to use the foods provided there. In the native school on Thursday Island twenty-three children were examined. They were living in homes in which a considerable part of the food was purchased at the company stores. The incidence of tooth decay was 12.2 percent of their 664 teeth. Many of these Thursday Island children had been born since their parents had begun using the commercial foods provided to the islanders. Among twenty-three individuals, 43.5 percent had abnormal dental arches.

While these investigations were planned and carried out primarily to obtain data on the condition of the native races in contact with modern white civilization, wherever possible, data were obtained on the whites also. In a school for whites on Thursday Island, fifty children were examined with regard to their dental arches, but an embarrassing situation was encountered with regard to the sensitiveness of the whites in the matter of having their children examined for dental caries. Figures were obtained for the facial development which reveal that, out of the fifty children examined, 64 percent had irregularities of facial and dental arch development. In the upper half of Fig. 62, will be seen a group of children photographed in the native school, and in the lower a group of white girls photographed at the white school. The difference in their facial development is readily seen. The son of the white teacher (Fig. 66, left) had marked under development of his face. The white population lived largely on canned food.

Hammond Island adjoins Thursday Island sufficiently close by to be easily reached in small boats. Accordingly, the people of this island have access to the stores of the white settlement on Thursday Island. Unlike Thursday Island, Hammond Island is quite fertile. Of twenty-seven individuals, all of native

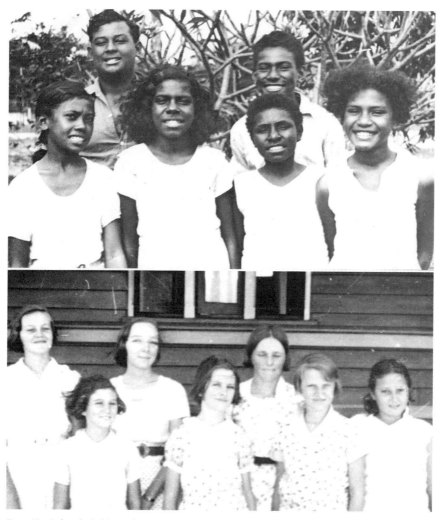

FIG. 62. School children from the two groups on Thursday Island. Note the beautifully proportioned faces of the natives, and the pinched nostrils and marked disturbance in proportions of the faces of the whites. The dental arches of the natives are broad, while many of the whites have very crowded teeth. The parents and children of the natives used native foods while the parents and children of the whites used the modern imported foods of commerce.

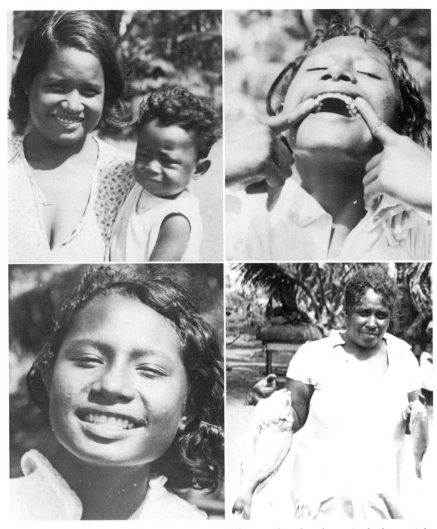

FIG. 63. These pictures tell an interesting story. The grandmother shown in the lower right knew the importance of sea food for her children and grandchildren and did the fishing herself. Note the beautiful teeth and well-formed faces of her daughters.

stock, 16.5 percent of their 732 teeth had been attacked by dental caries, and 40 percent of the individuals showed some deformity of the dental arches. After examining the children at the mission school, I inquired whether there were not families on the island that were living entirely isolated from contact with modern influences. I was taken to the far side of the island to an isolated family. This family had continued to live on their own resources. They were raising vegetables including bananas, pumpkins, and pawpaws. In the cases of the three girls in the family, one with a child five months of age, only six of their eighty-four teeth had been attacked by tooth decay, or 7.1 percent, as compared with 16.5 percent for the entire group on this island. These three girls all had normally developed dental arches and normal features. Three of the girls are shown in Fig. 63. We inquired about the mother and were told that she was out fishing, notwithstanding the fact that the sea was quite rough. While we were there, she came in with two fish (Fig. 63). Here was one of the principal secrets of their happiness and success in life. The Catholic priest who had charge of the mission on this island told me that this family practically never asked for assistance of any kind, and was always in a position to help others. They were happy and well nourished. It is important to note that the progressive degeneration in facial form which occurred in many of the families on the other islands was not found in this family.

The incidence of dental caries ranged from 20.6 percent of all of the teeth examined for the various age groups on Badu Island to 0.7 percent, on Murray Island. A group of individuals from this island will be seen in Fig. 64. Note the remarkable width of the dental arches. Note also in this connection that the natives of this island are conscious of the superior food of their locality and wish that their people were not required to purchase food from the government store. The island is situated on the Barrier Reef and has an abundant supply of small fish. The swarms of fish are often so dense that the natives throw a spear with several prongs into the school of fish and when the spear is drawn back, there are several fish on it. This condition provides abundant food for sharks, many of which could be seen surrounding the schools of small fish. Encircling the group, they dashed in, mouths open, and gorged themselves with the mass of fish from the water. It seemed quite remarkable that the people were willing to go into the water to spear the fish within the zone frequently approached by the sharks, but I was told by the natives that when the fish are so abundant the sharks never attack human beings. One of the natives rowed me in his canoe to a point where I could photograph the sharks at close range. To show his disdain for the shark, he had no hesitancy in standing up in the end of the canoe and hurling his spear into the side of the monster. The spear was immediately thrown out by the shark, which had not been frightened sufficiently to make it leave the scene of action. The sharks in my pictures were swimming so close to the shore that the upper part of the tail was forced out of the water, also the back fin, in order to clear the bottom. It was a great revelation to watch the movement of the tail. Instead of swinging it from side to side like other fish, with which I was familiar, the shark would rotate its tail half or three quarters of a turn in a motion like that of a propeller of a boat, then reverse the motion for the return trip. By a sudden increase of speed in this motion, the shark could dart ahead at a rapid rate, corral the small fish by encircling them, and finally make a dash through

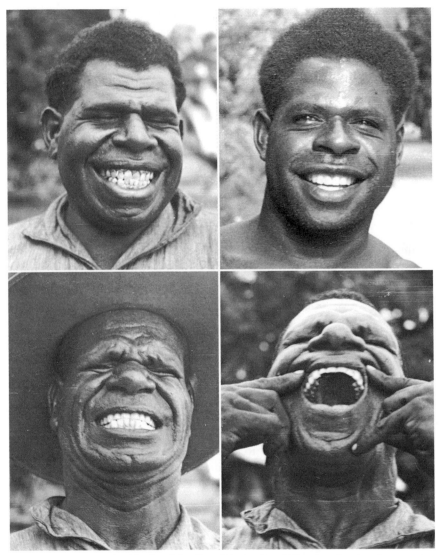

FIG. 64. Natives on the islands of the Great Barrier Reef. The dental arches here teach a high degree of excellence.

the school with its mouth open. Hundreds of the small fish, in order to escape, dart out of the water into the air. This exposes them to the birds, a flock of which follows the sharks when they are feeding on the fish. The birds dive down at the time they see the shark making his raid and catch the small fish as they dart out of the water. It is by the birds of prey that the native fishermen from their lookout locate the schools of fish. While there is a difference of opinion as to whether some species of shark will attack human beings, we saw one pearl diver who bore enormous scars received from the jaws of a shark.

The procedure on one island is to snare the sharks by calling them by means of special sounds made by clapping together two large half shells on the surface of the water. This attracts the shark, and then the men one at a time go into the water with a sharp stick with which they guard themselves against attack. A noose made of rope of coconut fiber is slipped over the shark's head and over the back fin. It is then allowed to tire out and is brought to shore. It was not unusual in a good season for the shark fishers to bring in three or four in a night's fishing. The strength of the native swimmers is almost beyond belief. The pearling boats are frequently in great danger of being dashed to pieces on a coral reef, since in those waters gales of fifty miles an hour are frequent. We experienced some such gales. On one occasion, when a pearling boat was wrecked some distance from an exposed rock, one strong swimmer rescued and helped two dozen of the crew to the rock, and was himself rescued after being in the water continuously for thirty-two hours. The pearling boats feed their crew largely on commercial provisions. When the men have been continuously on the boats for one or two years, or often when they have been at sea using this food for six months, they have rampant tooth decay. When the cavities approach or reach the pulp chambers the pain produced in the teeth by the high pressure in deep water produces such agony that they often have to give up pearling.

Physical characteristics of all these residents of the Torres Strait Islands, regardless of their tribal group, were, sturdy development throughout their bodies, broad dental arches, and for all of those who had always lived only on their native food, a close proximity to one hundred percent immunity to dental caries. These men are natural mariners. They do not hesitate to make long trips even in rough seas in their homemade crafts. They have an uncanny skill in determining the location of invisible coral reefs. They relate the height of the swell as it rolls over the reef to particular color tones in the water, all of which were too vague for me to see even when they were pointed out.

Among the inhabitants of the Torres Strait Islands, almost all individuals who had been born before the foods of modern civilization had become available were found to have dental arches normal in form. In many families, however, living on islands where a store had been established for some time, and on Thursday Island where imported foods had been available for several decades, many individuals were found who had been born since the use of imported foods. They had gross deformities of the dental arches. This fact is illustrated

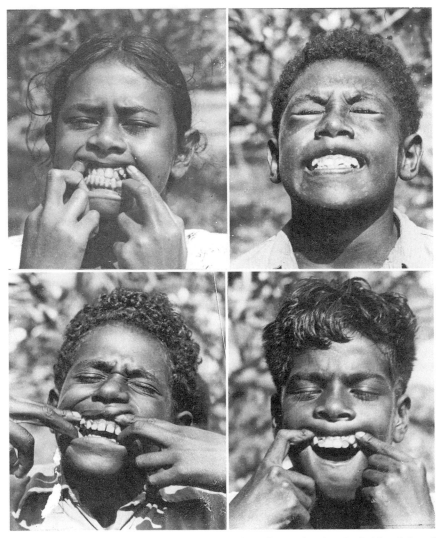

FIG. 65. The contrast between the primitive and modernized natives in facial and dental arch form is as striking here as elsewhere. These young natives were born to parents who had adopted our modern foods of commerce. Note the narrowed faces and dental arches with pinched nostrils and crowding of the teeth. Their magnificent heredity could not protect them.

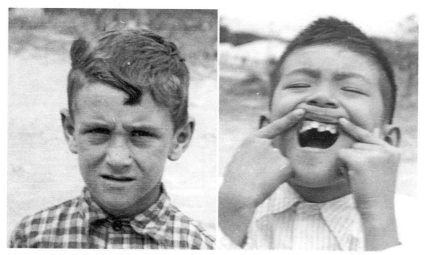

FIG. 66. These children are from the white colony on Thursday Island. Note the pinched nostrils and deformed dental arches with crowding of the teeth. The boy at the left is a mouth-breather.

in Fig. 65 in which typical depression of the laterals and narrowing of the upper arch and abnormal prominence of the cuspids due to the lack of space for the normal eruption may be seen. The facial deformity in two white boys is seen in Fig. 66. Rampant tooth decay in white children is shown in Fig. 67.

We are particularly concerned with data that will throw light on the nature of the forces responsible for the production of these deformities. Since they do not appear to their full extent until the eruption of the permanent teeth as part of the development of the adult, it is easy for the abnormality to be ascribed to the period of child growth. As a result, it has been related to faulty breathing habits, thumb-sucking, posture, or sleeping habits, of the child.

It would be difficult to find a more happy and contented people than the primitives in the Torres Strait Islands as they lived without contact with modern civilization. Indeed, they seem to resent very acutely the modern intrusion. They not only have nearly perfect bodies, but an associated personality and character of a high degree of excellence. One is continually impressed with happiness, peace and health while in their congenial presence.

These people are not lazy, but they do not struggle over hard to obtain food. Necessities that are not readily at hand they do not have. Their home life reaches a very high ideal and among them there is practically no crime.

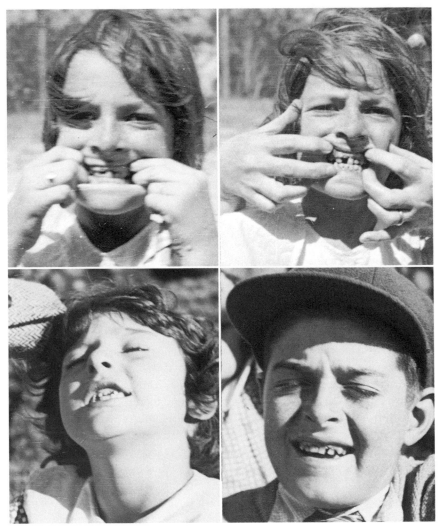

FIG. 67. As everywhere these whites prefer the modernized foods and pay the penalty in rampant tooth decay. They are in pathetic contrast with the superb unspoiled natives. They are within reach of some of the best foods to be found anywhere in the world and yet do not use them; a typical characteristic of modern whites.

In their native state they have exceedingly little disease. Dr. J. R. Nimmo, the government physician in charge of the supervision of this group, told me in his thirteen years with them he had not seen a single case of malignancy, and had seen only one that he had suspected might be malignancy among the entire four thousand native population. He stated that during this same period he had operated on several dozen malignancies for the white population, which numbers about three hundred. He reported that among the primitive stock other affections requiring surgical interference were rare.

The environment of the Torres Strait Islanders provides a very liberal supply of sea foods and fertile islands on which an adequate quantity of tropical plants are readily grown. Taro, bananas, papaya, and plums are all grown abundantly. The sea foods include large and small fish in great abundance, dugong, and a great variety of shellfish. These foods have developed for them remarkable physiques with practically complete immunity to dental caries. Wherever they have adopted the white man's foods, however, they suffer the typical expressions of degeneration, such as, loss of immunity to dental caries; and in the succeeding generations there is a marked change in facial and dental arch form with marked lowering of resistance to disease.

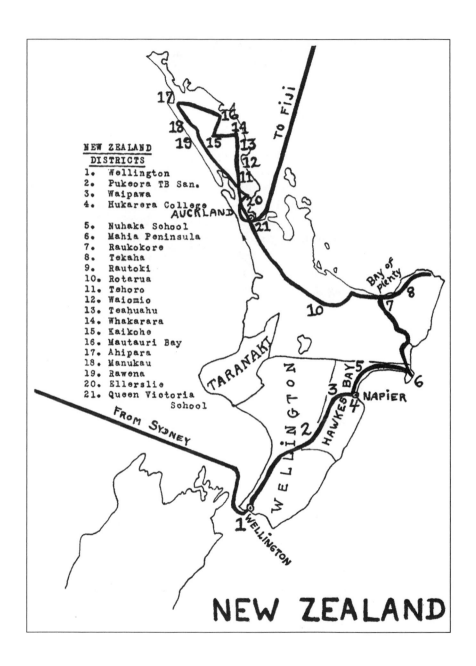

NEW ZEALAND
DISTRICTS
1. Wellington
2. Pukeora TB San.
3. Waipawa
4. Hukarera College

5. Nuhaka School
6. Mahia Peninsula
7. Raukokore
8. Tekaha
9. Rautoki
10. Rotarua
11. Tehoro
12. Waiomio
13. Teahuahu
14. Whakarara
15. Kaikohe
16. Mautauri Bay
17. Ahipara
18. Manukau
19. Rawena
20. Ellerslie
21. Queen Victoria
          School

NEW ZEALAND

Chapter 12

ISOLATED AND MODERNIZED NEW ZEALAND MAORI

BECAUSE of the fine reputation of the racial stock in its primitive condition, it was with particular interest that studies were made in New Zealand. Pickerill[1] has made a very extensive study of the New Zealand Maori, both by examination of the skulls and by examination of the relatively primitive living Maori. He states:

> In an examination of 250 Maori skulls—all from an uncivilized age—I found carious teeth present in only two skulls or 0.76 percent. By taking the average of Mummery's and my own investigations, the incidence of caries in the Maori is found to be 1.2 percent in a total of 326 skulls. This is lower even than the Esquimaux, and shows the Maori to have been *the* most immune race to caries, for which statistics are available.
>
> Comparing these figures with those applicable to the present time, we find that the descendants of the Britons and Anglo-Saxons are afflicted with dental caries to the extent of 86 percent to 98 percent; and after examining fifty Maori school children living under European conditions entirely, I found that 95 percent of them had decayed teeth.

It will be noted that the basis of computation in the above is percentage of individuals with caries. I am using in addition to these figures the percentage of teeth attacked by dental caries. Expressed in percentage of teeth affected, the figure for Pickerill's group would be 0.05 or 1 in 2,000 teeth.

We were deeply indebted to the government officials in New Zealand for their invaluable assistance. In anticipation of making these studies I had been in correspondence with the officials for over two years. When we arrived at Auckland, New Zealand, on our way to Australia, our ship was in port for one day. We were met by Colonel Saunders, Director of Oral Hygiene in the New Zealand Department of Public Health, who had been sent from the capitol at Wellington to offer assistance. A personal representative of the Government was sent as guide, and transportation to the various Maori settlements in which we wished to make our studies was provided.

New Zealand is setting a standard for the world in the care of growing children as well as in many other health problems. A large percentage of the schools in New Zealand are provided with dental service. A specially trained woman was in charge of the work in each school under Colonel Saunders' supervision.

The operations performed by these young women on children far exceeded in quality the average that I have seen by dentists in America. Their plan gives dental care to children twelve years of age and under, provided the parents express a wish that their children receive that care. The service was being extended rapidly to all communities. Since my return, I have learned that the work is being organized to provide for every community of New Zealand. The art of the Maori gives evidence of their great ability and skill in sculpturing. Boys and girls do beautiful carving and weaving. All native buildings and structures are embellished with carvings, often in fine detail.

It was most gratifying to find neat and well-appointed dental office buildings for both natives and whites, located beside a large number of the public schools throughout New Zealand. In many communities two or three schools were served by the same operator. Children were either brought to the central dental infirmary or provision was made for an operating room in the vicinity of each school. The operator went from district to district. A typical dental infirmary is shown in Fig. 68, with Colonel Saunders and one of his efficient women operators in the foreground. I had suggested that I should be glad to have observers from the Department of Health accompany us or arrange to be present at convenient places to observe the conditions and to

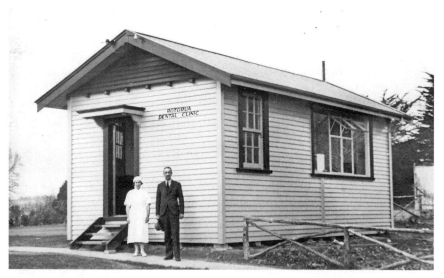

FIG. 68. The New Zealand government provides nearly universal free dental service for the children, regardless of color, to the age of twelve years. This is a typical dental clinic maintained in connection with the school system. They are operated by trained dental hygienists. The director of the system, Colonel Saunders, is seen in the picture.

note my interpretations of them. From two to five such observers were generally present, including the official representative of the department. The planning of the itinerary was very greatly assisted by a Maori member of Parliament, Mr. Aparana Ngata.

Although New Zealand is a new country with a relatively small population, there being approximately only a million and a half individuals, the building of highways has rapidly been extended to include all modernized sections. In order to reach the most remote groups it was often necessary to go beyond the zone of public improvements and follow quite primitive trails. Fortunately this was possible because it was the dry season. Even then, many streams had to be forded, which would have been quite impossible at other seasons of the year. We were able to average approximately a hundred miles of travel per day for eighteen days, visiting twenty-five districts and making examinations of native Maori families and children in native schools, representing various stages of modernization. This included a few white schools and tubercular sanitariums.

Since over 95 percent of the New Zealanders are to be found in the North Island, our investigations were limited to this island. Our itinerary started at Wellington at the south end of the North Island and progressed northward in such a way as to reach both the principal centers of native population who were modernized and those who were more isolated. This latter group, however, was a small part of the total native population. Detailed examinations including measurements and photographic records were made in twenty-two groups consisting chiefly of the older children in public schools. In the examination of 535 individuals in these twenty-two school districts their 15,332 teeth revealed that 3,420 had been attacked by dental caries or 22.3 percent. In the most modernized groups 31 to 50 percent had dental caries. In the most isolated group only 2 percent of the teeth had been attacked by dental caries. The incidence of deformity of dental arches in the modernized groups ranged from 40 to 100 percent. In many districts members of the older generations revealed 100 percent normally formed dental arches. The children of these individuals, however, showed a much higher percentage of deformed dental arches.

These data are in striking contrast with the condition of the teeth and dental arches of the skulls of the Maori before contact with the white man and the reports of examinations by early scientists who made contact with the primitive Maori before he was modernized. These reports revealed only one tooth in 2000 teeth attacked by dental caries with practically 100 percent normally formed dental arches.

My investigations were made in the following places in the North Island. The Pukerora Tubercular Sanatorium provided forty native Maori for studies. These were largely young men and women and being in a modern institution

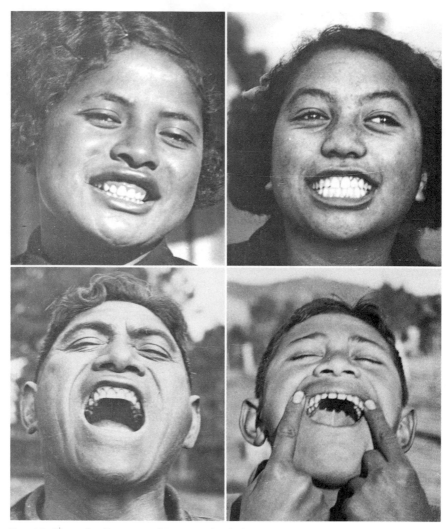

FIG. 69. Since the discovery of New Zealand, the primitive natives, the Maori, have had the reputation of having the finest teeth and finest bodies of any race in the world. These faces are typical. Only about one tooth per thousand teeth had been attacked by tooth decay before they came under the influence of the white man.

they were receiving the modern foods of the whites of New Zealand. Their modernization was demonstrated not only by the high incidence of dental caries but also by the fact that 90 percent of the adults and 100 percent of the children had abnormalities of the dental arches.

The Hukarera College for Maori girls is at Napier. These girls were largely from modernized native homes and were now living in a modern institution.

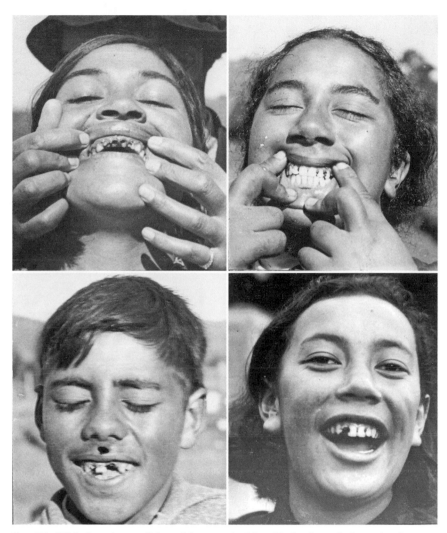

FIG. 70. With the advent of the white man in New Zealand, tooth decay has become rampant. The suffering from dental caries and abscessed teeth is very great in the most modernized Maori. The boy at the lower left has a deep scar in his upper lip from an accident.

Their modernization was expressed in the high percentage of dental caries and their deformed dental arches.

At the Nuhaka school an opportunity was provided through the assistance of the government officials to study the parents of many of the children. Tooth decay was wide-spread among the women and active among both the men and children.

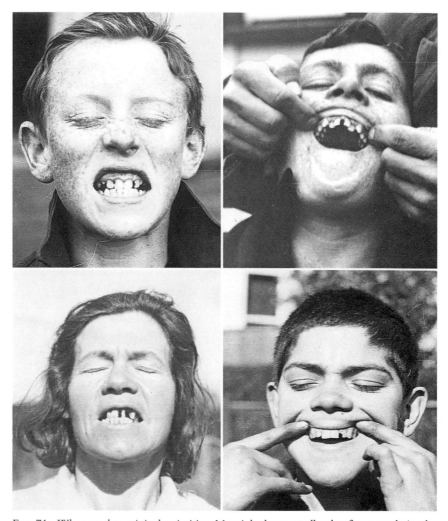

FIG. 71. Whereas the original primitive Maori had reportedly the finest teeth in the world, the whites now in New Zealand are claimed to have the poorest teeth in the world. These individuals are typical. An analysis of the two types of food reveals the reason.

The Mahia Peninsula provided one of the more isolated groups which showed a marked difference between the older generation and the new. These people had good access to sea foods and those still using these abundantly had much the best teeth. A group of the children who had been born and raised in this district and who had lived largely on the native foods had only 1.7 percent of their teeth attacked by dental caries.

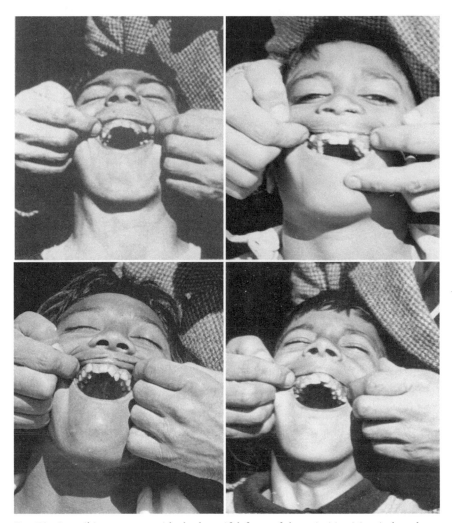

FIG. 72. In striking contrast with the beautiful faces of the primitive Maori, those born since the adoption of deficient modernized foods are grossly deformed. Note the marked underdevelopment of the facial bones, one of the results being narrowing of the dental arches with crowding of the teeth and an underdevelopment of the air passages. We have wrongly assigned these distorted forms to the mixture of racial bloods.

The other places studied were Raukokore, Tekaha, Rautoki, Rotarua, Tehoro, Waiomio, Teahuahu, Kaikohe, Whakarara, Mautauri Bay, Ahipara, Manukau, Rawena, Ellerslie, Queen Victoria School at Auckland and Waipawa.

New Zealand has become justly famous for its scenery. The South Island has been frequently termed the Southern Alps because of its snow-capped mountains and glaciers. Of the 70,000 members of the Maori race living in

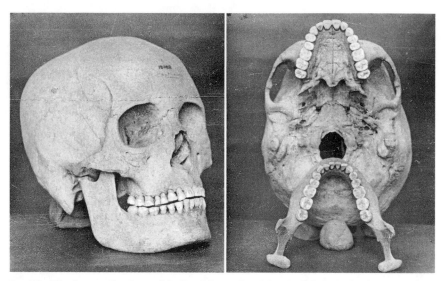

FIG. 73. The large collections of skulls of the ancient Maori of New Zealand attest to their superb physical development and to the excellence of their dental arches.

the two islands, about 2000 are on the South Island and the balance on the North Island. While snow is present on many of the mountains of the North Island in the winter season, only a few of the higher peaks are snow capped during the summer. Most of the shoreline of the seacoast of the South Island is very rugged, with glaciers descending almost to the sea. The coastline of the North Island is broken and in places is quite rugged. The approach to the Mahia Peninsula is along a rocky coast skirting the bay. The most important industries of New Zealand are dairy products, and sheep raising for wool.

The reputation of the Maori people for splendid physiques has placed them on a pedestal of perfection. Much of this has been lost in modernization. However, through the assistance of the government, I was able to see many excellent physical specimens. In Fig. 69 will be seen four typical Maori who retained much of the tribal excellence. Note their fine dental arches. A young Maori man who stands about six feet four inches and weighs 230 pounds was examined. The Maori men have great physical endurance and good minds. Many fine lawyers and government executives are Maori. The breakdown of these people comes when they depart from their native foods to the foods of modern civilization, foods consisting largely of white flour, sweetened goods, syrup and canned goods. The effect is similar to that experienced by other races after using foods of modern civilization. Typical illustrations of tooth decay are shown in Fig. 70. In some individuals still in their teens, half of the teeth were decayed. The tooth decay among the whites of New Zealand and Australia was severe. This is illustrated in Fig. 71. Particularly striking is the similarity between the deformities of the dental arches which occur in the Maori people who were born after their parents adopted the modern foods, and those of the whites. This is well illustrated in Fig. 72 for Maori boys. In my studies among other modernized primitive racial stocks, there was a very high incidence of facial deformity, which approached one hundred percent among individuals in tuberculosis sanatoria. This condition was found also in New Zealand.

Through the kindness of the director of the Maori Museum at Auckland, I was able to examine many Maori skulls. Two views are shown in Fig. 73. The skulls belong in the pre-Columbian period. Note the splendid design of the face and dental arches and high perfection of the teeth.

One of the most important developments to come out of these investigations of primitive races is the evidence of a rapid decline in maternal reproductive efficiency after an abandonment of the native foods and the substitution of foods of modern civilization. This is discussed in later chapters.

It was particularly instructive to observe the diligence with which some of the isolated Maori near the coast sought out certain types of food in accordance with the tradition and accumulated wisdom of their tribes. As among the various archipelagos and island dwellers of the Pacific, great emphasis was placed upon shell fish. Much effort was made to obtain these in large quantities. In Fig. 74 (lower), will be seen two boys who have been gathering sea clams found abundantly on these shores. Much of the fishing is done when the tide is out. Some groups used large quantities of the species called abalone on the West Coast of America and paua in New Zealand. In Fig. 74 (upper), a man, his wife and child are shown. The father is holding an abalone; the little girl is holding a mollusk found only in New Zealand, the tohaioa; the mother is holding a plate of edible kelp which these people use abundantly, as do many sea-bordering races. Maori boys enjoy a species of grubs which they seek with great eagerness and prize highly. The primitive Maori use large quantities of fern root which grows abundantly and is very nutritious.

Probably few primitive races have developed calisthenics and systematic physical exercise to so high a point as the primitive Maori. On arising early in the morning, the chief of the village starts singing a song which is accompanied by a rhythmic dance. This is taken up not only by the members of his household, but by all in the adjoining households until the entire village is swaying in unison to the same tempo. This has a remarkably beneficial effect in not only developing deep breathing, but in developing the muscles of the body, particularly those of the abdomen, with the result that these people maintain excellent figures to old age.

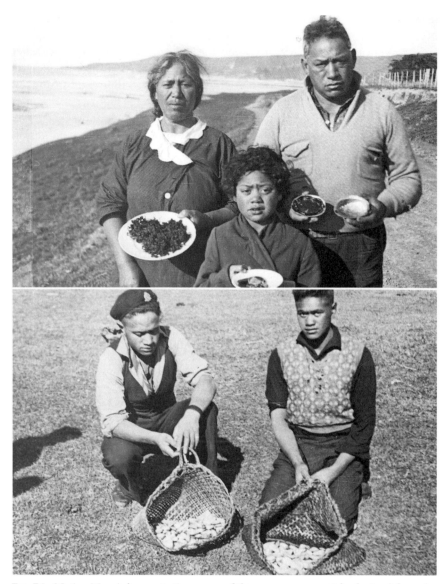

FIG. 74. Native Maori demonstrating some of the accessory essentials obtained from the sea. These include certain sea weeds and an assortment of shell fish. It is much easier for the moderns to exchange their labor for the palate-tickling devitalized foods of commerce than to obtain the native foods of land and sea.

Sir Arbuthnot Lane[2] said of this practice the following:

> As to daily exercise, it is shown here that every person capable of movement can benefit by it, and I am certain that the only natural and really beneficial system of exercise is that developed through long ages by the New Zealand Maori and their race-brothers in other lands.

The practical application of their wisdom is discussed in Chapter 21.

The Maori race developed a knowledge of Nature's laws and adopted a system of living in harmony with those laws to so high a degree that they were able to build what was reported by early scientists to be the most physically perfect race living on the face of the earth. They accomplished this largely through diet and a system of social organization designed to provide a high degree of perfection in their offspring. To do this they utilized foods from the sea very liberally. The fact that they were able to maintain an immunity to dental caries so high that only one tooth in two thousand had been attacked by tooth decay (which is probably as high a degree of immunity as that of any contemporary race) is a strong argument in favor of their plan of life.

REFERENCES

[1] PICKERILL, H. P. *The Prevention of Dental Caries and Oral Sepsis.* Philadelphia, White, 1914.

[2] LANE, A. Preface to *Maori Symbolism* by Ettie A. Rout. London, Paul Trench, Trubner, 1926.

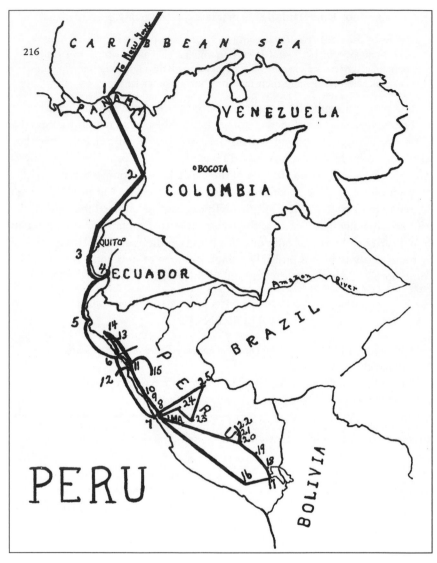

Key to Route Followed in Peru

1. Panama	10. Huaura	19. San Rosa
2. Buenaventura	11. Chimbote	20. Cuzco
3. Manta	12. Santa Island	21. Calca
4. Guayaquil	13. Chiclayo	22. Macchu Piccu
5. Talara	14. Eten	23. Huancayo
6. Trujillo	15. Huaraz	24. Oroya
7. Callao	16. Arequipa	25. Perene
8. Lima	17. Lake Titicaca	
9. Huacho	18. Juallanca	

Chapter 13

ANCIENT CIVILIZATIONS OF PERU

IN THE foregoing field studies among primitive races we have been dealing chiefly with living groups. Since the West Coast of South America has been the home of several ancient cultures, it is important that they be included with the living remnants of primitive racial stocks, in order to note the contributions that they may make to the problem of modern degeneration. The relationship between the Andes Mountain Range and the coast and the sea currents is such that there has been created a zone, ranging from forty to one hundred miles in width between the coast and the mountains, which for a distance of over a thousand miles is completely arid. The air currents drifting westward across South America from the Atlantic carry an abundance of moisture. When they strike the eastern foothills of the Andes they are projected upward into a region of constant cold which causes the moisture to be precipitated as rain on the eastern slopes, and as snow on the eastern Cordillera Range. Hence the name of the eastern range is the White Cordillera, and that of the western range, which receives little of this rain, is the Black Cordillera. Between these two ranges is a great plain, which in the rainy season is well watered. The great civilizations of the past have always utilized water from the melting snow through irrigation ditches with the result that a vast acreage was put to agricultural uses.

The Humboldt Current which sweeps northward from the southern ice fields and carries its chilly water almost to the equator has influenced the development of the West Coast of South America. The effect of the current on the climate is generally noticeable. One of the conspicuous results is the presence of a cloud bank which hovers over the coastal area at an altitude of from one thousand to three thousand feet above sea level for several months of the year. Back from the coast these clouds rest on the land and constitute a nearly constant fog for extended periods. When one passes inland from the coast up the mountains he moves from a zone which in winter is clammy and chilly, into the fog zone, and then suddenly out of it into clear sky and brilliant sunlight. It is of interest that the capital, Lima, is so situated that it suffers from this unhappy cloud and fog situation. When Pizarro sent a commission to search out a location for his capital city the natives commented on the fact that he was selecting a very undesirable location. Either on the coast or farther inland than Lima the climate is much more favorable, and these were the locations in which the ancient civilizations have left some very elaborate foundations of fortresses and extended residential areas. The great expanse of desert extending from the coast to the mountains, with its great moving sand dunes and with scarcely a sign of green life, is one of the least hospitable environments that any culture could choose. Notwithstanding this, the entire coast is a succession of ancient burial mounds in which it is estimated that there are fifteen million mummies in an excellent state of preservation. The few hundred thousand that have been disturbed by grave robbers in search of gold and silver, have been left bleaching on the sands. Where had these people come from and why were they buried here? The answer is to be found in the fact that probably few locations in the world provided such an inexhaustible supply of food for producing a good culture as did this area. The lack of present appreciation of this fact is evidenced by the absence of flourishing modern communities, notwithstanding the almost continuous chain of ancient walls, fortresses, habitations, and irrigation systems to be found along this coast. The Humboldt Current coming from the ice fields of the Antarctic carries with it a prodigious quantity of the chemical food elements that are most effective in the production of a vast population of fish. Probably no place in the world provides as great an area teeming with marine life. The ancient cultures appreciated the value of these sea foods and utilized them to the full. They realized also that certain land plants should be eaten with the sea foods. Accordingly, they constructed great aqueducts used in transporting the water, sometimes a hundred miles, for the purpose of irrigating river bottoms which had been collecting the alluvial soil from the Andes through past ages. These river beds are to be found from twenty to fifty miles apart and many of them are entirely dry except in the rainy season in the high Andes. In the river bottoms these ancient cultures grew large quantities of corn, beans, squash, and other plants. These plant foods were gathered, stored, and eaten with sea foods. The people on the coast had direct communication with the people in the high plateaus. It is of more than passing interest that some twenty-one of our modern food plants apparently came from Peru.

Where there is such a quantity of animal life in the sea in the form of fish one would expect to find the predatory animals that live on fish. One group of these attack the fish from the air and they constitute the great flock of guanayes, piqueros and pelicans. For a thousand miles along the coast, these fish-eating birds are to be seen in great winding queues going to and fro between the fishing grounds and their nesting places. At other times they may be seen in great clouds, beyond computation in number, fishing over an area of many square miles. On one island I was told by the caretaker that twenty-four million birds had their nests there. We passed through a flock of the birds fishing, which the caretaker estimated to contain between four and five million birds. On one island I found it impossible to step anywhere, off the path, without treading on birds' nests. It is of interest that a product of these birds has constituted one of the greatest sources of wealth in the past for Peru, namely, the guano, which is the droppings of the birds left on the islands along the coast where they have their nests. Through the centuries these deposits have reached to a depth of 100 feet in places. When it is realized that only one-fifth of the droppings are placed on the islands, it immediately raises the great question as to the quantity of fish consumed by these birds. As high as seventy-five fish have been found in the digestive tract of a single bird. The quantity of fish consumed per day by the birds nesting on this one island has been estimated to be greater than the entire catch of fish off the New England coast per day.

In addition to the birds, a vast number of sea lions and seals live on the fish. The sea lions have a rookery in the vicinity of Santa Island, which was estimated to contain over a million. These enormous animals devour great quantities of fish. It would be difficult to estimate how far the fish destroyed by this one group of sea lions would go toward providing excellent nutrition for the entire population of the United States. The guano, consisting of the partially digested animal life of the sea, constitutes what is probably the best known fertilizer in the world. It is thirty-three times as efficient as the best barnyard manure. At one time it was sent in shiploads to Europe and the United States, but now the Peruvian Government is retaining nearly all of it for local use. They have locked the barn door after the horse was stolen, figuratively speaking, since the accumulation of ages had been carried off by shiploads to other countries before its export was checked. At the present time all islands are under guard and the birds are protected. They are coming back into many of the islands from which they had been driven and are re-nesting. Birds are given two or three years of undisturbed life for producing deposits. These are then carefully removed from the surface of the islands and the birds are allowed to remain undisturbed for another period.

A very important and fortunate phase of the culture of the primitive races of the coast has been their method of burial. Bodies are carefully wrapped in many layers of raiment often beautifully spun. With the mummies articles of special interest and value are usually buried. Implements used by the individuals in their lifetime were also put in the grave. With a fisherman there were placed his nets and fishing tackle. Almost always, jars containing foods to supply him on his journey in the transition to a future life were left in the tomb. In some of the cultures the various domestic and industrial scenes were reproduced in pottery. These disclosed a great variety of foods which are familiar to us today. Even the designs of their habitations were reproduced in pottery. Similarly their methods of performing surgical operations, in which

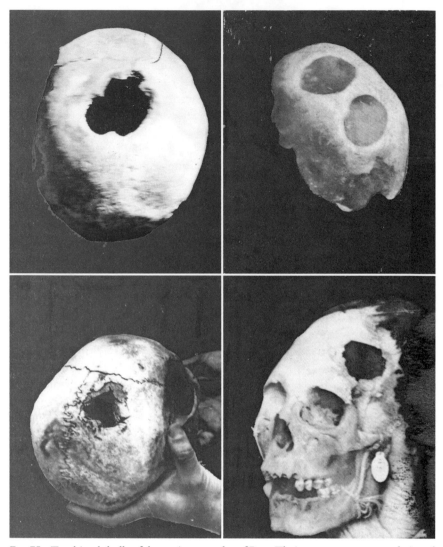

FIG. 75. Trephined skulls of the ancient peoples of Peru. Their war weapons were designed to produce skull fractures. Their surgeons trephined the skulls, thus removing the depressed area. The large percentage of operated skulls showing extensive healing indicates a large percentage lived for months and years afterwards. Their surgical flesh cutting knives were made of copper and bronze, the bone cutting of mounted crystals. They used cocoa leaves (cocaine) as a sedative as the natives do today.

they were very skillful, were depicted. Fortunately, the different cultures had quite different types of pottery as well as quite different types of clothing. This makes it possible to identify various groups and indicate the boundaries of their habitations.

Their engineering feats disclosed skill in planning fortresses. Their forts were probably impregnable from assault in that day. The materials used for building their temples, abodes, and fortifications differ somewhat in various locations. Throughout the greater extent of the coast of Peru, the walls of buildings were made of adobe often many feet thick and sometimes sixty feet high. They had walled cities protected by inner and outer lines of fortifications. It is particularly significant that the hardest metals that they are known to have had were copper and bronze. Silver and gold were quite plentiful. Their surgical instruments were flints and the operations that they were able to perform with these instruments were very remarkable. An important instrument in warfare consisted of a club with a star on the end made of copper or stone. With this the opponent's skull was crushed in. One of the amazing features in the various collections of skulls is the large number that show the results of surgical operations. These operations were apparently done for the purpose of saving the life of the individual. The procedure was to remove a section of bone in the center of the depressed area and raise the depressed edges surrounding that area. The fact that a large number of these show abundant evidence of healing and repair clearly indicates that the individual lived for an extended period following the operation. In some cases, the opening is apparently entirely closed in with new bone. Some of these trepanning operations removed a quantity of bone over an area large enough for a human hand to pass through. A group of these operated skulls are shown in Fig. 75. The owner of the one on the lower row, left, probably died following the operation, as there is no evidence of repair. The others show good healing, which in some is very extensive. A study of these trephined skulls reveals that 62 percent lived for months or years. In Fig. 75 (lower right), is seen a skull which shows a large operation. A part of the surgical procedure was to place a plate of gold over the opening in the skull for protection. One of these is shown in the upper half of Fig. 76. Below is shown the healed scar after removal of the gold plate.

The skill of the surgeons in amputations is illustrated by the pottery reproductions of amputated parts. One of these, for example, shows a man with an amputated foot holding the stump of his leg with one hand while putting on a sock over the end of the stump with the other hand. The technic of amputation is shown in pottery form in Fig. 77. A serious disease of the foot is suggested, requiring amputation of the leg, high up. Note how the thigh bone

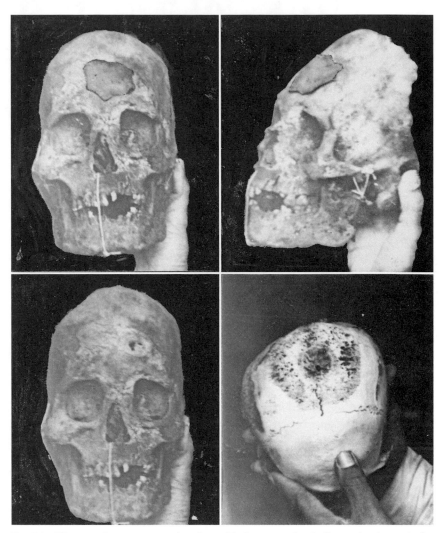

FIG. 76.   These ancient surgeons placed a gold plate over the skull opening beneath the
scalp to protect the brain. Above, two views are shown of a skull with a gold plate in position and below the same skull with the gold plate removed. Note that the skull opening
is nearly healed in. To the right below an extensive operation is shown.

was cut so as to provide a flesh-covered stump. Below in Fig. 77 is shown a
healed oblique fracture with good adaptation.

When the Spaniards arrived to carry forward the conquest of Peru they
found the entire coastal area and upper plateaus under the control of a culture organized under the Inca rulers. Prior to the domination of that culture,
which had its origin in the high plateau country, several other cultures had

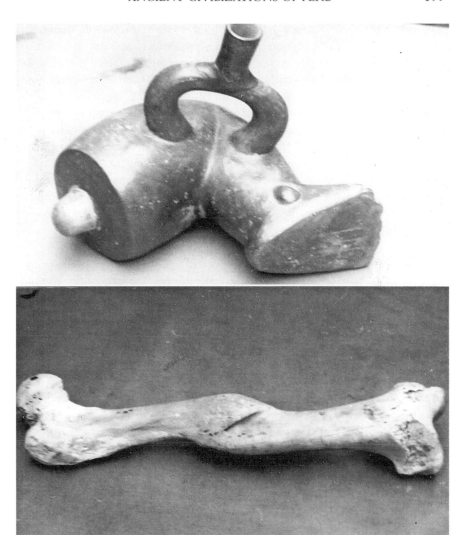

FIG. 77. The skill of the ancient surgeons in plastic and bone surgery is illustrated in the pottery jar above. In order to provide flesh for a pad over the amputated bone stump the flesh is cut lower than the bone by pushing the flesh up at the time the bone is cut. In the lower view good healing is shown of a difficult oblique fracture.

developed along the coast in succeeding eras of domination. In northern Peru the Chimus developed a great culture that extended over a long period of time. Their capital city was at Chan Chan, inland from the present coastal port of Saliverry and near Trujillo. This city is estimated to have contained a million people. The argument is sometimes presented that at the time these ancient cultures lived the coastal areas were not arid desert but well supplied with rain.

That this was not so is clearly evidenced by the fact that the walls were built of stucco made by mixing water with the available sand and rubble either in continuous molds or in blocks that were built into the fort. Since these blocks were only sun-dried they had very little resistance to rain. In this rainless desert land they have continued to stand through many centuries, many of them probably through several thousand years. There has been a vast change in the walls of the ruined city of Chan Chan within a decade and a half.

In 1925 this district was visited by a heavy downpour of rain which apparently exceeded any precipitation, not only through historic times, but for many centuries preceding. Temples, courtyards and military defenses which were in splendid preservation before that downpour were reduced to a mere semblance of their former structure. Clearly these great cities and their defenses could not have been built of this material in the period when downpours were even occasional, let alone frequent.

It was, of course, the wealth of the ancient cultures that spurred on the conquistadors. It is very difficult to estimate the per capita quantity of gold available in those early cultures. That gold and silver were abundant is evidenced by the extensive use that was made of these metals for covering the walls of rooms and decorating public buildings with massive plates, sometimes entirely encircling a building and the walls of its various rooms. A considerable quantity of gold and silver has been taken from the burial mounds. One burial mound is reported to have yielded between six and seven million dollars worth of gold. So great has been the activity of the grave robbers that the Peruvian Government has placed a ban on this enterprise though for a period it was allowed on condition that a stated percentage was given to the Government.

One of the principal characteristics of the Chimu culture of the coastal area of northern Peru is shown in the type of pottery they produced. All articles were realistic in design. The pots show hunting scenes, fishing and domestic scenes, as illustrated above. They were very skillful in reproducing features in nearly natural size. Many thousands of these portrait jars have been taken from the mounds of this district. The local museum in the vicinity of Chan Chan, under the skillful direction of Mr. Larco Herrera at Chiclyan was reported to contain over twenty thousand jars and specimens taken from the mounds.

To the south of the domain of the Chimu culture, a very strong culture was built up with very different characteristics known as the Naska. While many of their habits of life, including their methods of providing food, were similar to those of the Chimu culture, they were unique in the designs of their pottery, which were characterized by being allegorical. They used elaborate color designs and fantastic patterns. Very little is known as yet of the meaning of much that they have left. While sundials of ancient design and build have been found in many parts of Peru, it is not known to what extent they developed a knowledge of astronomy. The pilot of the plane that flew us from Lima to Arequipa took us over some very strange architectural designs of geometrical patterns which he had discovered and which he suggested had not been reported upon nor interpreted. I photographed some of these from the air. The straight lines constituting the sides of some of the geometric figures are over a thousand feet long and reveal a precision of the angles and a straightness of the ground structures which indicate the use of competent engineering equipment and a high knowledge of surveying.

One of the principal purposes of my trip to Peru was to study the effect of the Humboldt Current, with its supply of human food, on the ancient cultures which were buried along the coast. In other parts of the world, where Nature had provided the sea with an abundance of sea life which was being utilized by native races, I found quite routinely excellent physical development with typical broad, well-developed facial forms and dental arches with normal contours. In each of these groups, the people have reproduced quite closely the racial type in practically all members of the group. I have emphasized with illustrations this fact in connection with the Melanesians and Polynesians on eight archipelagos of the Pacific Ocean, the Malay races on the islands north of Australia, the Aborigines of Australia along the east coast; also the Gaelics in the Outer Hebrides, and the Eskimos of Alaska.

The activity of grave robbers in the ancient burial mounds has left skeletons strewn helter skelter where many of them have been weathering, probably for years. While many of these had apparently been deliberately smashed, large numbers were intact, and in a good state of preservation. Some of the ancient cemeteries apparently extended over areas covering a square mile; and as far as the eye could see the white bleaching bones, particularly the skulls, dotted the landscape. Since there were several distinct cultures, I endeavored to make a cross section study of a number of these burial grounds in order that a fair average of specimens might be obtained. The skulls were handled by me, personally, and large numbers of them were photographed. As I have mentioned, it was the ancient custom when making the burials to inter objects that were of special interest to the individuals, including the implements with which he had worked. Fishermen's skulls are shown in Fig. 78 with their nets. It will be noted that all these arches are broad and wide, that the third molars are well formed and almost always well developed, and in good masticating position. Notwithstanding the long period of interment the fabrics buried with these people were often in a remarkably good state of preservation. Even the hair was well preserved. A characteristic of the method of preparation for burial involved placing over the teeth a preparation that was held in position by a strip of cloth which cemented the teeth quite firmly to this strip with the result that when the mummy cases were torn open the removal of this bandage

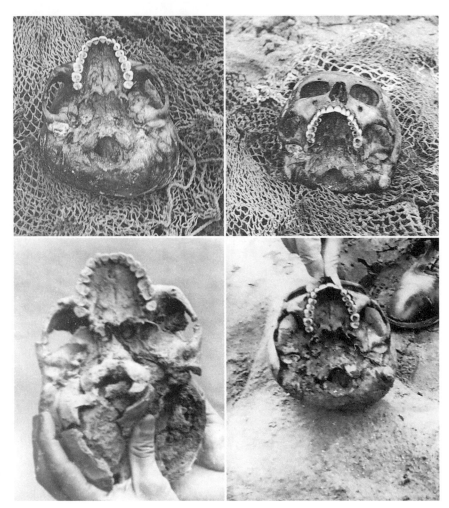

Fig. 78. The two skulls in the upper photograph apparently belonged to fishermen of the Chimu culture as evidenced by the flattened back of the head. Note the splendidly formed dental arches. In an examination of one thousand two hundred and seventy-six skulls in succession I did not find one with the typical deformities of our moderns.

removed the straight rooted teeth, and therefore large numbers of the skulls that were bleaching on the sandy wastes were without the straight rooted teeth. Of course, these would readily tumble out at the slightest jar, after the mummified tissues had decomposed from exposure. The teeth lost in this way would include practically all of the upper and lower incisors, some of the bicuspids and third molars.

Since our study was primarily concerned with the shape of the dental arches and facial form, these characteristics could be studied and recorded with the straight rooted teeth removed. Fortunately, there are some excellent collections of skulls in museums in Peru, with the skulls in position where they can be readily studied for the shape of the dental arches. When we have in mind that from 25 to 75 percent of individuals in various communities in the United States have a distinct irregularity in the development of the dental arches and facial form, the cause and significance of which constitutes one of the important problems of this study, the striking contrast found in these Peruvian skulls will be seen to constitute a challenge for our modern civilizations. In a study of 1,276 skulls of these ancient Peruvians, I did not find a single skull with significant deformity of the dental arches.

Since these investigations have apparently established the fact that this problem is related directly to nutrition, and chiefly to nutrition in the formative period, and, as we shall see, to a very early part of the formative period, we have here evidence of a system of living that is very closely in accord with Nature's fundamental laws of reproduction. Several studies have been made dealing with the incidence of dental caries or tooth decay among these ancient cultures. The author of *Bird Islands of Peru*[1] states that in his examination of fifty mummies in succession he found only four with a tooth with dental caries. This again is in striking contrast to our modernized communities in which from 95 to 100 percent of all the members of a community group suffer from dental caries. I have shown in connection with the Indians of the western coast of Canada that in six highly modernized communities where the Indians were using white man's foods, 40 percent of all the teeth had been attacked by dental caries. A similar high percentage was found in the Indians now living in Florida. The ancient burials in southern Florida revealed apparent, complete immunity. These were pre-Columbian burials.

The skill of the primitive cultures of Peru in engineering as evidenced by the irrigation systems has always been a subject of amazement to modern engineers. I visited in a valley fifteen miles from the Santa River an ancient aqueduct which was said to be a hundred miles long. Our guide informed me that he had walked in it for thirty-five miles. With its even grades, overflows and auxiliary channels for distribution, its adaptation to the area to be watered, and the skill with which it was cut through rock shoulders and its retaining walls built, it constitutes a monument to engineering ability. Modern engineers have estimated that this aqueduct could deliver sixty million cubic feet of water a day. In Fig. 79 will be seen a section where it has been carried through a rock cutting and beyond will be seen a retaining wall used to carry the flume along the sheer face of a rock. The modern inhabitants of this community have carried away this retaining wall for use in the foundations of their

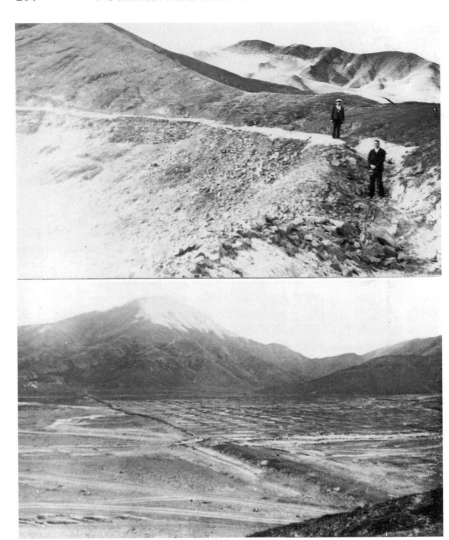

FIG. 79. The ancient civilizations of Peru had skilled engineers. In the upper view is seen one of the ancient aqueducts still intact for thirty-five miles which modern scientists estimate was capable of delivering sixty million cubic feet of water per day. They had no hardened tools or blasting powder, yet they cut this channel through boulders and rocks. Below is seen a valley covering thousands of acres once made fertile by irrigation but now an arid desert.

huts. Below, in Fig. 79, will be seen a district of many hundreds of acres, possibly a thousand, where the fields are laid out just as they were left hundreds
of years ago when the primitive people were driven from this habitat. All this
valley needs is water.

In order to reach the burial places it was necessary to drive many hundreds
of miles over the arid desert inland from the coast. We were exceedingly fortunate in having as our interpreter and guide Dr. Albert Giesecke, who for
fourteen years was the Chancellor of Cuzco University. With his excellent
knowledge of the country and its languages, with the credentials which gave
us entry to the secluded places, together with the kindness and helpfulness of
the Peruvian Government officials in almost all localities, we were able to obtain much valuable information. In an estimate of this culture not only their
arts, but their scientific skill should be included.

Since the primary object of this quest was to learn of the efficiency of
these primitive people in the art of living in harmony with Nature's laws and
their methods for accomplishing this, it was desirable to find, if possible, some
living descendants of these people to gain from them the information that
had been handed down. We were told that there were a few villages in an isolated section of the coast in northern Peru where the inhabitants claimed
descent from the ancient Chimu cultures of that area. This group was characterized by a flattening of the skull at the back which classified them as short
heads and is readily identified. We were very fortunate in having the assistance
of Commander Daniel Matto of the Peruvian Army. He was able to utilize
the police facilities for locating typical old residents who could tell us much
of the story of their race and its recent history as it had been handed down
by word of mouth. In Fig. 80 will be seen one of these nonagenarians. He told
us of incidents that had been related to him by his great-great-grandfather
and by the old people of that area, of the coming of Pizarro four hundred years
ago. The height of this man can be judged as he is seen standing beside Mrs.
Price, who is five feet three. His head is shown both front and side view, revealing the flattened surface at the back. An ancient skull with typical flattening is also shown. Fortunately these people are living very closely in accordance
with the customs of their ancestors. They are fisherfolk, with a hardihood and
skill that is in striking contrast with the lethargy of the modernized groups.
Their fine physical development, the breadth of their dental arches and the
regularity of their facial features are in striking contrast to the characteristics
noted among individuals in the modernized colonies. In Fig. 81 will be seen
typical members of these colonies.

The skill with which these men manage their fishing boats is inspiring. Even
though the surf was rolling in great combers they did not hesitate to go out
in either their small crafts carrying one individual or in their large sailboats

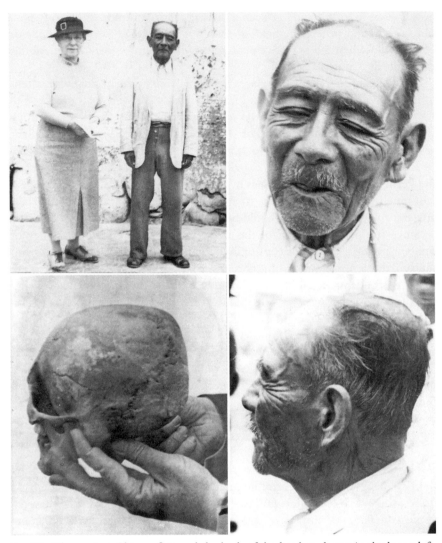

FIG. 80. The ancient Chimus flattened the back of the head, as shown in the lower left, by placing the infant on a board. A descendant of the Chimus is shown in the upper left with Mrs. Price, and in front and side views at the right. Note that the back of his head is similarly flattened.

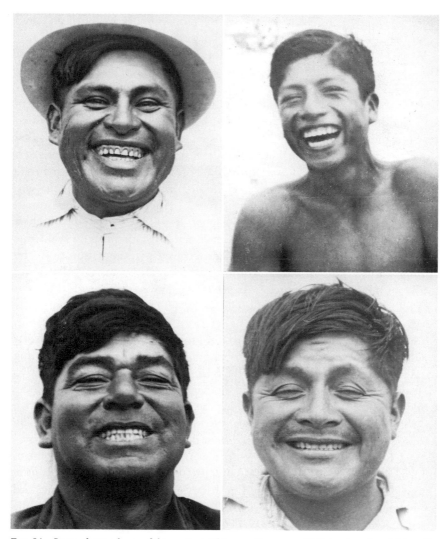

FIG. 81. Some descendants of the ancient Chimu culture are still living in a few fishing villages in the north of Peru. They live, as did their ancestors, largely on the sea food. Typical faces of this native stock are shown in this photograph. Note the breadth of the dental arches and full development of the facial bones.

carrying a dozen men. The abundance of the fish in this district is demonstrated by the large catch that each succeeding boat brought to shore.

At the time the Spanish Conquistadors arrived in Peru one of the most unique of the ancient cultures held sway over both the mountain plateaus and the coastal plains from Santiago of Chile northward to Quito, Equador, a distance of about 1200 miles. This culture took its name from the ruling emperors called Incas. The capital of their, great kingdom was Cuzco, a city located between the East and West Cordillera Ranges of the Andes. These parallel ranges are from fifty to two hundred miles apart. Between them is situated a great plateau ranging from 10,000 to 13,000 feet above the sea. The mountain ranges are snow-capped and include in Peru alone fifty peaks that are over 18,000 feet in altitude, ranging up to 22,185 feet in Mount Huascaran. Only Mount Aconcagua in Chile is higher. It is 23,075 feet—the highest mountain in the Americas. The air drift is across South America from east to west, carrying vast quantities of water received by evaporation from the Atlantic Ocean. This moisture is precipitated rapidly when the clouds are forced into the chill of the higher Andes. In the rainy season the great plateau area is frequently well watered, though not in sufficient quantity to meet the needs of agriculture for much of the territory. In the past the precipitation has been supplemented by vast irrigation projects using the water from the melting snows. It is estimated that the population ruled over by the reigning Incas at the time of the coming of the Spaniards reached five millions.

It is probable that few, if any, of the ancient or modern cultures of the world have ever attained a more highly perfected organization of society than had this Inca culture. The ruling Inca was a benevolent despot, and according to history unique in that he practiced most diligently all of the laws he promulgated for his people. There was no poverty, want or crime. Every man, woman and child was specifically provided with all necessities. The entire amount of tillable land was divided so that every man, woman and child had his assigned parcel. Everyone worked as assigned by the proper official. While it is not appropriate here to go into details, it is important that we have a bird's eye view of this great culture for which I will quote a paragraph from Agnes Rothery's *South America, The West Coast and The East*.[2]

> The people who erected this temple lived in order and health, under the most successful communism the world has ever seen. Their land was divided into three portions—one portion for the Inca, one for the Sun, and one for the people, with seventy square meters for every boy and thirty-five for every girl. The livestock and implements were similarly apportioned and the land was ploughed, planted, and the crops gathered in strict rotation. First the fields of the Sun were cultivated, and then the land of the aged, the sick, widows, and orphans was tended; then the lands of the people, neighbors assisting one another; and last of all the lands of the Inca, with songs of praise and joy, because this was the service of their King. To every living soul was

given his tasks, according to his physical and mental capacities. He was prevented from overwork, prohibited from idleness, cared for in illness and old age. Children were taken by the Government when they were five and trained to the profession where they were most needed. There was no hunger, no crime in the whole empire.

The Inca held his kingly office over the docile, industrious, and contented mass not only through his royal blood, but through his wisdom and kindness in caring for and guiding his subjects, his bravery in war, and his statesmanship at home. Although he set an example to his subjects by following every law which he promulgated (astonishing idea to our modern lawmakers!), he lived, as became his rank, in luxury. In his garden were rows of corn moulded from pure gold with leaves of pure silver, and a tassel of spun silver, as fine as silk, moving in the air. Llamas and alpacas, life-sized and cunningly fashioned from the same metal, stood upon his lawns, as they did in the courts of the Temple of the Sun.

Cuzco, the capital, is reported to have housed about two hundred thousand people at the time of the Spanish Conquest. It is situated on a branch of the Urabamba River in a beautiful valley surrounded by fertile mountain sides and towering snow-capped pinnacles. The Urabamba River drains a large area of the plateau lying to the south of Cuzco and has cut a magnificent gorge through the southern range of the Andes where it passes from the plateau to the eastern watershed and thence to the Amazon. A little to the south of Cuzco the eastern and the western ranges of mountains approach and combine in a cluster of magnificent pinnacles and intervening valleys and gorges, that are to be equalled by no mountain scenery in the world. Today, almost all travel from the Andean Plateau north of this region, as well as from all areas along the coast, must proceed to the coast, thence down the coast by boat to the port of Mollendo which is often dangerous or impossible of approach because of the heavy seas. The journey is made by train up through Arequipa and over the western Cordillera Range of the Andes into the plateau country and from there northward to Cuzco. So great is this natural barrier that the detour requires many days, and the crossing of several divides ranging from fourteen to sixteen thousand feet above the sea. This was not necessary for the Incas who had built roads and suspension bridges through these mountains from Cuzco to all parts of the great empire. It is in this mountain vastness that the Inca rulers had constructed their most superb fortresses. While the early Spanish conquerors of the country knew that the nobility had great defenses to which they might retreat, the location of the fortresses was not known. Their greatest fortress was discovered and excavated by Professor C. W. Bingham of Yale, under the auspices of Yale University and the American Museum of Natural History. This fortress and retreat is now world famous as Macchu Piccu, and probably represents the highest development of engineering, ancient and in some respects modern, on the American continent.

We are particularly concerned with the type of men that were capable of such great achievement, since they were required to carry forward their great undertakings without the use of iron or the wheel. While the great Inca culture dominated the Sierras and the coast for several centuries prior to the coming of the Spanish, and while they had their seat of government and vast agricultural enterprises in the high Sierras, it is of special interest that many of the most magnificent monuments remaining today in stone were not constructed by the Inca culture, but by the Tauhuanocan culture which preceded the Inca. The Incas were a part of the Quechu linguistic stock, while the Tauhuanocans were a part of the Aymara linguistic stock. The Incas had their capital in the high plateau country about the center of Peru. The earlier Tauhuanocan culture centered in southern Peru near Lake Titicaca where their most magnificent structures are to be found today. One of the largest single stones to be moved and put into the building of a great temple in the history of the world is to be found near Lake Titicaca. According to engineers, there is no quarry known in an easily reached locality where such a stone could be quarried. It is conjectured that it was brought two hundred miles over mountainous country. It is important to note that many magnificent structures, evidently belonging to this ancient Tauhuanocan culture, are found distributed through the Andean Plateau from Bolivia to Equador. Their masonry was characterized by the fitting together of large stones faced so perfectly that in many of the walls it was difficult to find a crevice which had enough space to allow the passage of the point of my pen knife, notwithstanding that these stones were many-sided with some of them fifteen to twenty feet in length. In Fig. 82 above will be seen a section of wall of the great fortress Sacsahuaman overlooking Cuzco. Modern engineers seem unable to provide a satisfactory answer as to how these people were able to cut these stones with the limited facilities available, nor is it explained how they were able to transport and hoist some of their enormous monoliths. The walls and fortress of Macchu Piccu, as well as the residences and temples, were built of white granite which apparently was taken from quarries in the bank of the river Urabamba, two thousand feet below the fortress. Without modern hoisting machinery, how did they raise those mammoth stones? In Fig. 82 below is shown a typical section of wall. One stone shown has twelve faces and twelve angles, all fitting accurately its boundary stones. It is as though the stones were plastic and pressed into a mould.

The country is rugged. Over it passes the highest standard-gage railroad in the world, about 16,000 feet above sea level. The banks of this river are protected for long distances by ancient stone retaining walls. The native Indians live and herd their flocks of llamas and alpacas up near the snow line, largely between 15,000 and 18,000 feet. The Incas and their descendants now occupying the high Sierras in the Andes have been thrifty agriculturists. They turn

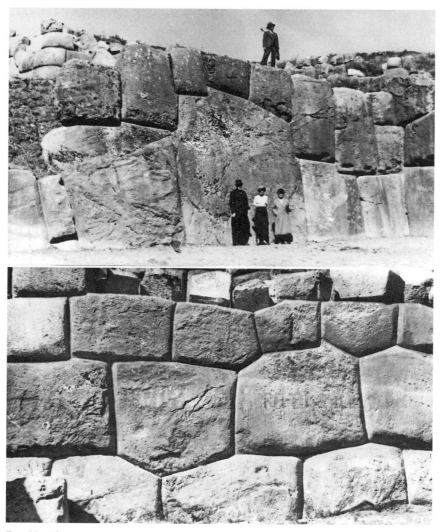

FIG. 82. The primitive peoples of the Andean Sierra built wonderful fortresses and temples of cut stones which are assembled without mortar and cut to interlock. The central stone, above, is estimated to weigh one hundred and forty thousand pounds. Below the largest stone has twelve faces and twelve angles.

the soil with a very narrow, long, slender bladed spade which they force into the ground, and with which they pry the ground up in chunks. They then break up the chunks. These spades were originally made of copper which they mined themselves. Cuzco is the archeological capital of South America, but its glory is in the ancient fortresses and temples, rather than in the modern structures. As one passes through the streets, he will note that in many instances the foundations and parts of the walls of many of the modern Spanish cathedrals and public buildings are of old Inca construction, of fine stone work surmounted by cheap rubble work and mortar superstructure. Whereas the original Cuzco had running water and an excellent sanitation system, modern Cuzco has deplorable sanitary conditions. The following is quoted from the West Coast Leader, published in Lima, dated July 20, 1937: "Of a total 3,600 houses in the city of Cuzco, 900 are without water or drainage; 2,400 are without light (windows) and 1,080 completely lack any sanitary systems." It is not surprising, therefore, that in some years the death rate exceeds the birth rate.

We are particularly concerned in studying these people to know the sources of their great capacity for developing art, engineering, government and social organization. Can such a magnificent culture be brought about unless founded on a superb physical development resulting from purely biologic forces?

Earthquakes are very frequent in the Andes. We experienced several while in Peru. One of these opened up a cave in the mountainside in the Urabamba Valley near which we were making studies. The cave had just been explored and a number of ancient burials found. I was able to examine a number of

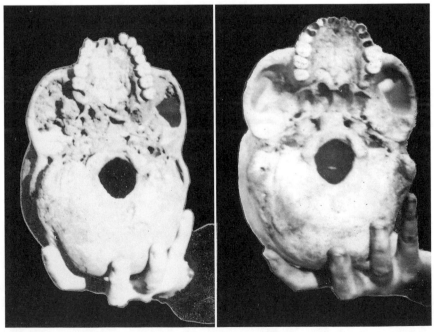

FIG. 83. Typical skulls of High Sierra Indians from a recently opened burial cave. Note the breadth of the dental arches provided by excellent development of the bones of the head.

skulls from this cave which apparently represented a pre-Spanish period. The date of the burials could not be determined. The skulls were interpreted as belonging to an early Indian period. In Fig. 83 may be seen two typical skulls. Note the broad sweep of the dental arches and freedom from tooth decay. The third molars (wisdom teeth) are well developed and in normal position for mastication. These are typical of the entire group found in this burial place. It is very evident that these individuals were provided with an adequate nutrition throughout the formative and growth periods, as well as during their adult life. This is significant because of the limited variety of foods easily obtainable for the people in the high plateau country of the Andes.

The ancient Peruvians of both the coastal area and high plateau country had developed superb physical bodies in each of the several cultures. This development had been brought about in spite of the bad conditions prevailing with arid desert land extending from the coast to the mountains, and in spite of the severe climate of the high Sierras. The people utilized the wide variety of animal life from the sea in conjunction with the excellent plant foods grown in the river basins with the aid of irrigation. Over twenty of our common plants had their origin in ancient Peru. In the high Sierras, their animal foods were largely limited to the llama, alpaca and wild animals. Each household, however, maintained a colony of guinea pigs. Owing to the difficulty of boiling in the high altitudes, they found it necessary to roast their cereals and meats. Their vegetable foods included potatoes, which were preserved in powder form by freezing and drying and pulverizing. Corn and several varieties of beans and quinoa were their principal cereals. The latter is a small seed of very high nutritive value.

REFERENCES

[1] MURPHY, R. C. *Bird Islands of Peru*. New York, Putnam, 1925.
[2] ROTHERY, A. *South America, The West Coast and the East*. New York, Houghton, Muffin, 1930.

Chapter 14

ISOLATED AND MODERNIZED PERUVIAN INDIANS

IN ORDER to understand the living descendants of the ancient residents of the high Andes it is essential that we know their environment. Their climate is cold at night the year around. While during the winter the snow is deep in the high mountains, there is very little on the plateau, since Peru is near the equator extending from 5 to 16 degrees south latitude. The sunshine is bright and warm even in winter. Consequently they have pasturage for their animals the year around.

The only native domesticated animals of the Andean Plateau are the llama and the alpaca. Both of these belong to the camel species, as does the vicuna. The llama is the Indians' beast of burden in the Andes. Only the males are used. The animals are very docile and respond with gentleness when treated with kindness. One continually marvels at the ease with which the Indian guides his loaded caravan with soft words or motions, never with harshness. The llama has many unique features as a beast of burden. It forages as it moves along and consequently must be driven very slowly. Each animal will carry a burden not exceeding a hundred pounds, and if more is placed on its back it will immediately lie down until the extra burden is removed. The llama has broad doubletoed feet like the camel which make it very sure-footed. It requires no shoeing and exceedingly little care. It can thrive, however, only in the high altitudes. The wool of the llama is coarse and is used for heavy, rough garments. The alpaca is a little smaller than the llama and produces a very heavy wool of fine quality. Accustomed as this animal is to the severe cold and the high altitudes, as well as to the rain and sun, its fleece is both durable and warm. It is used extensively throughout the world for suits for aviators. The native colors vary from white to bluish tints and from light to very dark browns. It accordingly provides very stable colors for weaving directly into ponchos and native apparel. The vicuna is a much smaller animal than either the llama or alpaca. It has one of the most highly prized coats of fur produced anywhere in the world. This animal has never been domesticated; vast herds have lived wild on the high slopes of the Andes mountains. The demand for vicuna fur became so great that a million and a half of these animals were slain in one year to obtain their fur pelts. The result is that the Peruvian Govern-

214

ment has now completely forbidden their destruction. The garments of the ruling class of the Incas were made of the vicuna wool.

One of the important objectives of my trip to Peru was to find and study, if possible, some descendants of these Andean stocks. Fortunately, large numbers of the Aymara linguistic stock, the descendants of the Tauhuanocan culture, are still residing in southern Peru and Bolivia where they are said to retain the essentials of their ancient methods of living. They constitute the principal native populations in the vicinity of Lake Titicaca and the high mountain plateaus of southern Peru and northern Bolivia. I have always encountered difficulty in persuading the native peoples to allow themselves to be photographed in their primitive costumes. They are usually willing to be photographed provided one will wait for them to put on some modern garment.

I am reminded of an experience on one of the South Sea Islands where there was need for roads, but no money with which to build them. Laws were passed by the chiefs that anyone approaching a highway in native garb where he might be seen by a foreigner was subject to arrest and to payment of a fine which had to be worked out as labor in building roads. Of course, on that island no one would allow himself to be photographed without some modern clothing. One boy presented himself wearing a single garment, a man's full dress vest, which had evidently reached the island in a missionary barrel.

The hats in the pictures in Fig. 84 are of native design and manufacture. They are made of fur and are like our modern derbies in construction.

It is important to note the roundness of the features of the Aymaras, the wide development of the nostrils for air intake and the breadth of the dental arches. Many of them had been transported several hundreds of miles to a coffee plantation because of their adeptness and skill in sorting imperfect coffee beans from the run. As I watched them I found it difficult to move my eyes fast enough to follow their fingers and pick out from the moving run the undesired or imperfectly formed kernels. This revealed a superb development of coordination. The wisdom of these Aymaras is discussed in Chapter 21.

I was very anxious to study the Incas in different parts of the high Andes, particularly some of the original type in the vicinity of Cuzco, their ancient capital. Throughout the Andean Plateau, the Indians from the higher elevations bring down their wares on market days to exchange with Indians from other localities, as well as to meet and visit with their friends. They are very industrious and one seldom sees a woman, either shepherding the stock or carrying a burden, who is not busily engaged in spinning wool. While their wool is obtained in part from sheep that have been imported, a great deal of it is obtained from the alpacas which, like the llamas, are raised in the high altitudes where the Indians always prefer to live. I was fortunate in making contact

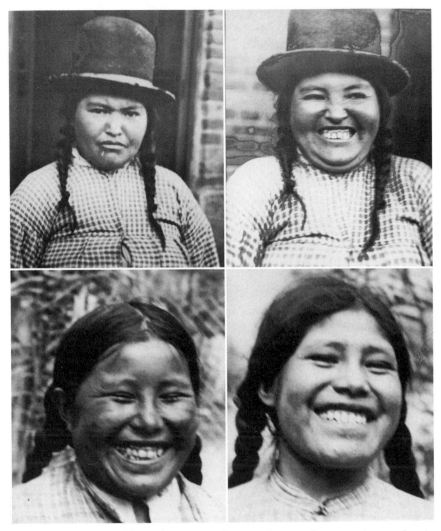

FIG. 84. Descendants of the Tauhuanocans who were the most famous ancient workers in stone. They live in the high Sierras of southern Peru and northern Bolivia. They belong to the Aymara linguistic division. They make fur felt hats and are skilled agriculturists.

with several groups of Indians in high altitudes through the kindness of the prefects. A group of Indians from the high mountains of the Urabamba Valley near Cuzco is shown in Fig. 85. An examination of this group of twenty-five revealed the fact that not one tooth had been attacked by dental caries and that, at all ages, the teeth normally due were present.

In Fig. 85, lower right, may be seen a typical Indian of the Andes carrying a heavy load. The Indians of this region are able to carry all day two hundred

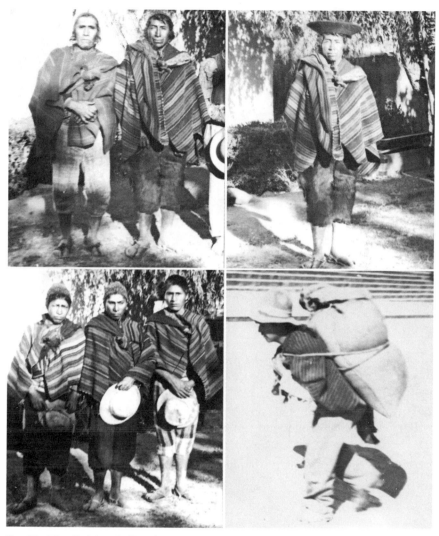

FIG. 85. The Quichua Indians living in the high Andes are descendants of the Incas. They live at high elevations, up to 18,000 feet, where they raise herds of llamas and alpacas. They weave their own garments and have great physical endurance. They can carry over 200 pounds all day at high altitudes in the manner shown at the lower right.

to three hundred pounds, and to do this day after day. At several of the ports, these mountain Indians have been brought down to the coast to load and unload coffee and freight from the ships. Their strength is phenomenal.

In approaching the study of the descendants of the Inca culture, it is important to keep in mind a little of their history and persecution under the Spanish rule. To this day they are bitter against the white man for the treachery

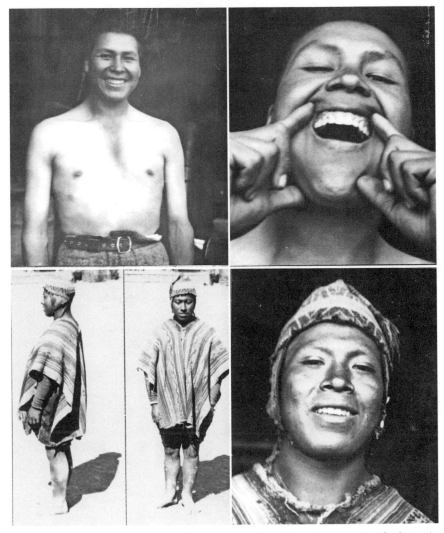

FIG. 86. The chest development, of necessity, must have large lung capacity for living in the rare atmosphere of the high Andes. The boy shown above has a magnificent physique, including facial and dental arch development. Below is seen the typical clothing worn up among the snows. Even in frosty weather they are bare below the knees.

that has been meted out to them on many occasions. Their leader was seized under treachery. The agreement to free him, if the designated rooms were filled with gold as high as a man could reach, was broken and their chief killed after the gold was obtained. It is recorded that some six million of them died in the mines under forced labor and poor foods under the lash of their Spanish oppressors. In many places they still keep themselves aloof by staying in the high mountains of the Andes with their flocks of llamas and alpacas. They come down only for trading. As in the past, they still weave their own garments. Indeed, they provide practically all of their necessities from the local environment. Their capacity for enduring cold is wonderful. They can sleep comfortably through the freezing nights with their ponchos wrapped about their heads and with their legs and feet bare. They wear two types of head cover, one inside the other. Several individuals are seen in Fig. 85. Many of them have faces that show strong character and personality.

The women of this district wear felt hats which can be turned up or down according to the weather. Fine examples of weaving were worn by the women.

In Fig. 86 will be seen two young men who had just come down from the high mountains to a government school. The one in the lower photograph is still wearing his native costume. The one in the upper has discarded his native costume for white man's trousers. Note the fine development of his chest, the splendid facial development and fine teeth and dental arches. It is important to keep in mind that these people are living in a rarified atmosphere and that, because of the high altitude, they need greater lung capacity and stronger hearts than do the people living at sea level. The ratio of oxygen content is reduced about half at 10,000 feet.

The broad dental arches of these Indians are shown in Fig. 87. Note the extensive wear of the teeth at the upper left. Much of the food is eaten cold and dry as parched corn and beans. Such rough foods as these wear the teeth down.

Market days which usually occur on Sunday present an interesting scene. The Indians travel long distances with their wares for exchange. They have no currency and exchanges are made by bargaining.

Where these Indians have become modernized, the new generation shows typical changes in facial and dental arch form as reported for the other groups. There is also a marked character reaction which will be discussed in detail in Chapter 19. In Fig. 88 are shown four typical modification patterns due to the influence of modernization after the foods of the white man have displaced the native dietary.

An important item in the life of the Andean Indians is the satisfaction they get from chewing cocoa leaves from which is made our modern cocaine. In order to extract the alkaloid they chew with these leaves the ash produced by the burning of a particular plant. This drug is chewed as tobacco; one large quid will last for several hours. Practically every Indian carries in a little pouch a quantity of these leaves in dried form. The effect of this drug is to increase their capacity for endurance. It makes them unconscious of hunger and fatigue. Through our interpreter we frequently asked them regarding the comfort or nourishment they obtained from the leaves and were told that they often preferred these leaves to food when they were on a journey and

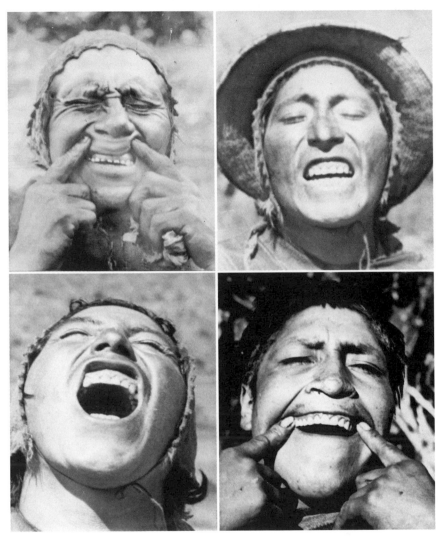

FIG. 87. The superb facial and dental arch development of these high Andean Indians is shown above. The man at the upper left was said to be very old yet he climbs the mountains up into the snows herding the llamas and alpacas. The teeth have a very high state of perfection. Long and vigorous use has worn the teeth of the old people.

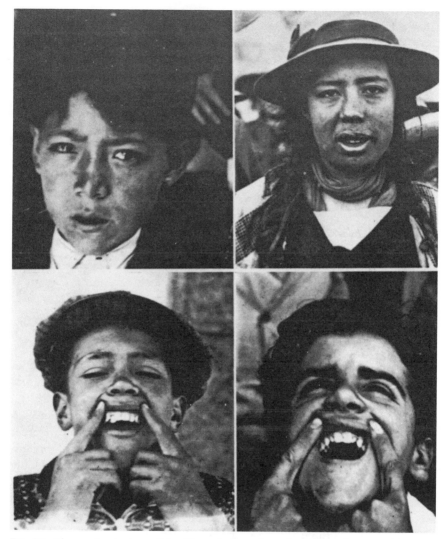

FIG. 88. The modernization of the Sierra Indians through the introduction of foods of modern commerce has produced a sad wreckage in physique and often character. The boy at the upper left is a mouth-breather because his nostrils are too small to carry sufficient air. The girl at the upper right has a badly underdeveloped chin and pinched nostrils. Both boys below have badly narrowed arches with crowding teeth.

carrying heavy loads. I was informed that they can increase the quantity of the drug used to a point at which they are quite unconscious of pain and able to endure injuries without suffering, and operations without discomfort. Since packets of these leaves were found in the burials near the coast, it is clear that the drugs were used throughout Peru in early times. It is also of interest that several of the skulls taken from the cave in the high Andes, were found with trephine operations in the skulls similar to those found in the burials along the coast.

The physical perfection and development of the present and past Andean population has been accomplished in spite of the difficulty of building and maintaining good bodily structure at the high altitude where dairy products have not been and are not at present a large part of the nutritional program. In this regard the ancient and contemporary peoples of the Andes differ radically from the present and past groups of people who live in the high valleys of Switzerland and Tibet where milk is plentiful. The cow, sheep, horse and pig have been imported into the high Andean countries during the last four hundred years since the Spanish Conquests, but they have not acclimatized easily. The earlier cultures were of course, dependent upon the llama, alpaca, wild deer, birds and guinea pig for animal foods. While there have been vast burial mounds built and preserved in the coastal regions where the absence of rain and the dry sand have added materially to their preservation, the rainy seasons have established very different conditions for skeletal preservation in the high altitudes. Nevertheless, a large number of skeletons in good state of preservation have been recovered.

The high Andean plateau extends throughout the length of Peru between the mountain chains. The present Indian stock was studied in four different places in the high plateau country, the farthest north being Huaras. In this area we were materially assisted by the governor of the province who very kindly sent messengers and brought down Indian families from high altitudes to the police headquarters at Huaras. This place is at an elevation of about 11,000 feet. We had an opportunity to study also many who had come from the higher altitudes to the markets to sell their wares. Huaras lies in a fertile valley that has been in contact with modern civilization for many decades. This vicinity, therefore, provided a wide range in classes of people, from Indians who are isolated to those who are living in highly modernized groups. In addition to the opportunity for studying the older people there were opportunities for studying adolescents in the two high schools, one for girls and one for boys. Some were pure-bloods who had been highly isolated in their formative and childhood periods. The mixed-bloods had been considerably modernized. There were some whites. I was told by the prefect and others who were well informed that there was quite a distinct difference between the Indians who were living in the high northern Cordillera, the western Andean range called the Black Mountains, and those living in the eastern range or White Mountains. The latter were physically much better built and were least modernized. Typical low immunity to caries and changes in facial and dental arch form were found in these modernized groups.

Another important area in which the native Indians were studied was Chiclayo. This district is unique in large part because of the influence of the modern civilization at Lima with which it is connected by the railroad. The native market here is very large and occupies about a mile of the main street of the town, through which no traffic except pedestrian traffic can pass while the market is in session. The town has been under the influence of the Spanish since the time of the Conquest. It has many colonial buildings and a large cathedral. It has not, however, accommodations for the influx of tourists who come out of curiosity for the purchase of Indian wares. With the aid of the prefect, even though no public accommodations were available, we were made very comfortable in the soldiers' barracks. As the Indians came down from the mountains to display and sell their wares, they were brought to us at the barracks. Since this district has been in quite intimate contact with the nutrition of the modernized capital, we found here many individuals showing typical degeneration of the teeth and dental arches.

The adaptation of racial characteristics to the environment in which they have developed is very strikingly illustrated in the Indian cultures of the Amazon Jungle district. We were very fortunate in being able to make studies of some groups living at present as did their ancestors through countless centuries in the Amazon basin. We were greatly pleased and impressed with the splendid physiques and fine personalities of many of the individuals of the groups.

The abundance of rain, the fertility of the soil and the warm climate make plant growth most luxuriant on the eastern slopes of the Andes. It is of interest that in passing from the capital, Lima, across the desert stretch between the ocean and the mountains and then up the wall of the Andes to an altitude of sixteen thousand feet and then down to the plateau at about twelve thousand feet and up again over the eastern range and down into the Amazon basin, one has passed through the tropics, temperate zone and sub-arctic zones with varieties of plant life corresponding to each. A distance of a few hundred yards will often divide the limits of particular birds and flowers. When one reaches the foothills of the Andes on the eastern side, he is in a region of rushing streams teeming with fish, a region of tropical fruits and vegetables. It is in this setting that some of the finest Indians we have seen were enjoying life in its

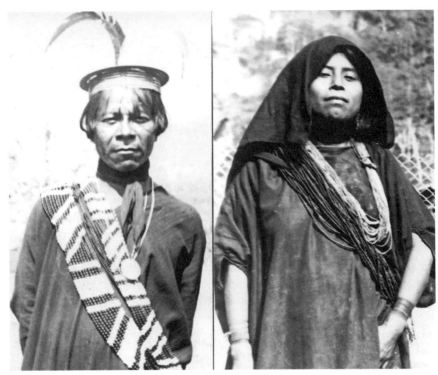

FIG. 89. Jungle Indians from the Amazon. This is the chief of a tribe who came prepared to have their pictures taken in their tribal regalia. Note the splendid features of both and the noble carriage of the woman.

fullness. The type of shelter is very simple, indeed, consisting as it does of a framework covered with banana and palm leaves. We were privileged to meet by special arrangement about thirty of this tribe who had been brought from some distance by the officials of the Perene Colony, owned and operated by the Peruvian Corporation. In Fig. 89 will be seen the chief and one of the noble women of his retinue. They understood that they would have their pictures taken and came dressed in royal regalia. Typical countenances are seen in Figs. 90 and 91. These people have very kind faces with broad dental arches, and a high sense of humor. They decorated their faces especially for their photograph. In the entire group associated with this chief I did not find a single tooth that had been attacked by dental caries. The fine dental arches are illustrated in Figs. 90 and 91. Many of these young men had really noble countenances, such as would rate them as leaders in modern science and culture.

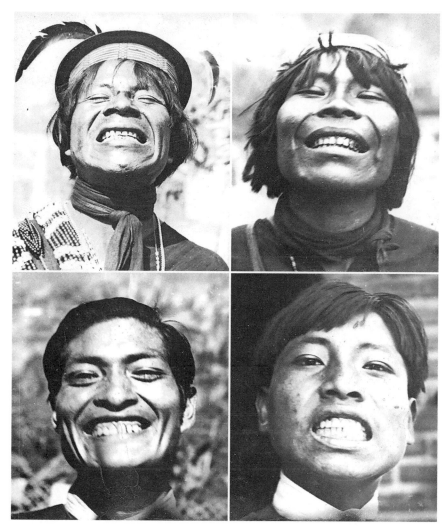

FIG. 90. The facial and dental arch development of the jungle Indians was superb and the teeth were excellent and free from dental caries. Note the complete development of the dental arches and nostrils.

In another tribe, however, of the same racial stock, efforts to modernize had been in operation for some time by a mission. The food of this latter group had been distinctly affected by their contact with the modern group. By reducing the animal foods, the change in physical efficiency, and appearance of tooth decay, is most marked. In Fig. 92 above will be seen typical cases of rampant tooth decay with extensive loss of the teeth. In Fig. 92 below are

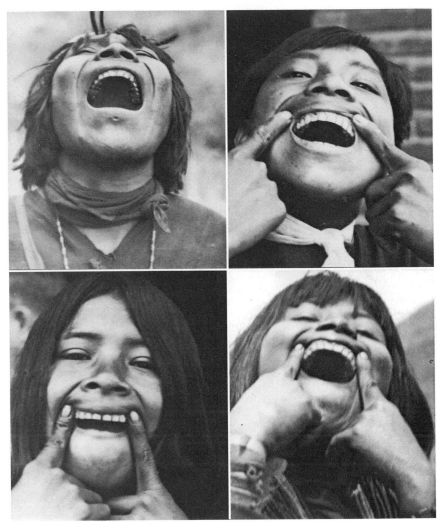

FIG. 91. The excellence of skeletal development of the jungle Indians as expressed in the faces and dental arches is illustrated in these views. Their foods were selected from the animal life of the streams and the bush together with native plants.

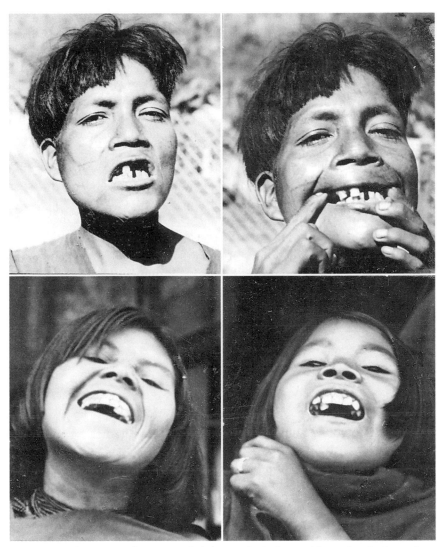

FIG. 92. At the point of contact of these jungle Indians with modernization where it included a change from their native diet tooth decay became rampant as shown. A marked change in facial form occurred accompanied by crowding of the teeth in the new generation.

shown two of the first generation following the adoption of the modernized type of diet in this group. Note the narrowing of the faces with crowding of the teeth. Note the deformed dental arches.

The native foods of these Amazon Jungle Indians included the liberal use of fish which are very abundant in both the Amazon and its branches, particularly in the foothill streams; animal life from the forest and thickets; bird life, including many water fowl and their eggs; plants and fruits. They use very large quantities of yucca which is a starchy root quite similar to our potato in chemical content. This is not the yucca of North America.

The Peruvian Indians, in the highlands and in the eastern watershed of the Andes, and also in the Amazon Basin, have built superb bodies with high immunity to dental caries and with splendidly developed facial and dental arch forms while living on the native foods in accordance with their accumulated wisdom. Whenever they have adopted the foods of modern civilization and have displaced their own nutrition, dental caries has been found to be wide-spread; and in the succeeding generations following the adoption of modern foods, a change in facial and dental arch forms has developed. The modernized foods which displaced their native foods were the typical white man's dietary of refined-flour products, sugar, sweetened foods, canned goods, and polished rice.

Chapter 15

CHARACTERISTICS OF PRIMITIVE AND
MODERNIZED DIETARIES

IF PRIMITIVE races have been more efficient than modernized groups in the matter of preventing degenerative processes, physical, mental and moral, it is only because they have been more efficient in complying with Nature's laws. We have two procedures that we can use for evaluating their programs: first, the interpretation of their data in terms of our modern knowledge; and second, the clinical application of their procedures to our modern social problems. Specifically, since the greater success of the primitives in meeting Nature's laws has been based primarily on dietary procedures, it becomes desirable first, to evaluate their dietary programs on the basis of known biologic requirements for comparison with the foods of our modern civilization; and second, to test their primitive nutritional programs by applying their equivalents to our modern families.

The advance in our knowledge of body-building and body-repairing materials from a biochemical standpoint makes it possible even with our limited knowledge of organic catalysts, to draw comparisons between the primitive and modernized dietaries. If we use the generally accepted minimal and optimal quantities of the various minerals and vitamins required, as indicated by Sherman,[1] we shall have at once a yardstick for evaluating the primitive dietaries.

Of the eighteen elements of which the human body is composed, all of which are presumably essential, several are needed in very small quantities. A few are required in liberal quantities. The normal adult needs to receive from the foods eaten one-half to one gram of calcium or lime per day. Few people receive more than one-half of the minerals present in the food. The requirements of phosphorus are approximately twice this amount. Of iron we need from one-seventh to one-third of a gram per day. Smaller amounts than these are required of several other elements.

In order to utilize these minerals, and to build and maintain the functions of various organs, definite quantities of various organic catalysts which act as activating substances are needed. These include the known and unknown vitamins.

Unlike some experimental animals, human beings have not the ability to create some special chemical substances (not elements) such as vitamins within their bodies. Several animals have this capacity. For example, scurvy, which is due to a lack of vitamin C, cannot be produced readily in rats because rats can manufacture vitamin C. Similarly, rickets cannot be produced easily in guinea pigs, because they can synthesize vitamin D. The absence of vitamin D and adequate minerals produces rickets in young human beings. Neither rickets nor scurvy can be produced readily in dogs because of the dogs' capacity to synthesize both vitamins C and D. We are not so fortunate. Similarly, the absence of vitamin B (B^1) produces in birds and man severe nervous system reactions, such as beri-beri. These symptoms are often less pronounced, or quite different, in other animals.

From our knowledge of the dietaries used by the various primitive racial stocks, we can calculate the approximate amounts of the minerals and vitamins provided by those dietaries for comparison with the amounts provided by modernized foods. Our problem is simplified by the fact that the food of the white man in various parts of the world being built from a few fundamental food factors, has certain quite constant characteristics. Hence the displacing diets are similar for the several modernized groups herewith considered.

As a further approach to our problem, it is important to keep in mind that, in general, the wild animal life has largely escaped many of the degenerative processes which affect modern white peoples. We ascribe this to animal instinct in the matter of food selection. It is possible that man has lost through disuse some of the normal faculty for consciously recognizing body requirements. In other words, the only hunger of which we now are conscious is a hunger for energy to keep us warm and to supply power. In general, we stop eating when an adequate amount of energy has been provided, whether or not the body-building and repairing materials have been included in the food. The heat and energy factor in our foods is measured in calories. In planning an adequate diet, a proper ratio between body building and energy units must be maintained. It is important to keep in mind that while the amount of body-building and repairing material required is similar for different individuals of the same age and weight, it is markedly different for two individuals, one of whom is leading a sedentary, and the other, an active life. Similarly, there is a great difference between the amount of body-building and repairing material required by a growing child or an expectant mother and an average adult.

There are certain characteristics of the various dietaries of the primitive races, which are universally present when that dietary program is associated with a high immunity to disease and freedom from deformities. In general, these are the foods that provide adequate sources of body-building and body-repairing material. The use by primitives of foods relatively low in calories has resulted in forcing them to eat large quantities of these foods in order to provide the heat and energy requirements of the body. The primitives have obtained, often with great difficulty, foods that are scarce but rich in certain elements. In these rare foods were elements which the body requires in small quantities, including minerals such as iodine, copper, manganese and special vitamins. In connection with the vitamins it should be kept in mind that our knowledge of these unique organic catalysts is limited. The medical profession and the public at large think of vitamin D as consisting of just one chemical factor, whereas, investigations are revealing continually new and additional factors. A recent review[2] describes in considerable detail eight distinct factors in vitamin D and refers to information indicating that there may be at least twelve. Clearly, it is not possible to undertake to provide an adequate nutrition simply by reinforcing the diet with a few synthetic products which are known to represent certain of these nutritional factors. By the mass of the people at large, as well as by members of the medical profession, activated ergosterol is considered to include all that is necessary to supply the vitamin D group of activators to human nutrition.

The various dietary programs of primitive races which appear to be successful in controlling dental caries and deformities may be divided into three groups based upon the sources from which they derive the minerals and fat-soluble activators. I do not use the term vitamins exclusively because as yet little is known about the whole group of organic catalysts, although we have considerable knowledge of the limited number which are designated by the first half dozen letters of the alphabet. Most lay people and members of the medical and dental professions assume that the six or eight vitamins constitute practically all that are needed in an adequate nutrition. These organic activators can be divided into two main groups, water-soluble and fat-soluble. An essential characteristic of the successful dietary programs of primitive races has been found to relate to a liberal source of the fat-soluble activator group.

When we discuss the successful dietary programs of the various groups from the standpoint of their ability to control tooth decay and prevent deformity we find that, for the people in the high and isolated Alpine valleys, their nutrition is dependent largely on entire rye bread and dairy products with meat about once a week and various vegetables, fresh in the summer season and stored for the winter season. An analysis in my laboratory of the dairy products obtained from the Löetschental Valley in Switzerland through a series of years has shown the vitamin content to be much higher than the average throughout the world for similar foods during the same seasons. The milk in these high valleys is produced from green pasturage and stored green hay of exceptionally high chlorophyll content. The milk and the rye bread provided minerals abundantly.

The diet of the people in the Outer Hebrides which proved adequate for maintaining a high immunity to dental caries and preventing deformity consisted chiefly of oat products and sea foods including the wide variety of fish available there. This diet included generally no dairy products since the pasture was not adequate for maintaining cattle. Oat grain was the only cereal that could be matured satisfactorily in that climate. Some green foods were available in the summer and some vegetables were grown and stored for winter. This diet, which included a liberal supply of fish, included also the use of livers of fish. One important fish dish was baked cod's head that had been stuffed with oat meal and chopped cods' livers. This was an important inclusion in the diets of the growing children. The oats and fish, including livers, provided minerals and vitamins adequate for an excellent racial stock with high immunity to tooth decay.

For the Eskimos of Alaska the native diet consisted of a liberal use of organs and other special tissues of the large animal life of the sea, as well as of fish. The latter were dried in large quantities in the summer and stored for winter use. The fish were also eaten frozen. Seal oil was used freely as an adjunct to this diet and seal meat was specially prized and was usually available. Caribou meat was sometimes available. The organs were used. Their fruits were limited largely to a few berries including cranberries, available in the summer and stored for winter use. Several plant foods were gathered in the summer and stored in fat or frozen for winter use. A ground nut that was gathered by the Tundra mice and stored in caches was used by the Eskimos as a vegetable. Stems of certain water grasses, water plants and bulbs were occasionally used. The bulk of their diet, however, was fish and large animal life of the sea from which they selected certain organs and tissues with great care and wisdom. These included the inner layer of skin of one of the whale species, which has recently been shown to be very rich in vitamin C. Fish eggs were dried in season. They were used liberally as food for the growing children and were recognized as important for growth and reproduction. This successful nutrition provided ample amounts of fat-soluble activators and minerals from sea animal life.

For the Indians living inside the Rocky Mountain Range in the far North of Canada, the successful nutrition for nine months of the year was largely limited to wild game, chiefly moose and caribou. During the summer months the Indians were able to use growing plants. During the winter some use was made of bark and buds of trees. I found the Indians putting great emphasis upon the eating of the organs of the animals, including the wall of parts of the digestive tract. Much of the muscle meat of the animals was fed to the dogs. It is important that skeletons are rarely found where large game animals have been slaughtered by the Indians of the North. The skeletal remains are found as piles of finely broken bone chips or splinters that have been cracked up to obtain as much as possible of the marrow and nutritive qualities of the bones. These Indians obtain their fat-soluble vitamins and also most of their minerals from the organs of the animals. An important part of the nutrition of the children consisted in various preparations of bone marrow, both as a substitute for milk and as a special dietary ration.

In the various archipelagos of the South Pacific and in the islands north of Australia, the natives depended greatly on shell fish and various scale fish from adjacent seas. These were eaten with an assortment of plant roots and fruits, raw and cooked. Taro was an important factor in the nutrition of most of these groups. It is the root of a species of lily similar to "elephant ears" used for garden decorations in America because of its large leaves. In several of the islands the tender young leaves of this plant were eaten with coconut cream baked in the leaf of the tia plant. In the Hawaiian group of islands the taro plant is cooked and dried and pounded into powder and then mixed with water and allowed to ferment for twenty-four hours, more or less, in accordance with the stiffness of the product desired. This is called poi. Its use in this form was comparable in efficiency with its use on other archipelagos as a boiled root served much as we use potatoes. For these South Sea Islanders fat-soluble vitamins and many of the minerals were supplied by the shell fish and other animal life from the sea.

The native tribes in eastern and central Africa, used large quantities of sweet potatoes, beans, and some cereals. Where they were living sufficiently near fresh water streams and lakes, large quantities of fish were eaten. Goats or cattle or both were domesticated by many tribes. Other tribes used wild animal life quite liberally. Some very unique and special sources of vitamins were used by some of these tribes. For example, in certain seasons of the year great swarms of a large winged insect develop in Lake Victoria and other lakes. These often accumulated on the shores to a depth of many inches. They were gathered, dried and preserved to be used in puddings which are highly prized by the natives and are well spoken of by the missionaries. Another insect source of vitamins used frequently by the natives is the ant which is collected from great ant hills that in many districts grow to heights of ten feet or more. In the mating season the ants develop wings and come out of the ant hills in great quantities and go into the air for the mating process. These expeditions are frequently made during or following a rain. The natives have developed procedures for inducing these ants to come out by covering over the opening with bushes to give the effect of clouds and then pounding on the ground to give an imitation of rain. We were told by the missionaries that one of the great luxuries was an ant pie but unfortunately they were not able to supply us with this delicacy. Parts of Africa like many other districts are often plagued by vast swarms of locusts. These are gathered in large quantities, to be cooked for immediate use or dried and ground into a flour for later use. They provide a rich source of minerals and vitamins. The natives of Africa used the cereals maize, beans, linga linga, millet, and Kafir corn, cooked or roasted. Most of these were ground just before cooking.

Among the Aborigines of Australia we found that those living near the sea were using animal life from that source liberally, together with the native plants and animals of the land. They have not cultivated the land plants during their primitive life. In the interior, they use freely the wild animal life, particularly wallaby, kangaroo, small animals and rodents. All of the edible parts, including the walls of the viscera and internal organs are eaten.

The native Maori in New Zealand used large quantities of foods from the sea, wherever these were available. Even in the inland food depots, mutton birds were still available in large quantities. These birds were captured just before they left the nests. They developed in the rockeries about the coast, chiefly on the extreme southern coast of the South Island. At this stage, the flesh is very tender and very fat from the gorging that has been provided by their parent. The value of this food for the treatment of tuberculosis was being heralded quite widely in both Australia and New Zealand. In the primitive state of the islands large quantities of land birds were available and because of the fertility of the soil and favorable climate, vegetables and fruits grew abundantly in the wild. Large quantities of fern root were used. Where groups of the Maori race were found isolated sufficiently from contact with modern civilization and its foods to be dependent largely on the native foods, they selected with precision certain shell-fish because of their unique nutritive value.

A splendid illustration of the primitive Maori instinct or wisdom regarding the value of sea foods was shown in an experience we had while making examinations in a native school on the east coast of the North Islands. I was impressed with the fact that the children in the school gave very little evidence of having active dental caries. I asked the teacher what the children brought from their homes to eat at their midday lunch, since most of them had to come too great a distance to return at noon. I was told that they brought no lunch but that when school was dismissed at noon the children rushed for the beach where, while part of the group prepared bonfires, the others stripped and dived into the sea, and brought up a large species of lobster. The lobsters were promptly roasted on the coals and devoured with great relish. Other sea foods are pictured in Fig. 74.

The native diet of the tribes living in the islands north of Australia consisted of liberal quantities of sea foods. These were eaten with a variety of plant roots and greens, together with fruits which grew abundantly in that favorable climate. Few places in the world have so favorable a quantity of food for sea-animal life as these waters which provide the richest pearl fisheries in the world. This is evidence of the enormous quantity of shell-fish that develop there. Here, as off the east coast of Australia, are to be found some of the largest shell-fish of the world. It was a common occurrence to see these shells being used by natives for such purposes as water storage and for bath tubs of a size approximately that of a wash tub. Australia and New Zealand are near enough to the Antarctic ice cap to have their shores bathed with currents coming from the ice fields, currents which abound in food for sea animals. The great barrier reef off the east coast of Australia extends north to within a few leagues of New Guinea. Murray Island is near the north end of this barrier. The fish in the water at times form such a dense mass that they can be scooped into the boats directly from the sea. Fishermen wading out in the surf and throwing their spears into the schools of fish usually impale one or several.

The incidence of tooth decay on this island was less than one percent of all of the teeth examined. Another important sea food in these waters was dugong, referred to as sea cow in northern waters. This animal is very highly prized but is becoming scarce. We found its meat very much like lamb. It lives on the vegetation of the sea floor in shallow water. As we flew over the bays of Eastern Australia going northward in search of colonies of native Aborigines, we could see these sea animals pasturing in the clear water among the ocean plants.

During these investigations of primitive races, I have been impressed with the superior quality of the human stock developed by Nature wherever a liberal source of sea foods existed. These zones of abundant marine life were largely in the wake of the ocean currents drifting from the ice fields of the poles. The Humboldt Current is probably the most liberal carrier of marine life of any of the ocean currents. It leaves the ice field of the Antarctic and bathes the west coast of South America from its southern tip nearly to the equator, where the coast line changes direction and the Humboldt Current is deflected out into the ocean. It meets here a warm current coming down from the coast of Central America, Panama and Columbia. If the superb physiques that Nature has established among the Maori of New Zealand, the Malays of the Islands north of Australia, the Gaelics of the Outer Hebrides and the natives on several of the archipelagos of the Pacific, owe their superior physical development to sea foods, we should expect to find that the tribes which have had contact with the great Humboldt Current food would also have superb physiques. Unfortunately, very little has been known of the ancient cultures that have developed along the coast of Chile and Peru. It has been reported that of all the Indian tribes of South America, those in Patagonia were the most stalwart. While the west coast of Peru is bathed by the Humboldt Current with its nearly inexhaustible supply of human nutrition, the lands bordering that shore are among the most desolate deserts of the world. The zone between the Andes Mountains and the coast for approximately a thousand miles is utterly barren, consisting of moving sand dunes and jagged promontories. Practically the only break in this waterless, treeless desert is to be found in the few ribbons of water that trickle down from the melting snows of the Andes Coastal Range. This coast has no rainy seasons. Any vegetation grown, now or in the past thousands of years, has had to be watered from the limited supply afforded by these rivers which seem so insignificant when compared with the vastness of the territory. These river bottoms contain the alluvial deposits from the Andes and are very rich when watered. It has been only by means of gigantic engineering undertakings that the water from these rivers has been carried through great irrigation ditches, sometimes fifty to a hundred miles long for the purpose of making it possible to utilize these river bottom lands for agriculture.

In many of the primitive tribes living by the sea we found emphasis on the value of fish eggs and on some animal forms for insuring a high physical development of growing children, particularly of girls, and a high perfection of offspring through a reinforcement of the mother's nutrition. It is also important to note that in several of the primitive tribes studied there has been a consciousness that not only the mother should have special nutrition, but also the father. In this group very great value was placed upon a product obtained from a sea form known locally as the angelote or angel fish, which in classification is between a skate and a shark. The young of the angelota are born alive, ready for free swimming and capable of foraging for themselves immediately at birth. Twenty to thirty young are born in one litter. The eggs of the female before fertilization are about one inch in diameter, slightly oval but nearly spherical. They are used as food by all, but the special food product for men is a pair of glands obtained from the male. These glands weigh up to a pound each, when they are dried. They have a recognized value among the natives for treating cases of tuberculosis, especially for controlling lung hemorrhages. The sea foods were used in conjunction with the land plants and fruits raised by means of irrigation in the river valleys. Together these foods provided adequate nutrition for maintaining high physical excellence.

In Chapter 13 I have discussed the probable order of these ancient cultures and the possible extent of their duration. Very little is known of their origin. Evidence has recently been discovered in Panama indicating that both the wealth and the culture of Peru were carried northward by maritime conquerors and that the cultures of Central America, including the Maya culture may have had their origins in these ancient cultures of Peru.

While the coastal area of Peru saw the development of many magnificent cultures through past ages, the highlands of Peru also have left much evidence of superior attainments and wisdom. The two great Indian linguistic groups of the Andean highlands of today are the Aymara of Southern Peru and Bolivia and the Quichus of central and northern Peru. The Aymara are credited with being the descendants of the Tauhuanocan culture which preceded the Incan culture in the highlands. The Quichu are credited with being the descendants of the Incan culture which had its zenith just prior to the coming of the Spaniards. In Chapter 14 I have shown photographs of these racial stocks as they are found today in the Andean Sierras. It may be possible that in former times the vast mountain ranges provided large herds of grazing wild animals of the deer family. Because of the vastness of the population and the extent to which all available land surfaces were utilized for agriculture, it does not seem possible that wild animal life could have been an adequate source of nutrition. The members of the camel family, the llamas, alpacas, and vicunas were utilized for food. Of these the first two were used to considerable extent as they are today. When it is recognized that in the Sierra the available water is largely that provided to the streams from the melting snows and from rains in the rainy season, it will be realized that these sources of fresh water could not provide the liberal quantity of iodine essential for human growth and development. It was, accordingly, a matter of great interest to discover that these Indians used regularly dried fish eggs from the sea. Commerce in these dried foods is carried on today as it no doubt has been for centuries. When I inquired of them why they used this material they explained that it was necessary to maintain the fertility of their women. I was informed also that every exchange depot and market carried these dried fish eggs so that they were always available. Another sea product of very great importance, and one which was universally available was dried kelp. Upon inquiry I learned that the Indians used it so that they would not get "big necks" like the whites. The kelp provided a very rich source of iodine as well as of copper, which is very important to them in the utilization of iron for building an exceptionally efficient quality of blood for carrying oxygen liberally at those high altitudes. An important part of their dietary consists today as in the past of potatoes which are gathered and frozen, dried and powdered, and preserved in the powdered form. This powder is used in soups with llama meat and other products. Since the vitamin D group of activators is absent from nearly all plant products but must be synthesized in animal bodies from the plant foods, where it is largely stored in organs, an adequate source had to be provided. The Indians of the highlands of Peru maintained colonies of guinea pigs which were used in their stews. The ancient burials also show that the guinea pig was a common source of food since mummified bodies of this animal were found. This is significant since of all the animals that are used for experimental work, the guinea pig is probably the most efficient in synthesizing vitamin D from plant foods. They are very hardy. They live on a great variety of green plant foods and twigs and are very prolific. They apparently played a very important part in the physical excellence of the ancient cultures.

It is unfortunate that as the white man has come into contact with the primitives in various parts of the world he has failed to appreciate the accumulated wisdom of the primitive racial stocks. Much valuable wisdom has been lost by this means. I have referred to the skill of the Indians in preventing scurvy and to the many drugs that we use which the white man has learned of from the primitives.

In this connection the Indians of British Columbia, who have been so efficient in preventing scurvy, have a plant product for the prevention and cure of diabetes. This has recently become known to the white man through the experience of a patient who was brought into the hospital at Prince Rupert, British Columbia, as reported in the Canadian Medical Journal, July 1938. Prince Rupert is near the boundary between British Columbia and Alaska on the coast. The patient came to that hospital for an operation and suddenly showed signs of diabetes, which required treatment with large doses of insulin. Dr. Richard Geddes Large asked him regarding the history of his affection and what he had been taking. He was told that for several years he had been using an Indian preparation which was a hot water infusion of a root of devil's-club which is a spiny, prickly shrub. This medicine was in common use by the British Columbia Indians. The material was obtained and used in this hospital for the treatment of diabetes and was found to be quite as efficient as insulin and had the great advantage that it would be taken by mouth whereas the insulin which is destroyed in the stomach by the process of digestion must be injected. They could see very little difference in the efficiency of this preparation whether taken internally or used hypodermically. This promises to be a great boon to a large group of individuals suffering from diabetes. It is also probable that its use will prevent the development of diabetes and since the Indians used it for other affections it may also become a very important adjunct in modern preventive medicine.

One of the sources that I have found to be helpful in studying primitive races is an investigation of knapsacks. I have asked for the privilege of seeing what is carried in their knapsacks. I found dried fish eggs and dried kelp in the knapsacks in the high Andes. It is also of interest that among this group in the Andes, among those in central Africa, and among the Aborigines of Australia, each knapsack contained a ball of clay, a little of which was dissolved in water. Into this they dipped their morsels of food while eating. Their explanation was to prevent "sick stomach." This is the medicine that is used by the native in these countries for combating dysentery and food infections. It is the treatment that was given me when I developed dysentery infection in central Africa while making studies there. The English doctor in Nairobi whom I called in said he would give me the native treatment of a suspension of clay. It proved very effective. An illustration of the way in which modern science is slowly adopting practices that have been long in use among primitive races, is to be found in the recent extensive use that is made of clay (kaolin) in our modern medicine. This is illustrated in the following:[3]

> In the course of an expedition to Lake Titicaca, South America, financed by the Percy Slade Trustees in which one of us (H.P.M.) took part, an interesting observation was made in regard to the diet of the Quetchus Indians on the Capachica Peninsula near Puno. These people are almost certainly descendants of the Incas and at the present time live very primitively. They exist largely on a vegetable diet of which potatoes form an important part. Immediately, before being eaten, the potatoes are dipped into an aqueous suspension of clay, a procedure which is said to prevent "souring of the stomach."
>
> We have examined this clay and found it to consist of kaolin containing a trace of organic material, possibly coumarin, and presumably a decomposition product of the grass from underneath which the clay is dug. The local name for the clay is Chacco, and the Indians distinguish between good and bad qualities. This dietetic procedure is universal among the Indians of the Puno district, and is probably of very ancient origin.
>
> Such a practice by a primitive people would appear rather remarkable in view of the comparatively recent introduction of kaolin into modern medicine as a protective agent for the gastric and intestinal mucosa and as a remedy for bacterial infections of the gut.

It is of interest that both the British and American Pharmacopeias have added kaolin to their list during the last two decades.

The Indians of the past buried, with their dead, foods to carry them on their journey. From an examination of these one learns that in many respects the Indians living in the high Sierras are living today very much as their ancestors did during past centuries. Items of importance now and in the past are parched corn and parched beans which are nibbled as the people walk along carrying their heavy burdens. Today these are the only foods eaten on many long journeys. We found the parched beans pleasant to taste and very satisfying when we were hungry.

The Indians of the Amazon Basin have had a history very different from either those of the high Sierras of the Andes or those of the coastal region. The fact that vast areas of the Amazon Basin have not only never been surveyed, but never even penetrated, indicates the nature of the isolation of these groups. Very little progress has been made in the effort to conquer or modernize these Indians. A few explorers have made expeditions into parts of the interior and have reported the characteristics of the plant and animal life, as well as of the native races. Our sole contact was with the tribe which came to the coffee plantation to assist in the gathering and the harvest of the coffee beans. In Chapter 14 I have described these people in considerable detail.

Since the Amazon Basin has vast quantities of rain as well as abundant streams from the eastern watershed of the Andes, the tribes live largely in tropical jungles where there is an abundance of water. They are expert, accordingly, in the use of river crafts and in fishing for the various types of marine life. Unlike the Indians of the high Andes or of the coast regions they are not agriculturists. They live on wild native foods almost entirely. They are expert with the blow gun, with the bow and arrow and in snaring with both nets and loops. They use very large quantities of a tuber root called yucca which has many qualities similar to the roots of the edible variety of the lily family. This plant is boiled and eaten much as are potatoes. They use also large quantities of fish from the streams, birds and small animals of the land, together with the native fruits including bananas. Their dietary provides a very liberal supply of minerals and vitamins together with an adequate quantity of carbohydrates, fats and proteins.

In evaluating the nutritive value of the dietary programs of primitive races and our modernized cultures, it is important that we have a yardstick adequately adjusted to make computation in terms of specific body needs for building good bodies and maintaining them in good health. The advance in modern chemistry has gone far toward making this possible.

The problem of estimating the mineral and activator contents, in other words the body-building and repairing qualities of the displacing foods used by the various primitive races, is similar in many respects to estimating these qualities in the foods used in our modern white civilizations, except that modern commerce has transported usually only the foods that will keep well. These include chiefly white flour, sugar, polished rice, vegetable fats and canned goods.

Very important data for typical American dietaries are now available provided by the Bureau of Home Economics, United States Department of Agriculture, and also by the Bureau of Labor Statistics, United States Department of Labor. These surveys provide a basis of estimating the nutrition of various income groups both with regard to the type of foods selected in our American communities and the quantities of each type used, together with the chemical content of these foods expressed quantitatively. Those who wish to have detailed reports are referred to the bulletins of the above departments. In my clinical studies of the mineral constituents of individuals, affected with dental caries and other disturbances of physical deficiency, I find a wide range of variation in the calcium, phosphorus and fat-soluble activator content of the dietaries used, although in general the calorie content is adequate. This latter factor is controlled by appetite. These computations reveal that the individuals studied have a calcium intake ranging from 0.3 to 0.5 grams; and a phosphorus intake of from 0.3 to 0.6 grams. The minimum adult requirements as provided by such an authority as Sherman, whose figures are used by the United States Department of Labor, are for the average adult 0.68 of a gram of calcium and 1.32 grams of phosphorus per day. It can be seen readily that the amounts given above are far short of the minimum even if individuals absorbed from the foods all of the minerals present. A question arises at this point as to the efficiency of the human body in removing all of the minerals from the ingested foods. Extensive laboratory determinations have shown that most people cannot absorb more than half of the calcium and phosphorus from the foods eaten. The amounts utilized depend directly on the presence of other substances, particularly fat-soluble vitamins. It is at this point probably that the greatest breakdown in our modern diet takes place, namely, in the ingestion and utilization of adequate amounts of the special activating substances, including the vitamins needed for rendering the minerals in the food available to the human system.

A recent report by the Council on Foods of the American Medical Association[4] makes this comment on spinach:

> Spinach may be regarded as a rich source of vitamin A and as a contributor of vitamin C, iron and roughage to the diet. It is therefore a valuable food. (But) the iron is not well utilized by infants . . . (and) the feeding of spinach is of no value during early infancy as a source of calcium.

Even though calcium is present in spinach children cannot utilize it. Data have been published showing that children absorb very little of the calcium or phosphorus in spinach before six years of age. Adult individuals vary in the efficiency with which they absorb minerals and other chemicals essential for mineral utilization. It is possible to starve for minerals that are abundant in the foods eaten because they cannot be utilized without an adequate quantity of the fat-soluble activators.

This is illustrated in the following case. A minister in an industrial section of our city, during the period of severe depression, telephoned me stating that he had just been called to baptize a dying child. The child was not dead although almost constantly in convulsions. He thought the condition was probably nutritional and asked if he could bring the boy to the office immediately. The boy was badly emaciated, had rampant tooth decay, one leg in a cast, a very bad bronchial cough and was in and out of convulsions in rapid succession. His convulsions had been getting worse progressively during the past eight months. His leg had been fractured two or three months previously while walking across the room when he fell in one of his convulsions. No healing had occurred. His diet consisted of white bread and skimmed milk. For mending the fracture the boy needed minerals, calcium, phosphorus and magnesium. His convulsions were due to a low calcium content of the blood. All of these were in the skimmed milk for the butter-fat removed in the cream contains no calcium nor phosphorus, except traces. The program provided was a change from the white flour bread to wheat gruel made from freshly ground wheat and the substitution of whole milk for skimmed milk, with the addition of about a teaspoonful of a very high-vitamin butter with each feeding. He was given this meal that evening when he returned to his home. He slept all night without a convulsion. He was fed the same food five times the next day and did not have a convulsion. He proceeded rapidly to regain his health without recurrence of his convulsions. In a month the fracture was united. Two views of the fracture are shown in Fig. 93, one before and one

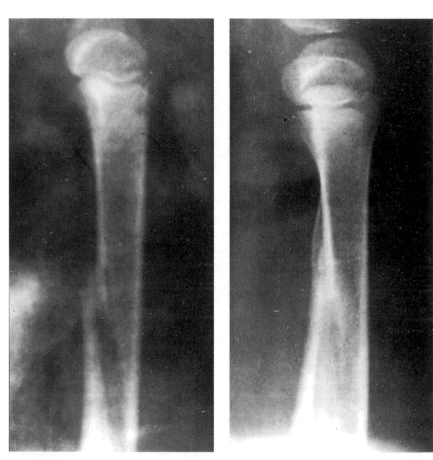

FIG. 93. This figure shows the rapid healing of a fractured femur of a boy four and one-half years of age suffering from convulsions due to malnutrition. His fracture occurred when he fell in a convulsion. There was no healing in sixty days. After reinforcing his nutrition with butter vitamins the healing at the right occurred in thirty days. Whole milk replaced skim milk and a whole wheat gruel made from freshly ground whole wheat replaced white bread.

after the treatment. Six weeks after this nutritional program was started the preacher called at the home to see how the boy was getting along. His mother stated that the boy was playing about the doorstep, but they could not see him. She called but received no answer. Presently they spied him where he had climbed up the downspout of the house to the second story. On being scolded by his mother, he ran and jumped over the garden fence, thus demonstrating that he was pretty much of a normal boy. This boy's imperative need, that was not provided in white bread and skimmed milk, was the presence of the vitamins and other activators that are in whole milk but not in skimmed milk, and in whole wheat, freshly ground, but not in white flour. He was restored to health by the simple process of having Nature's natural foods restored to him.

This problem of borrowing from the skeleton in times of stress may soften the bones so that they will be badly distorted. This is frequently seen as bow legs. An illustration of an extreme condition of bone softening by this process is shown in Fig. 94, lower section, which is the skeleton of a monkey that was a house pet. It became very fond of sweets and was fed on white bread, sweetened jams, etc., as it ate at the same table with its mistress. Note that the bones became so soft that the pull of the muscles distorted them into all sorts of curves. Naturally its body and legs were seriously distorted. In this condition my patient, whom I was serving professionally, asked me for advice regarding her monkey's deformed legs and distorted body. I suggested an improved nutrition and provided fat-soluble vitamins consisting of a mixture of a high-vitamin butter oil and high-vitamin cod liver oil with the result that minerals were deposited on the borders of the vertebrae and joints and on the surfaces of the bones as shown in the illustration. This of course, could not correct the deformity and the animal was chloroformed.

The necessity that the foods selected and used shall provide an adequate quantity of fat-soluble activators (including the known fat-soluble vitamins) is so imperative and is so important in preventing a part of our modern degeneration that I shall illustrate its need with another practical case.

A mother asked my assistance in planning the nutritional program for her boy. She reported that he was five years of age and that he had been in bed in hospitals with rheumatic fever, arthritis and an acute heart involvement most of the time for the past two and a half years. She had been told that her boy would not recover, so severe were the complications. As is so generally the case with rheumatic fever and endocarditis, this boy was suffering from severe tooth decay. In this connection the American Heart Association has reported that 75 percent of heart involvements begin before ten years of age. My studies have shown that in about 95 percent of these cases there is active tooth decay. The important change that I made in this boy's dietary program

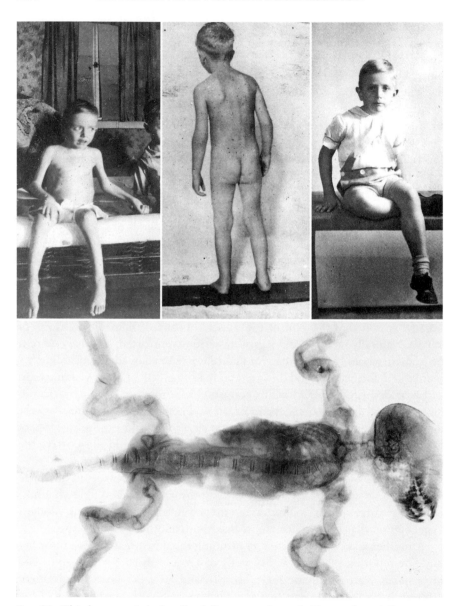

FIG. 94. This boy, age 5, had suffered for two and one-half years from inflammatory rheumatism, arthritis and heart involvement. Upper left shows limit of movement of neck, left wrist, swollen knees and ankles. The middle upper view shows the change in six months after improvement of his nutrition, and at right his change in one year. Below is shown the grossly demineralized and deformed skeleton of a pet monkey being fed on sweets and pastries.

was the removal of the white flour products and in their stead the use of freshly cracked or ground wheat and oats used with whole milk to which was added a small amount of especially high-vitamin butter produced by cows pasturing on green wheat. Small doses of a high-vitamin natural cod liver oil were also added. At this time the boy was so badly crippled with arthritis, in his swollen knees, wrists, and rigid spine, that he was bedfast and cried by the hour. With the improvement in his nutrition which was the only change made in his care, his acute pain rapidly subsided, his appetite greatly improved, he slept soundly and gained rapidly in weight. In the first view, to the left, in Fig. 94, the boy is shown sitting on the edge of the bed at the end of the first month on this program. His joints were still badly swollen and his spine so rigid that he could not rotate his head farther than shown in the picture. In the center view he is shown about six months later, and in the third view, one year later. This occurred six years ago. As I write this a letter has been received from the boy's mother. She reports that he is taller and heavier than the average, has a good appetite and sleeps well.

In the newer light regarding the cause of rheumatic fever, or inflammatory rheumatism (discussed in Chapter 21) there appear to be three underlying causes: a general lowered defense against infection in which the fat-soluble vitamins play a very important part; minute hemorrhages in joint tissues as part of the expression of deficiency of vitamin C, a scurvy symptom, and a source of infecting bacteria such as streptococcus. This could be provided by his infected teeth. These typical expressions of modern degeneration could not occur in most of the primitive races studied because of the high factor of safety in the minerals and vitamins of their nutrition. It is important to emphasize the changes that were made in our modern dietary program to make this boy's nutrition adequate for recovery. Sugars and sweets and white flour products were eliminated as far as possible. Freshly ground cereals were used for breads and gruels. Bone marrow was included in stews. Liver and a liberal supply of whole milk, green vegetables and fruits were provided. In addition, he was provided with a butter that was very high in vitamins having been produced by cows fed on a rapidly growing green grass. The best source for this is a pasturage of wheat and rye grass. All green grass in a state of rapid growth is good, although wheat and rye grass are the best found. Unless hay is carefully dried so as to retain its chlorophyll, which is a precursor of vitamin A, the cow cannot synthesize the fat-soluble vitamins.

These two practical cases illustrate the fundamental necessity that there shall not only be an adequate quantity of body-building minerals present, but also that there shall be an adequate quantity of fat-soluble vitamins. Of course, water-soluble vitamins are also essential. While I have reduced the diets of the various primitive races studied to definite quantities of mineral and calorie content, these data are so voluminous that it will not be appropriate to include them here. It will be more informative to discuss the ratios of both body-building and repairing material in the several primitive dietaries, in comparison with the displacing foods adopted from our modern civilization. The amount of food eaten by an individual is controlled primarily by the hunger factor which for our modernized groups apparently relates only to need for heat and energy. The dietaries adopted have all been built on the basis of the heat and energy requirements of the body for the groups living in the several districts and under their modes of life. These have been calculated for the principal foods eaten by the various groups. The figures will be published in detail in a more technical report. There are two simple ways in which these comparisons can be made. One is in terms of normal body requirements; and the other in terms of the ratio between the mineral and the vitamin content of the native foods and the displacing foods. If we use as a basis the ability of individuals to remove half of the minerals present even though their bodies need more than this, we will be more generous than the average individual's capacity will justify. This will require that we double the amount, as specified for minimum body use by the United States Department of Labor, Bureau of Labor Statistics, in their Bulletin R 409, that is, for calcium 0.68 grams; for phosphorus 1.32 grams; for iron 0.015 grams. The figures that will be used, therefore, are for twice the above amounts: 1.36 grams of calcium; 2.64 grams of phosphorus; 0.030 grams of iron.

Few people who have not been in contact with experimental data on metabolism can appreciate how little of the minerals in the food are retained in the body by large numbers of individuals who are in need of these very chemicals. We have seen that infants cannot absorb calcium from spinach. If we are to provide nutrition that will include an adequate excess as a factor of safety for overloads, and for such periods as those of rapid growth (for children), pregnancy, lactation and sickness, we must provide the excess to the extent of about twice the requirements of normal adults. It will therefore, be necessary for an adequate nutrition to contain approximately four times the minimum requirements of the average adult if all stress periods are to be passed safely.

It is of interest that the diets of the primitive groups which have shown a very high immunity to dental caries and freedom from other degenerative processes have all provided a nutrition containing at least four times these minimum requirements; whereas the displacing nutrition of commerce, consisting largely of white-flour products, sugar, polished rice, jams, canned goods, and vegetable fats have invariably failed to provide even the minimum requirements. In other words the foods of the native Eskimos contained 5.4 times as much calcium as the displacing foods of the white man, five times as much phosphorus, 1.5 times as much iron, 7.9 times as much magnesium, 1.8 times as much copper, 49.0 times as much iodine, and at least ten times that number of fat-soluble vitamins. For the Indians of the far North of Canada, the native foods provided 5.8 times as much calcium, 5.8 times as much phosphorus, 2.7 times as much iron, 4.3 times as much magnesium, 1.5 times as much copper, 8.8 times as much iodine, and at least a tenfold increase in fat-soluble activators. For brevity, we will apply the figures to calcium, phosphorus, magnesium, iron and fat-soluble activators in order. The ratio in the Swiss native diets to that in the displacing diet was for calcium, 3.7 fold; for phosphorus, 2.2 fold; for magnesium, 2.5 fold; for iron, 3.1 fold; and for the fat-soluble activators, at least tenfold. For the Gaelics in the Outer Hebrides, the native foods provided 2.1 times as much calcium, 2.3 times as much phosphorus, 1.3 times as much magnesium, and 1.0 times as much iron; and the fat-soluble activators were increased at least tenfold. For the Aborigines of Australia, living along the eastern coast where they have access to sea foods the ratio of minerals in the native diet to those in the displacing modernized foods was, for calcium, 4.6 fold; for phosphorus, 6.2 fold; for magnesium, 17 fold; and for iron 50.6 fold; while for the fat-soluble activators, it was at least tenfold. The native diet of the New Zealand Maori provided an increase in the native foods over the displacing foods of the modernized whites of 6.2 fold for calcium, 6.9 fold for phosphorus, 23.4 fold for magnesium, 58.3 fold for iron; and the fat-soluble activators were increased at least tenfold. The native diet of the Melanesians provided similarly an increase over the provision made in the modernized foods which displaced them of 5.7 fold for calcium, 6.4 fold for phosphorus, 26.4 fold for magnesium, and 22.4 fold for iron; while the fat-soluble activators were increased at least tenfold. The Polynesians provided through their native diet for an increase in provision over that of the displacing imported diets, of 5.6 fold for calcium, 7.2 fold for phosphorus, 28.5 fold for magnesium, 18.6 fold for iron; and the fat soluble activators were increased at least tenfold. The coastal Indians of Peru provided through their native primitive diets for an increase in provision over that of the displacing modernized diet of 6.6 fold for calcium, 5.5 fold for phosphorus, 13.6 fold for magnesium, 5.1 fold for iron; and an excess of tenfold was provided for fat-soluble vitamins. For the Indians of the Andean Mountains of Peru, the native foods provided an increase over the provision of the displacing modern foods of 5 fold for calcium, 5.5 fold for phosphorus, 13.3 fold for magnesium, 29.3 fold for iron; and an excess of at least tenfold was provided for fat-soluble vitamins. For the cattle tribes in the interior of Africa, the primitive foods provided an increase over the provision of the displacing modernized foods of 7.5 fold for calcium, 8.2 fold for phosphorus, 19.1 fold for magnesium, 16.6 fold for iron and at least tenfold for fat-soluble activators. For the agricultural tribes in Central Africa the native diet provided an increase over the provision of the displacing

modern diet of 3.5 fold for calcium, 4.1 fold for phosphorus, 5.4 fold for magnesium, 16.6 fold for iron and tenfold for fat-soluble activators. All the above
primitive diets provided also a large increase in the water-soluble vitamins
over the number provided in the displacing modern diets.

From the data presented in the preceding chapters and in this comparison
of the primitive and modernized dietaries it is obvious that there is great need
that the grains eaten shall contain all the minerals and vitamins which Nature
has provided that they carry. Important data might be presented to illustrate
this phase in a practical way. In Fig. 95 will be seen three rats all of which
received the same diet, except for the type of bread. The first rat (at the left)
received whole-wheat products freshly ground, the center one received a
white flour product and the third (at the right) a bran and middlings product. The amounts of each ash, of calcium as the oxide, and of phosphorus as
the pentoxide, and the amounts of iron and copper present in the diet of each
group, are shown by the height of the columns beneath the rats. Clinically
it will be seen that there is a marked difference in the physical development
of these rats. Several rats of the same age were in each cage. The feeding was
started after weaning at about twenty-three days of age. The rat at the left was
on the entire grain product. It was fully developed. The rats in this cage reproduced normally at three months of age. The rats in this first cage had very
mild dispositions and could be picked up by the ear or tail without danger of
their biting. The rats represented by the one in the center cage using white
flour were markedly undersized. Their hair came out in large patches and they
had very ugly dispositions, so ugly that they threatened to spring through the
cage wall at us when we came to look at them. These rats had tooth decay
and they were not able to reproduce. The rats in the next cage (illustrated by
the rat to the right) which were on the bran and middlings mixture did not
show tooth decay, but were considerably undersized, and they lacked energy.
The flour and middlings for the rats in cages two and three were purchased
from the miller and hence were not freshly ground. The wheat given to the
first group was obtained whole and ground while fresh in a hand mill. It is of
interest that notwithstanding the great increase in ash, calcium, phosphorus,
iron and copper present in the foods of the last group, the rats did not mature
normally, as did those in the first group. This may have been due in large part
to the fact that the material was not freshly ground, and as a result they could
not obtain a normal vitamin content from the embryo of the grain due to its
oxidation. This is further indicated by the fact that the rats in this group did
not reproduce, probably due in considerable part to a lack of vitamins B and
E which were lost by oxidation of the embryo or germ fat.

There is a misapprehension with regard to the possibility that humans may
obtain enough of the vitamin D group of activators from our modern plant

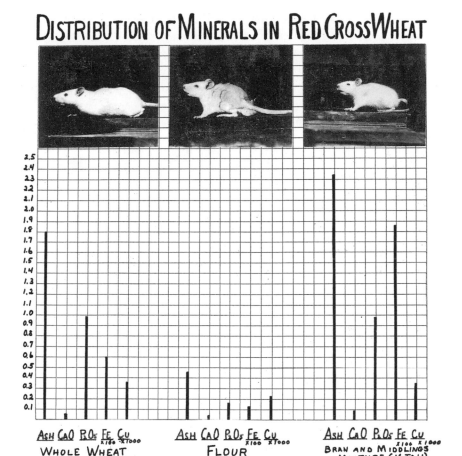

FIG. 95. Effect of different wheat products on rats. Left: whole wheat. Center: white flour. Right: bran and middlings mixture. The graphs record actual amount of indicated minerals present, as milligrams percent. Only the rats on the whole wheat developed normally without tooth decay. Those on white flour had tooth decay, were underweight, had skin infections and were irritable. They did not reproduce. The third group were undersize. The balance of the ration was the same for all.

foods or from sunshine. This is due to the belief viosterol or similar products by other names, derived by exposing ergosterol to ultraviolet light, offer all of the nutritional factors involved in the vitamin D group. I have emphasized that there are known to be at least eight D factors that have been definitely isolated and twelve that have been reported as partially isolated.

Coffin has recently reported relative to the lack of vitamin D in common foods as follows:[5]

1. A representative list of common foods was carefully tested, by approved technique, for their vitamin D content.
2. With the remote possibility of egg yolks, butter, cream, liver and fish it is manifestly impossible to obtain any amount of vitamin D worthy of mention from common foods.
3. Vegetables do not contain vitamin D.

It will be noted that vitamin D, which the human does not readily synthesize in adequate amounts, must be provided by foods of animal tissues or animal products. As yet I have not found a single group of primitive racial stock which was building and maintaining excellent bodies by living entirely on plant foods. I have found in many parts of the world most devout representatives of modern ethical systems advocating the restriction of foods to the vegetable products. In every instance where the groups involved had been long under this teaching, I found evidence of degeneration in the form of dental caries, and in the new generation in the form of abnormal dental arches to an extent very much higher than in the primitive groups who were not under this influence.

Many illustrations might be presented showing the special wisdom of the primitives in the matter of reinforcing their nutrition with protective foods.

Few people will realize how reluctant members of the primitive races are, in general, to disclose secrets of their race. The need for this is comparable to the need for secrecy regarding modern war devices.

The Indians of the Yukon have long known the cure for scurvy and history makes an important contribution to their wisdom in treating this disease. It is of interest that W. N. Kemp[6] of Vancouver states:

> The earliest recorded successful treatment of scurvy occurred in Canada in 1535 when Jacques Cartier, on the advice of a friendly Indian, gave his scurvy-prostrated men a decoction of young green succulent 'shoots' from the spruce trees with successful results. These happy effects apparently were not appreciated in Europe, for scurvy continued to be endemic.

Since that time untold thousands of mariners and white land dwellers have died with this dreaded disease.

Shortly before our arrival in Northern Canada a white prospector had died of scurvy. Beside him was his white man's packet of canned foods. Any Indian man or woman, boy or girl, could have told him how to save his life by eating animal organs or the buds of trees.

Another illustration of the wisdom of the native Indians of that far north country came to me through two prospectors whom we rescued and brought out with us just before the fall freeze-up. They had gone into the district, which at that time was still uncharted and unsurveyed, to prospect for precious metals and radium. They were both doctors of engineering and science, and had been sent with very elaborate equipment from one of the large national mining corporations. Owing to the inaccessibility of the region, they adopted a plan for reaching it quickly. They had flown across the two ranges of mountains from Alaska and when they arrived at the inside range, i.e., the Rocky Mountain Range, they found the altitude so high that their plane could not fly over the range, and, as a result, they were brought down on a little lake outside. The plane then returned but was unable to reach the outside world because of shortage of fuel. The pilot had to leave it on a waterway and trudge over the mountains to civilization. The two prospectors undertook to carry their equipment and provisions over the Rocky Mountain Range into the interior district where they were to prospect. They found the distance across the plateau to be about one hundred miles and the elevation ranging up to nine thousand feet. While they had provisions and equipment to stay two years they found it would take all of this time to carry their provisions and instruments across this plateau. They accordingly abandoned everything, and rather than remain in the country with very uncertain facilities and prospects for obtaining food and shelter, made a forced march to the Liard River with the hope that some expedition might be in that territory. One of the men told me the following tragic story. While they were crossing the high plateau he nearly went blind with so violent a pain in his eyes that he feared he would go insane. It was not snow blindness, for they were equipped with glasses. It was xeropthalmia, due to lack of vitamin A. One day he almost ran into a mother grizzly bear and her two cubs. Fortunately, they did not attack him but moved off. He sat down on a stone and wept in despair of ever seeing his family again. As he sat there holding his throbbing head, he heard a voice and looked up. It was an old Indian who had been tracking that grizzly bear. He recognized this prospector's plight and while neither could understand the language of the other, the Indian after making an examination of his eyes, took him by the hand and led him to a stream that was coursing its way down the mountain. Here as the prospector sat waiting the Indian built a trap of stones across the stream. He then went upstream and waded down splashing as he came and thus drove the trout into the trap. He threw the fish out on the bank and told the prospector to eat the flesh of the head and the tissues back of the eyes, including the eyes, with the result that in a few hours his pain had largely subsided. In one day his sight was rapidly returning, and in two days his eyes were nearly normal. He told me with profound emotion and gratitude that that Indian had certainly saved his life.

Now modern science knows that one of the richest sources of vitamin A in the entire animal body is that of the tissues back of the eyes including the retina of the eye.

In Chapter 18 I refer to the work of Wald on studies of vitamin A tissues. He states that extracts of eye tissue (retina, pigment, epithelium, and choroid) show the characteristic vitamin A absorption band and that they are potent in curing vitamin A deficient rats. He shows also that the concentration of vitamin A is constant for different mammals.

I have been impressed to find that primitive racial stocks in various parts of the world are familiar with the fact that eyes constitute an invaluable adjunct for nutrition. Even the one-time cannibals of the Fiji Islands, and the hereditary king of the Fiji Islands, told me in detail of the practices with regard to the use of eyes as an adjunct to diet. The chief, his father, and grandfather had the privilege of reserving the eyes of captives for their personal use. When among the natives of the islands north of Australia, I learned to enjoy greatly fish head soup made from certain selected tissues. After the fish had been cleaned, the heads were split and the eyes left in.

The space of the entire book might be used for discussing the nutritional wisdom of the various primitive races. It is a pity that so much of their wisdom has been lost through lack of appreciation by the whites who early made contact with them.

REFERENCES

[1] SHERMAN, H. C. *Chemistry of Food and Nutrition*. New York, Macmillan, 1933.

[2] BILLS, C. E. New Forms and Sources of Vitamin D. *J.A.M.A.*, 108:12, 1937, Nutrition Abstracts and Reviews, 1938.

[3] LAWSON, A. and MOON, H. P. A clay adjunct to potato dietary. *Nature*, 141: 40, 1938.

[4] Report Council on Foods. The nutritional value of spinach. *J.A.M.A.*, 109:1907, 1937.

[5] COFFIN, J. The lack of vitamin D in common foods. *J. Am. Dietet. A.*, 11:119, 1935.

[6] KEMP, W. N. The sources of clinical importance of the vitamins. *Bull. Vancouver Med. A.*, Dec., 1937.

Chapter 16

PRIMITIVE CONTROL OF DENTAL CARIES

THE ESSENTIAL differences in the diets of the primitive races and those of the modernized groups have been discussed in the preceding chapter. We are concerned now with discovering whether the use of foods, which are equivalent in body-building and repairing material to those used by the primitives will, when provided to our affected modernized groups, prevent tooth decay or check it when it is active.

There are two approaches to this problem of the control of tooth decay by nutritional means. One is by the presentation of clinical results and the other by the consideration of the characteristics of those nutritional programs which have been successful in producing a high immunity to tooth decay.

We may divide the primitive racial stocks into groups, classified according to the physical environment in which they are living and the manner in which the environment largely controls their available foods. It is significant that I have as yet found no group that was building and maintaining good bodies exclusively on plant foods. A number of groups are endeavoring to do so with marked evidence of failure. The variety of animal foods available has varied widely in some groups, and been limited among others.

In the preceding chapter we have seen that the successful dietaries included in addition to a liberal source of minerals, carbohydrates, fats, proteins, and water-soluble vitamins, a source of fat-soluble vitamins.

Vitamin D is not found in plants, but must be sought in an animal food. The dietaries of the efficient primitive racial stocks may be divided into groups on this basis: in the first place those obtaining their fat-soluble activators, which include the known fat-soluble vitamins, from efficient dairy products. This includes the Swiss in the high Alps, the Arabs (using camel's milk), and the Asiatic races (using milk of sheep and musk ox). In the second place there are those using liberally the organs of animals, and the eggs of birds, wild and domesticated. These include the Indians of the far North, the buffalo-hunting Plains Indians and the Andean tribes. In the third place there are those using liberally animal life of the sea. These include Pacific Islanders and coastal tribes throughout the world. In the fourth place there are those using small animals and insects. These include the Australian Aborigines in the interior, and the African tribes in the interior.

Many of the above groups use foods from two or more sources. Each of the groups has provided an adequate quantity of body-building material from both animal and plant tissues. It does not matter what the source of minerals and vitamins may be so long as the supply is adequate. In our modern life, the location of a group will determine the most efficient and most convenient source for obtaining the essential foods. Clearly, for those near the coast, the sea may be most convenient, while for those in the interior or in the far North, dairy products or the organs of animals may be the only available source. It would be fortunate indeed, if our problems were as simple as this statement might indicate. We have, however, in the first place, the need for a strength of character and will power such as will make us use the things our bodies require rather than only the foods we like. Another problem arises from the fact that our modern sedentary lives call for so little energy that many people will not eat enough even of a good food to provide for both growth and repair, since hunger appeals are for energy only, the source of heat and power, and not for body-building minerals and other chemicals. Still another problem confronts us, i.e., the sources of fat-soluble activators indicated above, namely: dairy products, organs of animals and sea foods, may vary through a wide range in their content of the fat-soluble activators or vitamins, depending upon the nutrition available for the animals. Cows fed on third grade hay, too low in carotene, not only cannot produce strong calves but their milk will not keep healthy calves alive. (Chapter 18.)

The League of Nations' Committee on Nutrition has estimated the amount of pasture land required per capita to provide adequate milk and meat. Owing to the density of population and cost of land near large cities, it is not possible to provide an adequate acreage for dairy cattle. This results in stall-feeding of shipped fodder. Only those cows can be kept in a herd whose production of milk and butterfat can pay in volume for their keep. Unfortunately milk may have a high cream line or butterfat content and still be low in essential fat-soluble vitamins. This constitutes an exceedingly important phase of our modern problem. Butter ships best when hard and this quality can be largely controlled by the fodder given to the cattle and hence becomes an important factor in the wholesale butter industry. Since 1927, I have been analyzing samples of dairy products, chiefly butter, from several parts of the world for their vitamin content. These samples are received every two to four weeks from the same places, usually for several years. They all show a seasonal rise and fall in vitamin content. The high level is always associated with the use of rapidly growing young plant food. This tide in plant life, fluctuating with the seasons, controlled the migration of the buffalo southward in the autumn and winter and northward in the spring. They moved at the rate of about twelve miles per day, travelling with the sun in order to provide the highest-vitamin milk for the young calves born in the south. No doubt these tides in nutrition control also the migration of birds. By far the most efficient plant food that I have found for producing the high-vitamin content in milk is rapidly growing young wheat and rye grass. Oat and barley grass are also excellent. In my clinical work small additions of this high-vitamin butter to otherwise satisfactory diets regularly checks tooth decay when active and at the same time improves vitality and general health.

Similarly the value of eggs for providing fat-soluble vitamins depends directly upon the food eaten by the fowl. The fertility of the eggs also is a direct measure of the vitamin content, including vitamin E.

Since the sea foods are, as a group, so valuable a source of the fat-soluble activators, they have been found to be efficient throughout the world not only for controlling tooth decay, but for producing a human stock of high vitality. Unfortunately the cost of transportation in the fresh state often constitutes a factor limiting distribution. Many of the primitive races preserved the food value, including vitamins, very efficiently by drying the fish. While our modern system of canning prevents decomposition, it does not efficiently preserve some of the fat-soluble activators, particularly vitamin A.

Since the organs, particularly the livers of animals, are storage depots of the vitamins an important source of some of the fat-soluble activators can be provided by extracting the fat of the livers and shipping it as liver oils. Modern methods of processing have greatly improved the quality of these oils. There are some factors, however, which can be provided to great advantage for humans from dairy products of high efficiency.

I have shown in the preceding chapter the quantities of several of the minerals that are essential in suitable chemical form to maintain an adult in good health and make possible tissue repair. The dietaries of the various primitive groups have all been shown to have a mineral content several times higher than that found in the inadequate food eaten by modernized primitives and the people of our modernized cultures.

Modern commerce has deliberately robbed some of nature's foods of much of their body-building material while retaining the hunger satisfying energy factors. For example, in the production of refined white flour approximately eighty percent or four-fifths of the phosphorus and calcium content are usually removed, together with the vitamins and minerals provided in the embryo or germ. The evidence indicates that a very important factor in the lowering of reproductive efficiency of womanhood is directly related to the removal of vitamin E in the processing of wheat. The germ of wheat is our most readily available source of that vitamin. Its role as a nutritive factor for the pituitary gland in the base of the brain, which largely controls growth and organ function, apparently is important in determining the production of mental types. Similarly the removal of vitamin B with the embryo of the wheat, together with its oxidation after processing, results in depletion of body-building activators.

Refined white sugar carries only negligible traces of body-building and repairing material. It satisfies hunger by providing heat and energy besides having a pleasant flavor. The heat and energy producing factors in our food that are not burned up are usually stored as fat. In the preceding chapter we have seen that approximately half of the foods provided in our modern dietaries furnish little or no body-building or repairing material and supply no vitamins. Approximately 25 percent of the heat and energy of the American people is supplied by sugar alone which goes far in thwarting Nature's orderly processes of life. This per capita use is unfortunately on the increase. Therefore we must begin by radically reducing the foods that are so deceptive, and often injurious in overloading the system. Even this much change in our modern nutrition will raise the factor of safety sufficiently to check tooth decay in a large percentage of people. It will not, however, be adequate for most children in whom the additional demands of rapid growth must be satisfied. I have found the highest incidence of tooth decay in the high school and boarding school girls, and the next in the boarding school boys. These groups suffer even more than the childbearing mothers.

In discussing the technical aspects later I shall consider the defensive factors in the saliva as controlled by the nutrition through the blood stream, and also the role of oral prophylaxis.

It is appropriate at this point to note some characteristics of a decaying tooth. The process of tooth decay never starts from within but always from without and is most likely to start at the contact points between the teeth or in the pits and grooves, especially when these are incompletely formed. Teeth never have caries while they are covered with flesh but decay most easily soon after eruption, when conditions are unfavorable. If the saliva is normal the surfaces of the teeth progressively harden during the first year after eruption. While there are many theories regarding the relative importance of different factors in the process of decay practically all provide for a local solution of the tooth substance by acids produced by bacteria. The essential difference in the various theories of tooth decay is the difference in theories relative to the control of these decalcifying organisms, and relative to their quantity and activity. The dental profession has been waiting for decades for this question to be solved before taking active steps to prevent the whole process. The primitive approach has been to provide a program that will keep the teeth well, that is, prevention of dental caries by adequate food combinations. I have just stated that teeth harden after eruption if the saliva is normal. This occurs by a process of mineralization much like the process by which petrified wood is produced.

The tooth is made up of four structures. The first is the pulp within, which carries blood vessels and nerves. This structure is surrounded in both the root and crown by the dentine or tooth bone which is nourished from within. The dentine of the root is covered by cementum which receives nourishment from the membrane which attaches the root to the jaw bone. The dentine of the crown or exposed part of the tooth is covered with enamel. Tooth decay proceeds slowly through the enamel and often rapidly in the dentine, always following the minute channels toward the pulp, which may become infected before the decay actually reaches the pulp to expose it; nearly always the decay infects the pulp when it destroys the dentine covering it. When a tooth has a deep cavity of decay, the decalcified dentine has about the density of rotten wood. With an adequate improvement in nutrition, tooth decay will generally be checked provided two conditions are present: in the first place, there must be enough improvement in the quality of the saliva; and in the second, the saliva must have free access to the cavity. Of course, if the decay is removed and a filling placed in the cavity, the bacteria will be mechanically shut out. One of the most severe tests of a nutritional program, accordingly, is the test of its power to check tooth decay completely, even without fillings. There are, however, two further tests of the sufficiency of improvement of the chemical content of the saliva. If it has been sufficiently improved, bacterial growth will not only be inhibited, but the leathery decayed dentine will become mineralized from the saliva by a process similar to petrification. Note that this mineralized dentine is not vital, nor does it increase in volume and fill the cavity. When scraped with a steel instrument it frequently takes on a density like very hard wood and occasionally takes even a glassy surface. When such a tooth is placed in silver nitrate, the chemical does not penetrate this demineralized dentine, though it does rapidly penetrate the decayed dentine of a tooth extracted when decay is active. This process is illustrated in Fig. 96 which shows two deciduous teeth extracted from the same child, one before, and the other a few months after improving the nutrition. These deciduous molars were replaced by the bicuspids of the second dentition. The tooth at the left had deep caries and was removed before the treatment was begun. Note that the silver nitrate has blackened the tissue to the depth of the decay. The tooth at the right was removed about three months after the nutrition was changed. Note that the decayed dentine is so dense that the silver nitrate has not penetrated deeply and discolored it.

There is still another test that demonstrates Nature's protective mechanisms. Ordinarily, when the pulp of a tooth is exposed by dental caries, the pulp becomes not only infected, but dies opening up a highway of infection

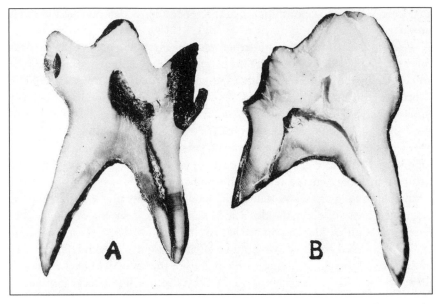

FIG. 96. A, illustrates the permeability of decayed dentin to silver nitrate. B, illustrates the decreased permeability of decayed dentin to silver nitrate due to mineralization, after saliva has been improved by correcting the nutrition.

direct from the infected mouth to the inside of the fort at the end of the root. One expression of this is a dental abscess, the existence of which is usually unknown to the individual for sometime and the infecting germs pass more or less freely throughout the body by way of the blood stream and lymph channels. This infection may start the degeneration of organs and tissues of other parts of the body.

Among some of the primitive races, whose nutritional programs provided a very high factor of safety, even though the teeth were worn down to the gum line and into what was formerly the pulp chamber, the pulp was not exposed. Nature had built a protecting zone, not in the cavity of the tooth in this case, but within the pulp chamber. This entirely blocked off a threatened exposure and kept the walls of the fort sealed against bacteria. This process does not occur in many instances in people of our modern civilization. Pulp chambers that are opened by wear provide exposed pulp which becomes infected with subsequent abscess formation. If a reinforced nutrition as efficient as that of many of the primitive races is adopted, the pulp tissue will seal

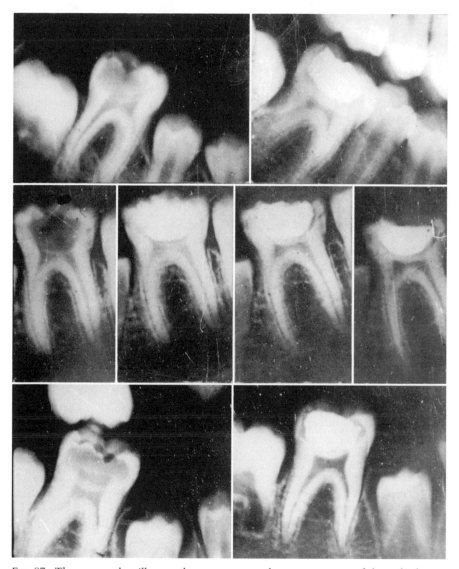

FIG. 97. Three cases that illustrate how nature can close an exposure of the pulp due to dental caries by building a protecting wall within the pulp chamber when the nutrition is adequately improved.

up the opening made by decalcification of the dentine, by building in a new layer of normal dentine which is vital and quite unlike the petrified decay exposed to the saliva, thus completely walling off the impending danger. This is illustrated in Fig. 97 with three cases. At the left are shown x-rays of teeth of three children in one of my experimental clinics in a poor district in Cleveland. The pulp chambers and pulp tissues of the root canals are shown as dark streaks in the center of the tooth. The very large cavities which had decalcified the tooth to the pulp chamber are shown as large dark areas in the crown. Temporary fillings had to be placed because of pain produced by the pressure of food on the pulp below the decayed dentine. After the nutrition was improved, the tissues of the pulp built in secondary dentine thus reincasing itself in a closed chamber. This process is shown in each of the three cases presented in Fig. 97, in the views to the right.

Under the stress of the industrial depression the family dietary of the children shown in Fig. 97 was very deficient. They were brought to a mission where we fed them one reinforced meal at noon for six days a week. The home meals were not changed nor the home care of the teeth. The preliminary studies of each child included complete x-rays of all of the teeth, a chemical analysis of the saliva, a careful plotting of the position, size and depth of all cavities, a record of the height, and weight, and a record of school grades, including grades in deportment. These checks were repeated every four to six weeks for the period of the test, usually three to five months. It is important to note that the home nutrition which had been responsible for the tooth decay was exceedingly low in body-building and repairing material, while temporarily satisfying the appetite. It usually consisted of highly sweetened strong coffee and white bread, vegetable fat, pancakes made of white flour and eaten with syrup, and doughnuts fried in vegetable fat.

The nutrition provided these children in this one meal included the following foods. About four ounces of tomato juice or orange juice and a teaspoonful of a mixture of equal parts of a very high-vitamin natural cod liver oil and an especially high-vitamin butter was given at the beginning of the meal. They then received a bowl containing approximately a pint of a very rich vegetable and meat stew, made largely from bone marrow and fine cuts of tender meat: the meat was usually broiled separately to retain its juice and then chopped very fine and added to the bone marrow meat soup which always contained finely chopped vegetables and plenty of very yellow carrots; for the next course they had cooked fruit, with very little sweetening, and rolls made from freshly ground whole wheat, which were spread with the high-vitamin butter. The wheat for the rolls was ground fresh every day in a motor driven coffee mill. Each child was also given two glasses of fresh whole milk. The menu was varied from day to day by substituting for the meat stew, fish chowder or organs of animals. From time to time, there was placed in a two quart jar a helping similar to that eaten by the children. This was brought to my laboratory for chemical analysis, which analysis showed that these meals provided approximately 1.48 grams of calcium and 1.28 grams of phosphorus in a single helping of each course. Since many of the children doubled up on the course, their intake of these minerals was much higher. I have shown in the preceding chapter that the accepted figures for the requirements of the body for calcium and phosphorus are 0.68 grams of calcium and 1.32 grams of phosphorus. It is obvious that this one meal a day plus the other two meals at home provided a real factor of safety. Clinically this program completely controlled the dental caries of each member of the group.

The chemical analysis of the saliva[1,2] revealed a marked improvement which progressively increased. At the beginning of the test the average for the group showed a very low factor of safety, so low that we should expect tooth decay to be active. In six weeks the average changed to a condition which we should expect would be accompanied by a cessation of tooth decay. The saliva factor of safety continued to improve for five months at which time the special program was discontinued for the summer.

Several incidents of special interest occurred. Two different teachers came to me to inquire what had been done to make a particular child change from one of the poorest in the class in capacity to learn to one of the best. Dental caries is only one of the many expressions of our modern deficient nutritions.

I have referred to the importance of a high-vitamin butter for providing the fat-soluble activators to make possible the utilization of the minerals in the foods. In this connection, it is of interest that butter constitutes the principal source of these essential factors for many primitive groups throughout the world. In the high mountain and plateau district in northern India, and in Tibet, the inhabitants depend largely upon butter made from the milk of the musk ox and the sheep for these activators. The butter is eaten mixed with roasted cereals, is used in tea, and in a porridge made of tea, butter and roasted grains. In [Anglo-Egyptian] Sudan, I found considerable traffic in high-vitamin butter which came from the higher lands a few miles from the Nile Basin. This was being exchanged for and used with varieties of millet grown in other districts. This butter, at the temperature of that area, which ranged from 90° to 110° Fahrenheit, was, of course, always in liquid form. Its brilliant orange color testified to the splendid pasture of the dairy animals. The people in Sudan, including the Arabs, had exceptionally fine teeth with exceedingly little tooth decay (Chapter 9). The most physically perfect people in northern India are probably the Pathans who live on dairy products largely in the form of soured curd, together with wheat and vegetables. The people are very tall and are free of tooth decay.

Probably every housewife is familiar with the low melting quality of the butter produced in early summer when the cows have been put on the green pastures. This is particularly true of butter that has the grassy flavor and the deep yellow to orange color. This butter is usually several times as high in fat-soluble activators including vitamins A and D as butter produced from stall-fed cattle or cattle on poorer pasturage. In Chapter 15, I have explained why this butter is not favorable for shipping and why dairymen so frequently give the cows a ration that will produce less of these qualities. One of the principal foods used for accomplishing this is made of cotton seed meal and cereals.

There are many illustrations of the low efficiency of this type of fodder for providing vitamins essential for dairy products. In one of the recent severe droughts in the Mississippi Valley several thousand cattle were shipped to Ohio for water and green pasture as a means of saving their lives. They were fed enroute on concentrates said to consist of cotton seed meal and grain. Professor Oscar Erf of the Department of Dairying of Ohio State University has given me the following detailed information:

> With reference to the cattle from the south-western and central-northern states of the drought area which were brought into Ohio in the fall of 1935 on a 600-acre farm north of Delaware, will say that I had the privilege of viewing some of these cattle previous to the time that they were brought to Ohio in 1935. Because of the extreme drought period and the hot sun, it was rare to see green grass on the prairies. The sedges were nearly all dried up. The tumbleweed was about the only thing that was available for the cattle in some instances. The corn was dried up and very little green was in evidence. In the particular location that I was in we found the cattle suffering terribly. Many had infected eyes.
>
> There were a good many deaths on the plains which were literally dried up. Sometimes there was even a small amount of decomposition after death. In the fall, those that survived on the plains, were loaded up and driven to the corrals, loaded into cars and sent east. Only the good ones were loaded and even a large number of these passed out in transit.
>
> I was informed that the crop of grass the year before was very scant. Consequently, a large number of calves were born with weak eyes and these were the early ones to pass out on the plains. The low vitality of the individuals which I considered was due to the lack of vitamin A or the green grass factors was the cause of the serious infection, however their being secondary to the primary cause.
>
> The first train load of the twenty-eight hundred cattle that were brought to this ranch were fed on green corn stalks. There was a nine acre patch of corn in this area. The fences were taken down one afternoon at 3 o'clock and by 9 o'clock there was no evidence of stubbles or roots. This had all been eaten in a very short space of time. We had quite a time getting hays

and green stuff which we demanded because of its carotin content and its green grass factor. There was not enough grass available in the beginning so we had to buy about 400 tons of hay a day to keep the animals fed. They got no grain of any kind because it was a question of bringing the cattle to a more or less normal condition with no intention of fattening the animals.

After they had made arrangements for feeding operations and made feed racks in sufficient numbers, we went over the herd to estimate the numbers that were blind and had sore eyes, which I assume from past experience, was due to a vitamin A deficiency. As near as we can estimate, nearly 812 animals were affected (29 percent). There were 157 calves born and approximately 50 percent were deformed and not normal. We did not get the complete figures but they probably ranged a little higher than that. The worst infected cows were calves and animals that were 18 to 20 months old. I could not get the story of these individuals but they must have been in the area of dry grass for 2 years. There was a slight improvement in those that were not seriously infected after they were fed here. They improved decidedly in October and November and were practically all slaughtered before the middle of December.

The milk of these vitamin deficient cows would not properly nourish either their calves or human beings.

Many children have tooth decay even while using whole milk, in part because the milk is too low in vitamin content, due to the inadequacy of the food given the cows. The means for improving this condition have been discussed in Chapter 15.

Some of the current theories of the chemistry of tooth decay place the responsibility on the local condition in the mouth as affected by the contributing factors provided by sugars and starches which enhance the growth of acid producing organisms. A phase of this has been closely related to the slogan that a clean tooth cannot decay. Among the difficulties in applying this interpretation is the physical impossibility of keeping teeth bacteriologically clean in the environment of the mouth. Another difficulty is the fact that many primitive races have their teeth smeared with starchy foods almost constantly and make no effort whatsoever to clean their teeth. In spite of this they have no tooth decay. In many of the primitive groups that I have studied the process of modernization includes teaching oral hygiene and prophylaxis. Yet, even with the addition of this important adjunct to health, they have in most cases lost their immunity to tooth decay and dental caries has become active. This will be seen in many of the illustrations of the primitive races in the preceding chapters. Of course everyone should clean his teeth, even the primitives, in the interest of and out of consideration for others.

In my clinical work I have sought for extreme cases of active tooth decay in order to test the primitive wisdom. Many of these cases have been furnished by members of the dental profession in other cities and states. By the simple procedure of studying the nutrition of the individual, obtaining a sample of saliva for analysis, seeing x-rays of the individual's teeth and supporting bone, and getting a history of the systemic overloads, I have been able to outline a nutritional program which, in well above 90 percent of the cases has controlled the dental caries. Improvement in the condition of the teeth has been confirmed by later x-rays and reports by the patients' dentists. In a few cases where I had contact with the patients only through correspondence the cooperation was not adequate for accomplishing complete improvement. While it is true that there is a marked difference in the susceptibility of different individuals to dental caries, even those who would ordinarily be classed as highly susceptible, have generally received permanent benefit from the treatment.

These principles of treatment have now been applied to many hundreds of patients as indicated by the fact that over 2,800 chemical analyses of the saliva have been made. The dietary programs that have been recommended have been determined on the basis of a study of the nutrition used by the patient, the data provided by the x-rays, from the saliva analysis and case history. The diets have been found to be deficient in minerals, chiefly phosphorus. Fat-soluble vitamins have been deficient in practically every case of active tooth decay. The foods selected for reinforcing the deficient nutritions have always included additional fat-soluble vitamins and a liberal source of minerals in the form of natural food. Human beings cannot absorb minerals satisfactorily from inorganic chemicals. Great harm is done, in my judgment, by the sale and use of substitutes for natural foods.

One of our greatest difficulties in undertaking to apply the wisdom of the primitives to our modern problems involves a character factor. The Indians of the high Andes were willing to go hundreds of miles to the sea to get kelp and fish eggs for the use of their people. Yet many of our modern people are unwilling to take sufficient trouble to obtain foods that are competent to accomplish the desired results.

Jobbers and middlemen as well as supply depot managers want butter sold in accordance with its label rather than in accordance with its vitamin content. One large distributor whom I asked to cooperate by maintaining a stock of high-vitamin butter to which I could refer people, told me frankly that he wished I would stop telling people about the difference in the vitamins in butter. He did not wish them to think of butter in terms of its vitamin content. Another large concern told me that when I had worked up a sufficiently large market they would become interested in supplying the demand. I counsel people to put in storage some of that butter which has the grassy flavor and which melts easily and is produced when the cows go onto the rapidly growing young grass. Unfortunately, cows that have been on a stable fodder low in carotene and under the stress of gestation often are so depleted in their own body vitamins that it takes them three or four weeks to replenish their own bodies when they get on good pasture. Then the vitamins will appear in liberal quantity in their milk. This has made it necessary for me to assist many patients in obtaining a supply by analyzing butter for its vitamin content and then putting this material in storage and making it available for special cases as needed.

The program that I have found most efficient has been one which includes the use of small quantities of very high-vitamin butter mixed in equal parts with a very high-vitamin cod liver oil. A simple method of preparing the butter is by melting it and allowing it to cool for twenty-four hours at a temperature of about 70° F, then centrifugalizing it which provides an oil that remains liquid at room temperature. When this butter oil is mixed in equal parts with a very high-vitamin cod liver oil, it produces a product that is more efficient than either alone. It should be used within a couple of weeks of the time it is mixed. It is desirable that this material be made available in various parts of the country. Even the high-vitamin butter produced on the early summer growth of grass put in storage and used during the winter will go far toward solving our great national problem of shortage of fat-soluble vitamins. The quantity of the mixture of butter oil and cod liver oil required is quite small, half a teaspoonful three times a day with meals is sufficient to control wide-spread tooth decay when used with a diet that is low in sugar and starches and high in foods providing the minerals, particularly phosphorus. A teaspoonful a day divided between two or three meals is usually adequate to prevent dental caries and maintain a high immunity; it will also maintain freedom from colds and a high level of health in general. This reinforcement of the fat soluble vitamins to a menu that is low in starches and sugars, together with the use of bread and cereal grains freshly ground to retain the full content of the embryo or germ, and with milk for growing children and for many adults, and the liberal use of sea foods and organs of animals, produced the result described.

I have previously reported[3] seventeen cases of extensive dental caries. In these patients there were found 237 open cavities of apparently active caries. Most of the individuals were between twelve and twenty years of age and accordingly had twenty-eight permanent teeth each, or a total of 476. It will be noted that if one cavity is allowed per tooth, approximately half of the total number of teeth were affected, or precisely 49.7 percent of all the teeth had open cavities. This group includes only persons of whom I have been making critical examination every six to twelve months over a three-year period.

In practically all cases, Roentgen-ray examinations were made in addition to clinical examinations of the teeth. While these persons have been on the reinforced nutritional program during the winter and spring months of the past three years, only two new cavities have developed in the group, or 0.4 percent. The length of time during which the cavities previously found had been developing is not known beyond the fact that all of the patients were receiving frequent and thorough dental service, most of them twice a year and many of them more frequently. It is accordingly probable that the cavities found had developed in less than a year. That dental caries was not a new problem with these persons was indicated by the very extensive and numerous dental restorations that had been made in their mouths. It is, therefore, apparent that 250 times as many cavities developed in the period preceding the starting of the nutritional program as in the three years following its adoption. If these data were reduced to a yearly basis, the comparison would show a much wider variation.

In a group of fifty persons, including the above mentioned seventeen, who had been on the special nutritional program for from one to six years, most of them three years or more, only two new cavities developed. Allowing these persons to have an average of twenty-eight teeth per person, or a total of 1,400 teeth, this would represent an incidence of dental caries in a period of three years of 0.14 percent. In this group of fifty, there are many instructive and striking cases.

For example, H. F. did not have a single cavity from October, 1932, to June, 1933, while taking additional vitamins and high mineral foods. From June, 1933, to May, 1934, while not taking the special vitamins, she developed ten new cavities.

S. K., prior to 1931 had rampant tooth decay with pulps nearly exposed in all first permanent molars. The remaining deciduous teeth had been reduced to shells. She was on the special nutritional program from December, 1931, to June, 1932, during which time caries was completely arrested. She discontinued taking the special oil in June, 1932, and did not take it again until October, 1933, during most of which time she was taking viosterol under a physician's prescription to prevent dental caries. She came in October, 1933, with fourteen new cavities. She was immediately placed again on the special program, from October, 1933, to May, 1934. During this period, the dental caries was completely under control. During the time that she was not on the special program, there developed on many of the surfaces of the permanent teeth white patches of decalcifying enamel. Under the reinforced nutritional program, these largely disappeared, and those that did not regain their translucency turned dark.

Among the group of seventeen J. H., sent in from another city, had thirty-eight open cavities in June, 1931. In addition to active caries, he had quite disturbing heart symptoms, which curtailed his activity, and he also had a marked sense of lassitude and weariness. He has been on the reinforced nutritional program during the fall, winter and spring of each year since that time. During this time, he has not developed a single new cavity. The density of all the teeth has progressively improved as evidenced by Roentgen-ray records. His physical condition has been greatly improved so that he is able to carry on his college activities and heavy outside work to earn money to maintain his college expenses. He is not conscious of a heart limitation. When asked what the principal change was that he had noticed, he said that in addition to not feeling tired, he was more rested with six hours of sleep than formerly with ten hours.

A. W. had thirty-two new cavities in the two years previous to beginning the special nutritional reinforcement. She continued this regularly during the winter and spring months for three years and has not had a single new cavity since that time.

In a group of children whose mothers had the special nutritional reinforcement during gestation and lactation and who had been provided with the same dietary adjuncts during the winter and spring months of infancy and early childhood, not a single carious cavity has developed. A number of these children are now in public schools. Their physical development is distinctly above that of the average children of their age, as is also their efficiency in school work.

It is important that I emphasize here some dangers that are not usually recognized or properly emphasized in the literature. When fish oils including cod liver oils are given in too large doses to some patients they experience quite definite symptoms of depression. The available evidence indicates that fish oils that have been exposed to the air may develop toxic substances. My work and that of others with experimental animals has demonstrated that paralysis can be produced readily by over-dosing. Serious structural damage can be done to hearts and kidneys. I have reported this in considerable detail.[4] My investigations have shown that when a high-vitamin natural cod liver oil is used in conjunction with a high-vitamin butter oil the mixture is much more efficient than either alone.[4] This makes it possible to use very small doses. Except in the late stages of pregnancy I do not prescribe more than half a teaspoonful with each of three meals a day. This procedure appears to obviate completely the undesirable effects. As stated elsewhere fish oils should be stored in small containers to avoid exposure to the air. Rancid fats and oils destroy vitamins A and E,[5] the former in the stomach.[6]

I am frequently reminded that ancient skulls are often found with extensive dental caries thus disproving that the primitive groups were more free from dental caries than the modern groups. It must be kept in mind that the fundamental laws of Nature have been in operation as long as animals and men have been on the earth. In my investigations among primitive races, I have been concerned particularly with the study of changes that have taken place both in immunity to dental caries and in the environment, including the foods used. It has been important that I find large groups with relatively high immunity to dental caries to be used as controls. There is great need, accordingly, that additional data be provided. Fortunately, this need is being met. There have just come to my desk two interesting reports; one, from Dr. Arne Hoygaard[7] and the other from Dr. P. O. Pedersen.[8] These two distinguished scientists have spent a year in East Greenland among the Eskimos in that very barren and isolated region. The percentage of teeth found attacked by dental caries among the isolated Eskimos of East Greenland is exceedingly low, less than 1 percent. Where the Eskimos were in contact with modernized store foods at the port, tooth decay was active. The conditions which they have found were apparently not quite so favorable as in the groups I studied in Alaska. The Greenland Eskimos apparently are living in a more difficult environment. The data provided by these investigations are in accord with the data I have obtained among isolated Eskimos and other primitive racial stocks. Eastern Greenland, by international agreement, is administered by the Danish Government and no one is permitted even to visit the coast of Greenland without special permission. This permission is very difficult to obtain. Even Danish citizens are not free to travel there. We are, accordingly, very grateful to Dr. Hoygaard and Dr. Pedersen for their contribution from studies made in that protected field. We shall look forward with interest to their detailed reports.

Unfortunately, the public is very much at sea because of the extravagant claims that are made for many of the products advertised over the radio, in journals, and by door to door solicitation. A dependable and helpful booklet on the vitamin content of foods has been published by the United States Department of Agriculture, Miscellaneous Publications, No. 275. The fact should always be emphasized that foods as Nature makes them have much more nutritional value than after they are processed so that insect life cannot live on them. When foods cannot support insect life they cannot support human life.

A report has just appeared in the September number of the *New Zealand Dental Journal* by H. H. Tocker on behalf of the Hawkes Bay Branch of the New Zealand Dental Association in which he reports the results of the application of my suggestions in the Hukarera School for native Maori girls at

Napier. I have reported my studies there in Chapter 12. They used only one part of my suggestions for checking the activity of dental caries. The diet of both their control group and tested group was the same except for one item, i.e., "one heaped teaspoonful twice daily of malt and cod liver oil." In a group of sixty-six native girls the thirty-three with the best teeth were used as a control group. The remaining thirty-three were given the additional fat-soluble vitamins. In six months' time "resistance of this group was raised by 41.75 percent" as compared with the control group. The nutrition of the test group was not adequately reinforced to obtain the best results. There was a marked inadequacy of mineral carrying foods in proportion to the energy and heat providing factors in the foods. An adequate quantity of such efficient foods should be as readily available today as before the white men came to New Zealand.

It is important to summarize at this point some of the data that I have developed in other chapters because of their direct relation to the control of dental caries and other degenerative processes. Since human life like other animal life has been developed in Nature's laboratory to fit Nature's natural foods we run a great risk when we undertake to modify seriously these foods. Bakers' so-called whole wheat bread is not comparable to Nature's foods that provide entire wheat and other cereals, because of the factors that have been removed from the wheat either mechanically or by oxidation. This is so large a problem that adequate changes in the available grain foods cannot be made until there is sufficient public demand to produce them through the normal channels of supply and demand. It is primarily a problem for our Federal and State governments. Packaged foods containing dry cereals can undergo important changes, even while the material is being processed or while in packages on the shelves. The determinations of the loss of vitamins in packaged foods as reported in 1938 by the Agricultural Experimental Station of Oklahoma Agricultural and Mechanical College, reveal that a material loss occurs in two weeks' time and a very serious loss in one to two months' time in certain stock rations.

An important source of misapprehension is the literature and teachings of fadists. Such, for example, as the misapprehension of many people that they must use only alkaline producing foods and that a great danger is associated with the use of acid producing foods. In the primitive races I have found practically no difference between the acid balance meat diet of the isolated Eskimos of the far north and the less acid vegetable and milk diet of other groups as efficient factors in control of caries. It is important to keep in mind that our bodies have a mechanism for maintaining proper acid and alkali balance in the blood and this varies through only a very narrow limit whether the balance of the total food eaten is acid or alkaline. It is also important to have in mind that there are certain fat-soluble vitamins provided in dairy products in adequate quantity that cannot all be supplied in fish oils. Also that overdosing with cod liver oil and other fish oils can be definitely detrimental. When packages of cod liver oil are purchased from the trade the material should be received in full containers not exposed to air and when opened should be transferred to small units so it is not progressively oxidized during the period of its use.

The excess of calories over body-building minerals is exceedingly high in sweets of various kinds regardless of their special branding and the methods of manufacture and storage. There is very little of the body-building minerals in maple syrup, cane syrup from sugar or honey. They can all defeat an otherwise efficient dietary. The problem is not so simple as merely cutting down or eliminating sugars and white flour though this is exceedingly important. It is also necessary that adequate mineral and vitamin carrying foods be made available. It is also necessary to realize that many of our important foods for providing vitamins are very low in body-building material. For example, one would have to eat nearly a bushel of apples a day or half a bushel of oranges to obtain a liberal factor of safety for providing phosphorus; similarly one would be required to eat nine and one half pounds of carrots or eleven pounds of beets each day to get enough phosphorus for a liberal factor of safety, while this quantity would be provided in one pound of lentils or beans, wheat or oats. I have discussed elsewhere the availability of phosphorus depending upon its chemical form. Since the calories largely determine the satisfying of the appetite and since under ordinary circumstances we stop when we have obtained about 2,000 to 2,500, very little of the highly sweetened fruits defeats our nutritional program. We would have to consume daily the contents of thirty-two one-pound jars of marmalade, jellies or jams to provide a two-gram intake of phosphorus. This quantity would provide 32,500 calories; an amount impossible for the system to take care of.

Milk is one of the best foods for providing minerals but it may be inadequate in several vitamins. Of all of the primitive groups studied those using sea foods abundantly appear to obtain an adequate quantity of minerals particularly phosphorus with the greatest ease, in part because the fat-soluble vitamins provided in the sea foods (by which I mean animal life of the sea) are usually high. This enables a more efficient utilization of the minerals, calcium and phosphorus.

As I study routinely the sample dietaries being used by people suffering from dental caries, usually associated with other disturbances, I find large numbers who are not getting in their food even half the minimum require-ments of calcium, phosphorus and magnesium and iron and usually only a fraction of the minimum requirements of the fat-soluble vitamins. These lat-ter have a role which in many respects is like the battery of an automobile which provides the spark for igniting the fuel. Even though the tank is filled with gasoline there is no power without the igniting spark.

There are two programs now available for meeting the dental caries prob-lem. One is to know first in detail all the physical and chemical factors in-volved and then proceed. The other is to know how to prevent the disease as the primitives have shown and then proceed. The former is largely the prac-tice of the moderns. The latter is the program suggested by these investigations. Available data indicate that the blood and saliva normally carry defensive fac-tors which when present control the growth of the acid producing organisms and the local reactions at tooth surfaces. When these defensive factors are not present the acid producing organisms multiply and produce an acid which dissolves tooth structure. The origin of this protective factor is provided in nutrition and is directly related to the mineral content of the foods and to known and unknown vitamins particularly the fat-soluble. Clinical data dem-onstrate that by following the program outlined, dental caries can be prevented or controlled when active in practically all individuals. This does not require either permission or prescription but it is the inherent right of every individual. A properly balanced diet is good for the entire body.

REFERENCES

[1] TISDALL, F. F. and KRAMER, B. Methods for the direct quantitative determination of sodium, potassium, calcium, and magnesium in urine and stools. *J. Biol. Chem.*, 48:1, 1921.

[2] KUTTNER, T. and COHEN, H. Micro colorimetric studies. I. A molybdic acid, stannous chloride reagent. *J. Biol. Chem.*, 75: 517, 1927.

[3] PRICE, W. A. Eskimo and Indian field studies in Alaska and Canada. *J. Am. Dent. A.*, 23:417, 1936.

[4] PRICE, W. A. Control of dental caries and some associated degenerative processes through reinforcement of the diet with special activators. *J. Am. Dent. A.*, 19:1339, 1932.

[5] MATTILL, H. A. The oxidative destruction of vitamins A and E. *J.A.M.A.*, 89:1505, 1927.

[6] LEASE, E. J., et al. Destruction of vitamin A by rancid fats. *J. Nutrition*, 16:571, 1938.

[7] HOYGAARD, A. Some investigations into the physiology and nasology of Eskimos from Angmagsslik in Greenland. Oslo, Dybwad, 1937.

[8] PEDERSEN, P. O. Investigations into dental conditions of about 3000 ancient and modern Greenlanders. *Dent. Rec.*, 58:191, 1938.

Chapter 17

ONE ORIGIN OF PHYSICAL DEFORMITIES

R ACES are classified on the basis of physical characteristics and appearances which identify them as having a common ancestry. The constant reproduction of ancestral patterns constitutes one of the fundamental laws of heredity. We are concerned here with the divergences from the normal course of reproduction.

The precision with which Nature reproduces widely distributed racial stocks demonstrates how deeply seated and controlling are the Mendelian laws. In Fig. 98 may be seen four young men of the Melanesian race born on four different islands. They have never seen each other, yet they look like brothers. Similarly, in Fig. 99 are shown four Polynesian girls. Here again they look so much alike that they might readily be taken for sisters. Yet, they live in four different groups of Polynesian islands; the Hawaiian, the Samoan, the Tahitian, and the Rarotongan.

The blending of different racial stocks produces typical characteristics of either or both ancestral patterns. When, however, marked divergences appear without mixing of racial stocks, the result is not due to heredity, but occurs in spite of heredity. In the previous chapters, I have shown that in the modernized groups of various primitive racial stocks, certain individuals developed marked changes in facial and dental arch form from the racial pattern. We are interested to know the nature of the forces responsible for this distortion of the ancestral pattern. In a study of 1,276 skulls of the ancient civilizations of Peru, I did not find one with a typical divergence from normal such as we find in modern whites or in children of primitive racial stocks after the parents have adopted the foods of our modern civilization. It is important that we study this phase in further detail.

In Fig. 100 are shown two Indian fathers and their sons, whom we studied in Peru. The father and son shown above lived at Talara, in a highly modernized Indian colony. The father worked in the oil fields on the coast. This district is an arid desert into which practically all food has to be shipped for the large colony engaged in the oil industry. The father was born while his parents were using the native foods of the coast, including an abundance of

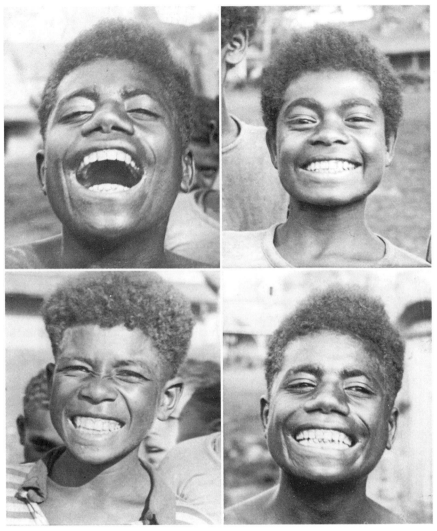

FIG. 98. These four Melanesian boys born on different islands look like brothers but are not blood relations. They illustrate the role of heredity in reproducing racial type. Heredity, however, can only operate normally when the germ cells have not been injured.

sea foods. The son was born to his parents after they had adopted the foods of modern civilization. The father and son shown below, lived in the high Sierras. The father is an Indian descendant of the Incas and was born while his parents were living on the native dietary of the high plateau country, near Cuzco. After the adoption of the modern foods by the parents, the son shown

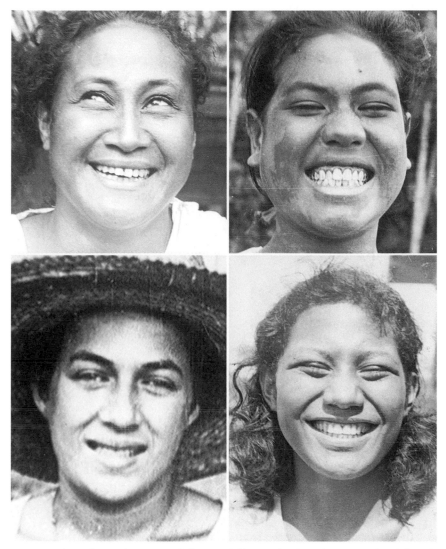

FIG. 99. These four Polynesian girls live on different islands and are not related though they look like sisters. They record their racial type by undisturbed heredity.

to the right was born. It is important to keep in mind that the marked change in these fathers and sons has occurred in the first generation after the parents have adopted the white man's foods, and has occurred in spite of heredity.

In Fig. 101 above is shown a Wakamba father in central Africa, a man who is working for the railroad company which contributed largely to the food

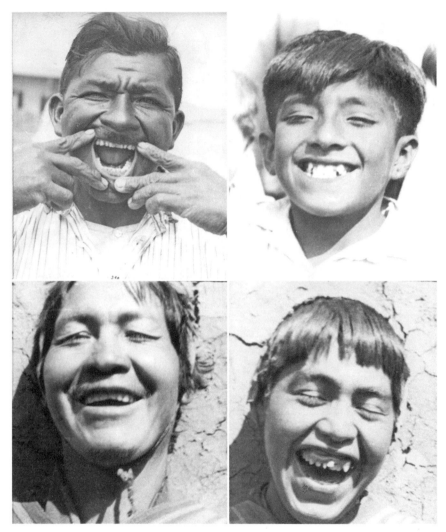

FIG. 100. Disturbed heredity. Above, father a primitive coastal Indian of Peru with normal facial and dental arch development. Son at right presents distortions of both facial and dental arch form. Below, father a primitive Andean Indian with excellent facial and dental arch form. His son at right has not reproduced the racial pattern. Both sons are full blood.

supply for the laborers. The boy shown at the right was born after the parents had adopted the imported foods. In the lower picture, in Fig. 101, is seen a Fiji Islander and his son. The father was born to parents living on the native foods, and his son was born after the adoption of the white man's foods. All these are typical cases of the inhibition of Nature's normal procedure. We have additional data which indicate that our problem is associated with a pro-

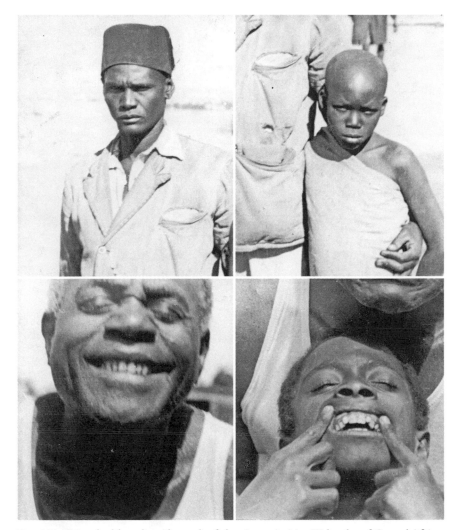

FIG. 101. Disturbed heredity. Above, the father is a primitive Wakamba of Central Africa. His son at right has not reproduced the tribal pattern. Below, the father presents the typical Fijian primitive facial and dental arch form. His son at right has a narrowed arch and change in facial form. Both sons are full blood.

gressive lowering of reproductive capacity on the part of one or both of the parents.

In photographing the members of modernized families, regardless of racial stocks, we frequently find that changes in facial expression appear in the younger members of the family. This change in facial contour within a family does not occur in the primitive races, while on their native dietary.

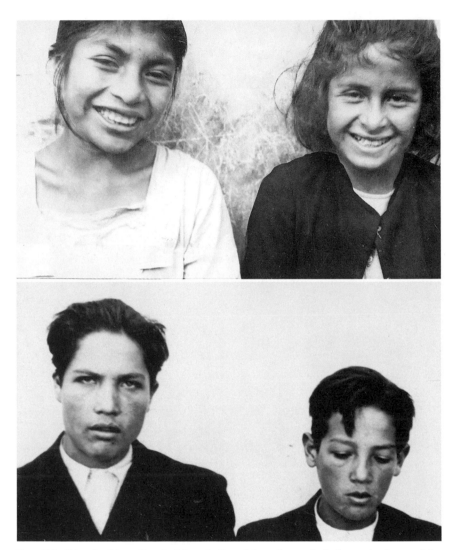

FIG. 102. Disturbed heredity. Quichua Indians. Note the marked change in shape of the face and dental arches of the younger sister at the right. Also of the younger brother at the right. These families demonstrate a lowering of reproductive capacity of the parents with the later born children.

In contrast with this we see, in Fig. 102, two sisters and two brothers. In each pair there is a marked change in the facial form of the younger. The arches and the nostrils of the younger child are narrower and there is a marked lack of development in both the middle and lower thirds of the face.

Very striking illustrations of this progressive degeneration in the children of a given family were found among the modernized Aborigines of Australia.

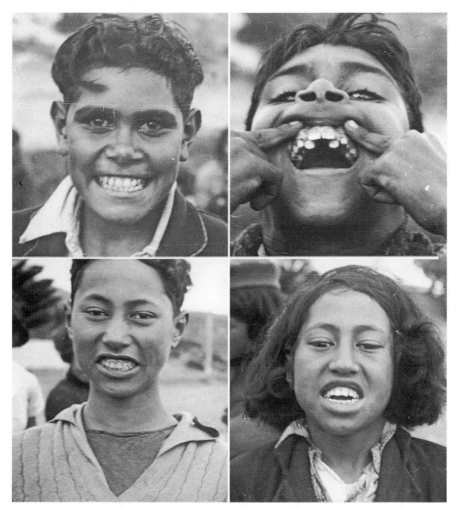

FIG. 103. Disturbed heredity. These children are Australian Aborigines. Note the marked change in facial and dental arch form in the younger child at the right in both families. This is depressed reproductive capacity of the parents.

Two views of brothers are shown in Fig. 103 (upper). The father and mother of these two boys were born in the Bush. They were living, when photographed, in one of the reservations, on the imported modern foods which were provided by the government. This is also illustrated in the lower photograph. Note the marked underdevelopment of the middle third of the face of the girl.

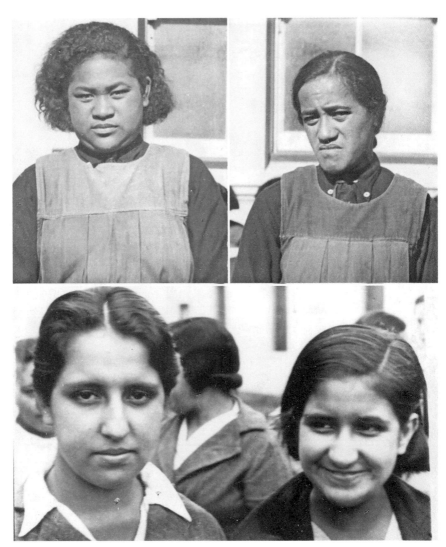

FIG. 104. Above, two Maori girls in New Zealand and below, two white girls in Peru. Note the facial change in the girls at the right compared with their older sisters.

Striking instances were frequently seen among the modernized Maori of New Zealand. Two sisters presenting two extremes of facial form are shown in the upper section of Fig. 104. The girl to the left is the older. She has the typical tribal pattern which has been completely lost in her younger sister to the right.

If the change in facial form were the result of racial admixture, we should not have the types of deformity patterns that these cases show. Indeed, in the same family we should not find several different deformity patterns. The lack of development downward of the upper anterior incisors and the bone supporting them is illustrated for the younger child, in Fig. 103 lower right. It will be noted that when this girl's molar teeth are in contact her front teeth still miss occluding by a considerable distance.

Members of the white race are affected in a similar manner. In Fig. 104 (lower) are shown two sisters; the younger to the right reveals strikingly the lack of development of the middle and lower third of the face. The fact that this condition so frequently shows a progressively severe injury in the younger members of the family is a matter of great importance in tracing the causative factors. It is important to keep in mind that when the injury shows in the face of the young child it becomes worse when the adult face forms. This increase in deformity occurs at the time of the development of the permanent dentition, at from ten to fourteen years of age.

In the islands north of Australia where contact with modern civilization is just being made, the adult individuals showed a constant reproduction of the tribal pattern, while those born since contact was made, had many divergences from normal. In Fig. 105 will be seen a family of six individuals. Four were born before the modern store was put on that island and two after the parents had come into contact with the influence of the imported foods. It will be seen that the four older brothers show marked uniformity of facial design, and that all have reproduced the tribal pattern. The two younger members show definite change in facial pattern. This is also illustrated in Fig. 106 above, in which the oldest brother was born before the store was put on Badu Island, and the three younger, after the establishment of the store twenty-three years ago.

This problem of progressive degeneration in the younger members of the family is again illustrated by the group shown in Fig. 107. The older girl has reproduced the tribal pattern of the race with normal broad, dental arches. The second girl shows marked narrowing and lengthening of the face. The third child, a boy, shows very marked divergence from the tribal pattern. This group is shown below with their teeth exposed. It will be seen that the oldest girl has broad dental arches typical of Nature's normal design. The second girl has a marked depression laterally in the molar and bicuspid region producing a narrowing of the palate. The third child has in addition to the narrowing of the face a marked deficiency in bone growth so that the cuspids both above and below are forced entirely outside the arch. The total circumference as well as the breadth of the upper arch is so reduced that space is not

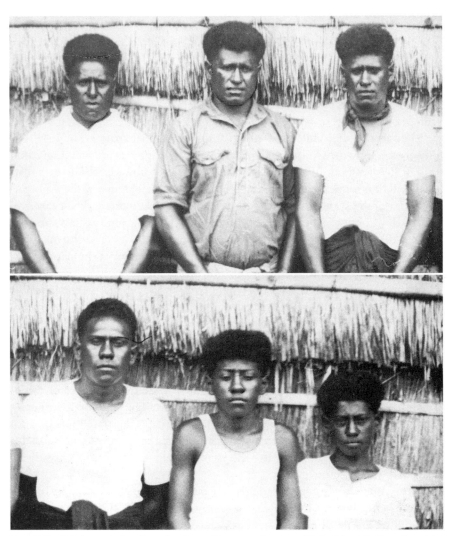

FIG. 105. Of these six brothers the four older were born on Badu Island before the white man's store was established. The two younger at right below, after. Note change in facial form.

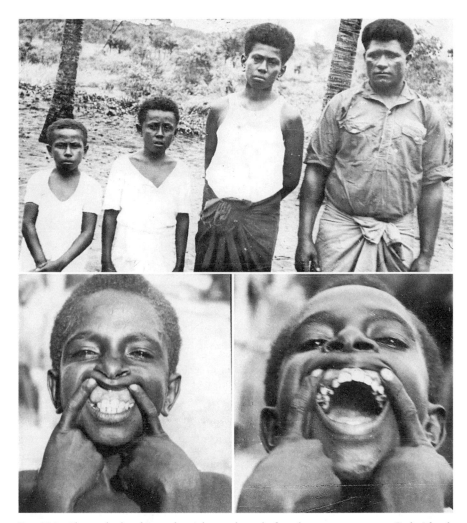

FIG. 106. Above, the brother at the right was born before the store was put on Badu Island, the three younger, after. Note the change in facial form. Below, note that the dental arches are too constricted to provide space for the erupting cuspids. This boy is the one shown at the left in Figure 107.

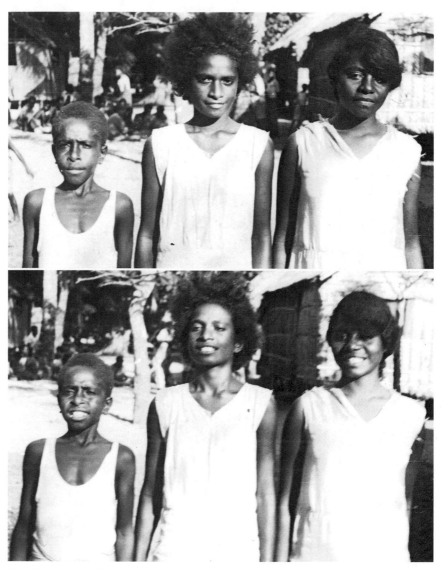

FIG. 107. Natives from islands north of Australia. Above, note the progressive facial change in the younger sister and brother with lengthening and narrowing of the face and body. Below, note the broad arches of the oldest girl at the right, lateral depression of the bicuspids and molars of the next girl and inadequate bone development of the boy's face. These are on an island north of Australia.

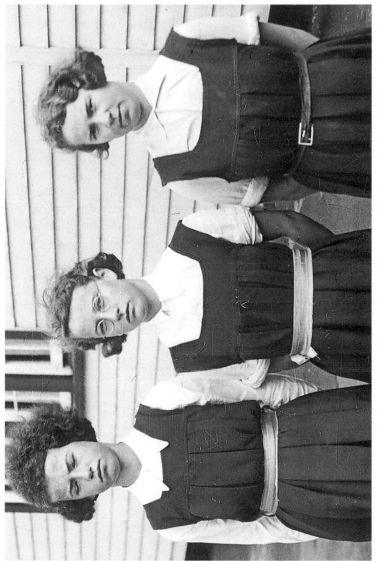

FIG. 108. White Girl Scouts, New Zealand. Note the progressive lengthening and narrowing of the face and narrowing of the hips in the younger girl at the left.

available for the cuspids. They will be seen imbedded high in the tissue, as illustrated in the lower picture of Fig. 106.

Fig. 108 shows three white girl scouts in New Zealand. Note that progressive narrowing of the body including both shoulders and hips has occurred in the younger members of the family. This is also shown in Fig. 107.

It would be remarkable if these disturbances in the physical pattern were limited to the face and dental arches. An illustration of other deficiency injuries is shown in Fig. 109, which shows children in a modernized Maori family. It will be seen that while the oldest girl has the typical Maori racial pattern of face, there is a marked lack of development of the middle third of the face, with progressive severity of distortion in her two younger brothers. On observing the feet it will be seen that she has splendidly formed feet while the second child has flat feet, and the third child has clubbed feet.

I have found similar examples in several of the modernized primitive racial stocks. The severity of the disturbing factors may be different under different circumstances. Drought, industrial depression, unemployment, and the like, all have their influence. In Fig. 110 will be seen three Maori children of New Zealand; the second child is smaller in stature than the third and gives more evidence of facial injury. While his older sister and younger brother have normal feet, his quite severe disturbance in facial growth is associated with club feet.

I have one patient who was the seventh of a family of eleven children. All the children in the family have good facial development, except this patient. She was born in the midst of a severe financial depression when the total amount of money available for the food for the family was reduced to a very low level. The other children were born before or after the depression, and were not injured. In addition to this patient's severe facial deformity, she has had some arthritis and a general rheumatic tendency. Her facial injury is marked and is characterized by a lack of development of the middle third.

Deformities of the feet associated with facial deformity have been found in several modernized groups of primitive racial stocks. A typical case among the modernized Indians of Peru is shown in Fig. 111. The face of this boy shows abnormal development with narrowing of the upper arch and displacement of the teeth. This is associated with gross deformity of one foot and shortening of the leg. He lives in the high country. This phase is strikingly illustrated in Fig. 112 where the face is very badly injured and both feet are seriously clubbed. This boy is a Coastal Indian.

The serious expressions of physical deformities which we found had occurred in several primitive racial stocks, after they have become modernized sufficiently to be using the foods of our modern civilization, are occurring in our modern American families with equal severity and great frequency.

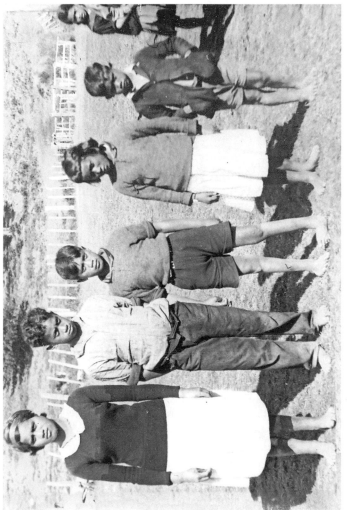

FIG. 109. New Zealand Maori. Note the progressive change in facial form of the two younger boys on the left as compared with their older sister. Then note the progressive change in their feet. Normal feet, flat feet and club feet. (*Editor's Note:* The original picture of these children was evidently cropped to fit the page at the time of the first publication and only included the three children on the left. This is the original which includes all five children. There is marked improvement in the physical structure of the youngest two on the far right who were born after the parents returned to their native diet. This demonstrates how positive changes in succeeding generations can be made by use of the proper foods.)

One method for determining the cause of these deformities is through an examination of birth and death certificates to note the recorded data relative to physical deformities. An outstanding contribution to this approach has been made by Dr. D. P. Murphy, of the University of Pennsylvania. In an examination of 130,132 individual death certificates that have been recorded between 1929 and 1933, he found physical deformities recorded in 1,476 cases. Dr. Murphy sent field workers to make a personal study of the family histories by contacting the mothers or grandmothers, of whom they were able to locate 890. From this group he was able to select 405 with sufficiently complete family histories to allow tabulation in a form that would throw light upon the birth rank and other data. His studies strongly emphasize the presence of a period of low reproductive activity. In concluding one of his reports he states:[1]

> Miscarriages, stillbirths, and premature births occurred more often than would be expected by chance in the pregnancies immediately preceding and immediately following the pregnancy which resulted in the birth of a defective child, and less often than would be expected by chance in the remaining pregnancies. Miscarriage, stillbirth, and premature birth occurred most often in the pregnancy immediately preceding that of the defective child.
>
> From the above observations, it is concluded that the birth of a congenitally malformed child may be only one expression of a prolonged decrease in functional reproductive activity, the other expressions being miscarriages, stillbirths, and premature births.
>
> It is suggested that the obstetrician has unusual reason to suspect the possible existence of a congenital malformation in the pregnancy which follows immediately after a miscarriage, a stillbirth, or a premature birth.

Shute, of the University of Western Ontario, London, Canada, in a personal communication, states that he has been impressed, in his studies of aborted fetuses, with the large percentage that are malformed. This seems to link the malformations with the causative factors which have resulted in decreased reproductive activity.

In connection with the production of imperfect infants, the period in the formative process at which the injury occurs and also its origin are important. Murphy has thrown important light on this phase in his study of the cause of the defectives in forty families with two or more malformed.[2] He concludes: "Many if not most of the congenital malformations met with in this study resulted from defects in the germ plasm, which were present before fertilization."

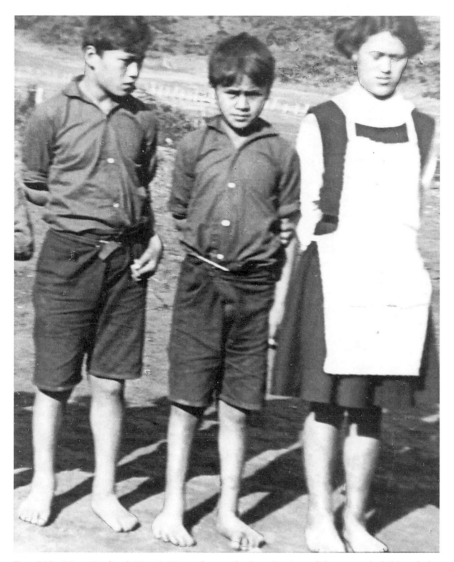

FIG. 110. New Zealand Maori. Note the marked undersize of the second child and the underdevelopment of the face associated with marked deformity of the feet.

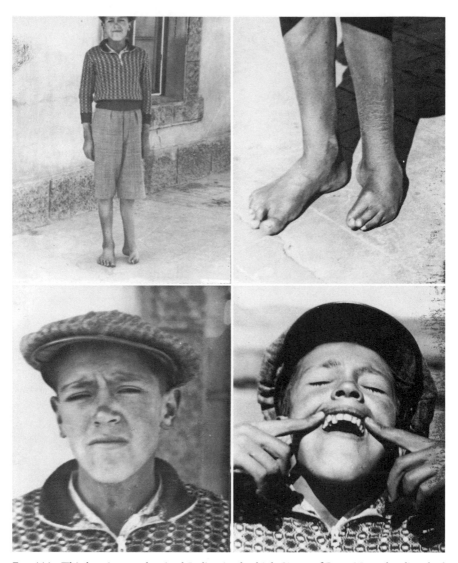

FIG. 111. This boy is a modernized Indian in the high Sierra of Peru. Note the disturbed development of the face associated with the deformity of one foot.

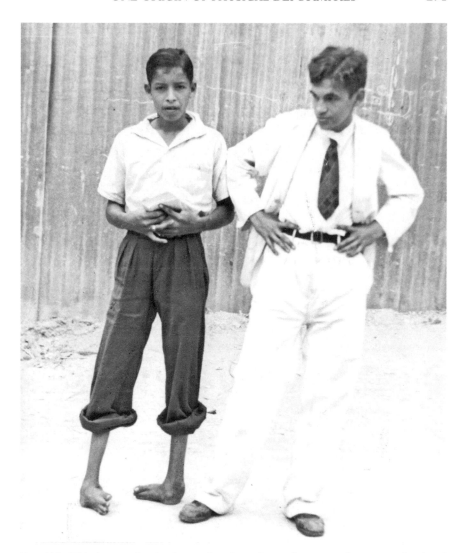

FIG. 112. This is a modernized coastal Indian of Ecuador. Note the serious facial and dental arch distortion associated with club feet.

Among the important questions that arise is the relative responsibility of the two parents. As an approach to this phase Murphy[2] has made a study which deals with a consecutive series of 884 families in each of which there appeared at least one congenitally malformed child. In forty of these families, there were two or more malformed brothers and sisters. He presents extensive data in tabular form from which he takes examples to illustrate his interpretation. He states under the "Clinical Value of Study" the following:

> It is evident from the above data (tables) that there is a strong tendency for congenital malformations to duplicate in siblings that belong to a consecutive series of families. And also that such defects tend to appear rather frequently among their more distant relatives. This duplication of malformations is to be observed in the case of the more serious types of defects, just as it is noticed in the less serious ones. These findings lend support to the theory that congenital malformations are primarily the result of influences which affect the germ cells prior to, rather than after, fertilization. The validity of this theory is emphasized by three examples taken from Tables I and II. Family 17 in Table I contained 3 children with pyloric stenosis, two of which were twins. Family 6 in Table II possessed 2 siblings with cleft palate, conceived by the same father, but born to different mothers. Family 8 in Table II contained 2 children both exhibiting an absence of the right half of the diaphragm. It does not seem likely that such sequences of events as these could be the result of any forces that did not operate until after fertilization had taken place. . . .
>
> Since, as has been shown in a previous report, congenital malformations are 24 times more common in siblings of defective children than in the population at large, the present observations should be of added clinical interest.

Summary and Conclusions

1. A consecutive series of 40 families having 2 or more congenitally malformed children has been studied with respect to the duplication of defects in siblings.
2. The defect observed in the first malformed child reappeared in a subsequent malformed sibling in about 50 percent of all cases; the 50 percent remaining including all other possible defects.
3. In a second group of 39 consecutive families, in which a malformed child possessed a malformed relative, the malformation in the child and in the relative were identical in about 41 percent of cases.
4. In 19 non-consecutive families with 2 or more malformed children, the defect of the first child repeated in a subsequent child in over half of the families.

It is significant that while these important factors are just coming to light in our modernized civilization, the evidence clearly indicates that several so-called primitive races have been conscious of the need for safeguarding motherhood from reproductive overloads which would reduce the capacity for efficient reproduction. For example, G. T. Basden[3] in his book *Among the Ibos of Nigeria* states:

> It is not only a matter of disgrace but an actual abomination, for an Ibo woman to bear children at shorter intervals than about three years.... The idea of a fixed minimum period between births is based on several sound principles. The belief prevails strongly that it is necessary for this interval to elapse in order to ensure the mother being able to recuperate her strength completely, and thus be in a thoroughly fit condition to bear another child. Should a second child be born within the prescribed period the theory is held that it must inevitably be weak and sickly, and its chances jeopardized.

Similarly, the Indians of Peru, Ecuador and Columbia have been familiar with the necessity of preventing pregnancy overloads of the mother. Whiffen[4] in his book *North-West Amazons* states:

> The numbers (of pregnant women) are remarkable in view of the fact that husbands abstain from any intercourse with their wives, not only during pregnancy but also throughout the period of lactation—far more prolonged with them than with Europeans. The result is that two and a half years between each child is the minimum difference of age, and in the majority of cases it is even greater.

It may also be important to note that the Amazon Indians have been conscious of the fact that these matters are related to the nutrition of both parents. Whiffen states that:

> These Indians share the belief of many peoples of the lower cultures that the food eaten by the parents—to some degree of both parents—will have a definite influence upon the birth, appearance, or character of the child.

This problem of the consciousness among primitives of the need for spacing children has been emphasized by George Brown[5] in his studies among Melanesians and Polynesians in which he reports relative to the natives on one of the Solomon Islands as follows:

> After the birth of a child the husband was not supposed to cohabit with his wife until the child could walk. If a child was weak or sickly, the people would say, speaking of the parents, "Ah, well, they have only themselves to blame."

These new data have a very important bearing on the problems of degeneration in our modern civilization. Since it is true that a racial pattern can be changed in a single generation, our modern concept and teaching with regard to the role of heredity must be modified in its relationship to cause and effect. A deformity arising from intercepted heredity is just as truly biologic as a deformity arising from accumulated impacts as expressed in heredity. Instead of blaming the past generations for the distortions or frailties of our modern generation and thus relieving our own generation of responsibility, these new data indicate that the social organization that is creating these divergences from normal must alone accept the responsibility.

This completely changes some aspects of the theories and practice of modern social education. Instead of planning the care and management of distorted personality as though the lesion were the result of environmental influences upon a normally organized individual, it should be looked upon as a distortion affecting one link in the chain of heredity which is neither the result of the distortions of previous links nor a controlling factor for future links in the chain. The prognosis, in other words, while being bad for the individual is not necessarily bad for his or her descendants.

While many of the individuals who have suffered physical distortions have apparently practically normal brain development, we shall see in the following chapter that a certain percentage have so great a disturbance in brain organization that they cannot and should not be considered as individually responsible for their behavior.

It is urgent therefore that the data presented in this chapter be looked upon as an important key to the progressive degeneration that is taking place in many parts of the world under the influence of our so-called modern civilization. It is a matter of profound significance that the most primitive races were originally able to avoid the physical degeneration so general in many communities today. It is also a matter of importance that the primitives recognized not only these dangers but were conscious of and practiced adequate means for preventing them. They had sufficient character to achieve the ends which they deemed essential. Weakness in character may constitute the greatest barrier in the reorganization and conservation of our modern civilization.

Two serious defects from which many individuals in our modernized civilization suffer are impacted teeth and the absence of teeth due to their failure to develop. It is significant that in the arches of the primitive races practically all teeth form and erupt normally, including the third molars. In the modernized primitives and among our modern whites with deformed dental arches many teeth are impacted and often several of the permanent teeth have never formed. The evidence indicates that this, like the facial and dental arch deformities, is due to an absence of vitamin A in the diet of the mother during the gestation period or of one or both of the parents prior to conception. The cause is discussed in the next chapter.

REFERENCES

[1] MURPHY, D. P. Reproductive efficiency and malformed children. *Surg. Gynec. and Obst.*, 62:585, 1936.

[2] MURPHY, D. P. The duplication of congenital malformations in brothers and sisters and among other relatives. *Surg. Gynec. and Obst.*, 63:443, 1936.

[3] BASDEN, G. T. *Among the Ibos of Nigeria*. Phila., Lippincott, 1921.

[4] WHIFFEN, T. *North-West Amazons*. N.Y., Duffield, 1915.

[5] BROWN, G. *Melanesians and Polynesians*. London, Macmillan, 1910.

Chapter 18

PRENATAL NUTRITIONAL DEFORMITIES
AND DISEASE TYPES

A RELATIONSHIP between physical types and certain disease susceptibilities has been recognized by diagnosticians for centuries. The skill of many physicians in reading intuitively and from external signs the nature of their patients' troubles when these could not be classified with precision played an important part in the successful warfare against disease in the period preceding the advance in modern laboratory technique. For many of the old-time physicians, these constitutional qualities were expressed as diathesis. An individual would be recognized as having a phthisical diathesis (a susceptibility to tuberculosis). Similarly, the arthritis group had a rheumatic diathesis. While modern science has undertaken to express its findings numerically, the problem of reducing the diatheses to mathematical formulas has required so many overlappings that it has been impossible to establish definite limiting boundaries.

In my investigations regarding the types of individuals who develop rheumatic group lesions as a result of dental focal infections,[1] I found that individuals could be divided into very definite groups in which 15.05 percent with severe lesions belonged to families in which similar disease symptoms had occurred. Evidence was disclosed of a systemic factor that played a controlling role in determining whether or not the individual would be seriously injured from dental focal infections. It became very clear that the soil was quite as important a determining factor as was the type of infection. This finding led me to broaden the scope of my investigations to include a search for control cases that were free from the degenerative processes. I was not able to find these controls in the clinical material afforded by our modern civilization, and therefore extended the search to isolated primitive racial stocks.

Associated with a fine physical condition, the isolated primitive groups have a high level of immunity to many of our modern degenerative processes, including tuberculosis, arthritis, heart disease, and affections of the internal organs. When, however, these individuals have lost this high level of physical excellence, a definite lowering in their resistance to the modern degenerative processes has taken place. To illustrate, the narrowing of the facial and dental arch forms of the children of the modernized parents, after they had adopted the white man's food, was accompanied by an increase in susceptibility to pulmonary tuberculosis.

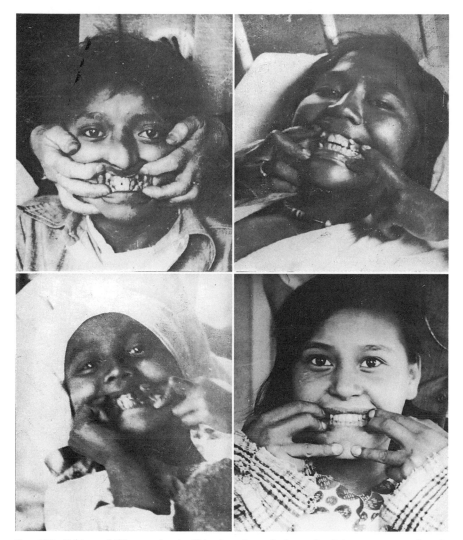

FIG. 113. Eskimo children seriously ill in the tuberculosis wards of the government hospital at Juneau, Alaska. They were too ill to be moved to good light for photographing. Every tubercular child in these wards had disturbed facial development and deformed dental arches. The parents were living on modern foods.

In Fig. 113 will be seen four young people, examined in the tuberculosis wards of the Juneau (Alaska) Hospital for Indians and Eskimos. All exhibited marked evidence of prenatal injury. Note the cuspids erupting outside the line of the arch. The teeth of the upper arch of the boy at the upper left, pass inside the teeth of the lower arch. His upper arch is so narrow that even a finger could

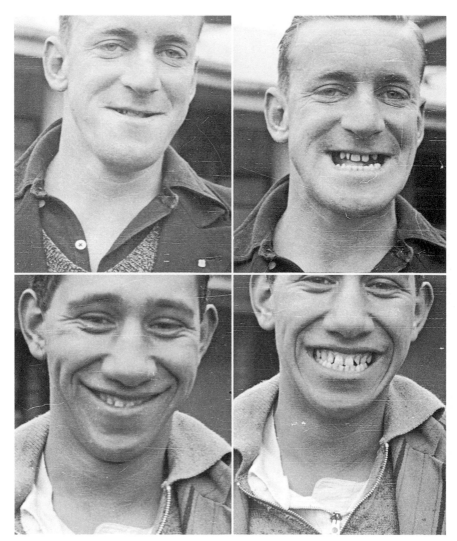

FIG. 114. These are patients in the Maori Hospital for tuberculosis in New Zealand. Note the very marked underdevelopment of the middle third of the face above and of both middle and lower thirds of the face below. Every patient under thirty years of age in these wards had deformed dental arches and disturbed facial development.

not be passed between the lateral walls. These pictures had to be taken with short exposures in the poor light of the wards. They reveal, however, the conditions.

In Figs. 114 and 115 are shown several individuals photographed in the tuberculosis hospital in New Zealand. Note the lack of development of the middle third of the face and the narrowing and lengthening of the face. In several indi-

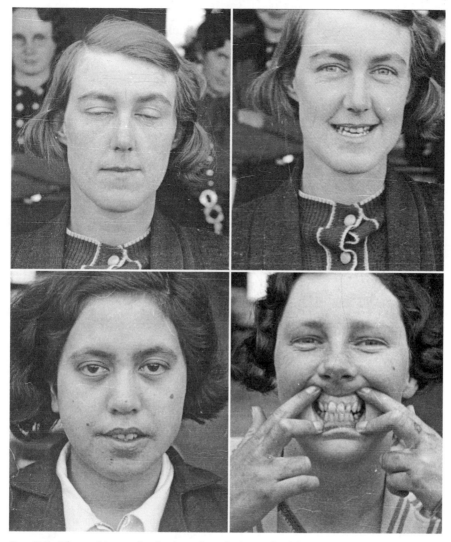

FIG. 115. These girls are also in the tuberculosis ward of the New Zealand Hospital for Maori. Note the marked disturbance in development of the face and dental arches. All have pinched nostrils.

viduals the teeth of the upper arch closed inside the teeth of the lower arch, instead of outside, as in normal persons. Here again, 100 percent of the young people with tuberculosis gave evidence of injury in the formative period, and 91.2 percent of the total number of patients were found to have disturbed dental arches.

In Fig. 116 are shown four typical individuals in the tuberculosis hospitals in Hawaii; one in Hilo and the other in Honolulu. In each of these hospitals 100 percent of the individuals had abnormal development of the face and dental arches.

While we know many of the factors contributing to the nature of diatheses, I have found no data dealing with the forces which determine diatheses, except the influence of heredity. The data I am presenting in this volume, deal with forces other than heredity.

An outstanding advance in organizing the data which relate the physical characteristics of individuals to their disease susceptibilities has been made by the Constitutional Clinic of Columbia University and the Presbyterian Hospital of New York, under the able direction of Dr. George Draper. He has found it necessary in order to study man as a whole, to view him from four different angles: "his form, his function, his immunity mechanism and his psychology." These four attributes he has designated as the "four panels of personality."

Dr. Draper has published several communications including two textbooks, one entitled, *Human Constitution*,[2] and the other, *Disease and the Man*[3]. Dr. Draper has approached this problem from the data provided in the medical clinics, and therefore, from the characteristics of affected individuals, whereas my approach has been through a study of the primitive groups and the physical changes and disease susceptibilities which occur as a result of their modernization. The similarity of our conclusions greatly emphasizes the importance of the findings of each. Dr. Draper has emphasized the importance of the face and of the dental arches in the general matter of susceptibility to disease. He closes one of his chapters, entitled "The Relation of Face, Jaws and Teeth to Human Constitution and Its Bearing on Disease," as follows:

> The lessons which we have learned from these observations, however, is that the face and jaws hold much information of value to the student of the human being. As clinicians in the field of internal medicine we have been taught to observe the gums and teeth in order to detect possible foci of infection. But for the student of clinical organismalism, the teeth and jaws hold much valuable information about the total personality. For the worker in the dental branch of medicine it would seem that an unusual opportunity is offered for extending such observations and correlations. It may very well be that the dental student who becomes interested in the relation of the mouth to the organism may form a most important link with the responsibilities of internal medicine.
>
> The more we come to view man as a totality, as an organism which functions as a whole and not as a collection of separate elements, the more do all the special branches of medicine become fused with the general concept which forms the basis of this discussion, namely, the relation of the human organism as a whole to those various reactions of maladjustment with environment which we call disease.

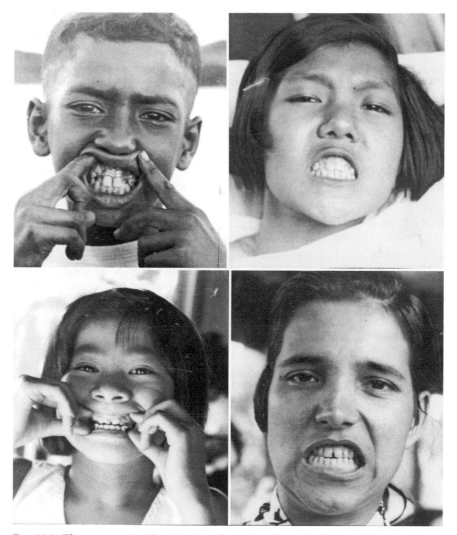

FIG. 116. These are native Hawaiians in tuberculosis hospitals. Every child in the wards showed marked disturbance of facial development and dental arch form.

It is clear that a definite association of abnormal facial patterns with specific disease susceptibilities exists. From my studies it is also clear that these abnormal facial patterns are associated with influences resulting from a change in the nutrition of the parents of the individual. We are at this point concerned with the forces that underlie these phenomena.

In approaching this problem as it applies to human beings, much can be learned from a study of domestic and wild animals. Until recent years it has been common knowledge among the superintendents of large zoos of America and Europe that members of the cat family did not reproduce efficiently in captivity, unless the mothers had been born in the jungle. Formerly, this made it necessary to replenish lions, tigers, leopards and other felines from wild stock as fast as the cages were emptied by death or as rapidly as new stock should be added by enlargement.

The story is told of a trip to Africa made by a wild animal specialist from the London zoo for the purpose of obtaining additional lions and studying this problem. While in the lion country, he observed the lion kill a zebra. The lion proceeded then to tear open the abdomen of the zebra and eat the entrails at the right flank. This took him directly to the liver. After spending some time selecting different internal organs, the lion backed away and turned and pawed dirt over the carcass which he abandoned to the jackals. The scientist hurried to the carcass and drove away the jackals to study the dead zebra to note what tissues had been taken. This gave him the clue which when put into practice has entirely changed the history of the reproduction of the cat family in captivity. The addition of the organs to the foods of the captive animals born in the jungle supplied them with foods needed to make reproduction possible. Their young, too, could reproduce efficiently. As I studied this matter with the director of a large lion colony, he listed in detail the organs and tissues that were particularly selected by animals in the wilds and also those that were provided for animals reproducing in captivity. He explained that, whereas the price of lions used to be fifteen hundred dollars for a good specimen, they were now so plentiful that they would scarcely bring fifteen cents. If we observe the parts of an animal that a cat eats when it kills a small rodent or bird, we see that it does not select exclusively the muscle meat.

During my biological investigations using animals, I have had barn rats gnaw their way into the room where the rabbits were kept and kill several animals during a night. On two different occasions, only the eyes of the rabbits had been eaten, and the blood may have been sucked. On another occasion the brains had been eaten. It was evident that these rats had a conscious need for special food elements that were provided by these tissues.

No phases of the problem of physical degeneration can be as important as knowledge of the forces that are at work and the methods by which they operate. It is clear from the data presented in previous chapters that these forces can become operative with sufficient speed to make a difference in two generations, one succeeding the other. It is also clear from preceding data that these forces originate in the change of the nutrition of the parents.

A chemical analysis of the food (Chapter 15) discloses a marked reduction in the intake of some of the vitamins and minerals in individuals who are undergoing a degenerative process.

Many investigators have presented important data dealing with the role of vitamin A in prenatal as well as postnatal growth processes. It is known that the eye is one of the early tissues to develop injury from the absence of vitamin A, hence the original name for this vitamin was the xerophthalmic vitamin. The importance of vitamin A to the eye, and the fact that this vitamin is stored in eye tissue have been emphasized by several investigations.

Wald[4] in discussing vitamin A in eye tissues states:

> Extracts of eye tissue (retina, pigment epithelium and choroid) showed the characteristic vitamin A absorption band at 620 mu. with the SbC13 test and were also potent in curing vitamin A deficient rats. The concentration of vitamin A was very constant for different mammals, at about 20 Y per g. dry tissue. Values for frog tissues were much higher.

This comment is of interest in connection with the observation that I have previously quoted regarding the raid of barn rats on the rabbit cages in the stress of deep winter. While it has been shown that vitamin A is essential for the normal function of eyes, its role in the formation of eye tissues has not been clearly understood. Probably the most sensitive procedure for testing the depletion of vitamin A in domestic animals today is by observing their behavior in semi-darkness.

Edward Mellanby[5] has presented important new data dealing with vitamin A deficiency and deafness. He states in an abstract of a paper read before the Biochemical Society, in London in November 1937, the following:

> In previous publications I have shown that a prominent lesion caused by vitamin A deficiency in young animals, especially when accompanied by a high cereal intake, is degeneration of the central and peripheral nervous systems. In the peripheral system it is the afferent nerves which are principally affected, including the eighth nerve, both cochlear and vestibular divisions. It has now been possible to show that vitamin A deficiency produces in young dogs degenerative changes in the ganglia, nerves and organs of both hearing and balance inside the temporal bone. All degrees of degeneration have been produced, from slight degeneration to complete disappearance of the hearing nerve. The nerves and ganglion cells supplying the organ of Corti are more easily damaged than those of the vestibular division. As might be expected when once the spiral ganglion cells have disappeared, additions of vitamin A to the diet have no effect, and the organ of Corti remains completely denervated. The "inattention" of dogs on these diets which I previously ascribed to cerebral defect is undoubtedly due to deafness. It now remains to determine whether these results may be extended to explain certain forms of deafness in man.

The serious effects of deficiency in vitamin A on pregnant rats has been investigated and reported by Mason[6] as follows:

> Abnormalities are described in the pregnancies of rats maintained on diets deficient in vitamin A in varying degree. Prolongation of the gestation

period up to 26 days in severe cases and a long and difficult labour which might last 2 days and often resulted in death of both mother and young were characteristic.

Defects due to deficiencies in vitamin A in the diet of dairy animals, (pregnant cows, their offspring and normal calves fed on the milk from those cows) have been reported upon by Meigs and Converse[7] as follows:

> In 1932 we reported from Beltsville evidence that farm rations frequently fed to calves may be dangerously low in vitamin A, and that milk produced by cows fed hay which has lost its green color may be an unsafe source of vitamin A in the calf ration. This preliminary paper reported results dealing with four cows which had been fed over two years on a good grain mixture and late-cut low-color timothy hay. Of six calves born of these cows, two were dead, one was unable to stand and died shortly after birth, and three were both weak and blind. The fact that cows so fed were unable to properly nourish their calves before birth led to the question whether the milk from these cows might not be deficient for normal growth of calves from other cows fed on rations adequate in vitamin A. This preliminary report included results on three normal calves fed milk from those cows fed low-color timothy hay. The three calves died at fifty-seven, sixty-two, and seventy-one days of age respectively.

Since growth, prenatal and postnatal, is related directly to the pituitary body, we are specially interested in the knowledge available on the functioning of this gland.

The work of Barrie[8] throws important light on this subject. She has reported as follows:

> Partial deficiency of vitamin E as shown in the female rat fed on a diet containing only a trace of vitamin E but which is otherwise complete, results in the prolongation of gestation, which may be continued as long as 10 days beyond the normal period. The offspring under these conditions are abnormal. These young may develop slowly and be thin and undersized in spite of sufficiently profuse lactation, or they may become extremely fat and develop a leg weakness and carpopedal spasm about 18 days after birth. Animals of both types have thin skulls and short silky fur. Complete E deficiency in the adult also produces the soft fur and imperfectly calcified skull. Partially E deficient animals occasionally give birth to a litter but fail to lactate.
>
> The changes observed are similar in several ways to those produced by hypophysectomy (surgical removal of pituitary gland). Marked degranulation of the anterior pituitary is found in both the abnormal young and the adult sterile animals. Lack of vitamin E therefore produces a virtual nutritional hypophysectomy in the young rat.

The inability of various species to complete gestation when vitamin E is not provided in adequate quantity has been reported by many investigators.

A. L. Bacharach, E. Allehorne and H. E. Glynn have used their study of this factor as a means of estimating the quantity of vitamin E in the diet.[9] They state:

> A diet suitable for work on vitamin E causes female rats, fed on this diet from weaning, to show a gestation-resorption rate not significantly differing from 100 percent; when the diet is supplemented with adequate amounts of vitamin E, also administered from weaning, the live litter rate does not differ significantly from 100 percent. It is found that, on such a diet, the percentage of implantations (conceptions) is markedly different between animals that have been submitted to a single gestation-resorption, owing to lack of vitamin E, and animals that are mated for the first time. The authors suggest that the process of undergoing gestation-resorption brings about some deep-seated changes in the reproductive mechanism of the rat, of a kind not hitherto recognized as characterising the vitamin E deficiency syndrome.

One of the outstanding changes which I have found takes place in the primitive races at their point of contact with our modern civilization is a decrease in the ease and efficiency of the birth process. When I visited the Six Nation Reservation at Brantford, Ontario, I was told by the physician in charge that a change of this kind had occurred during the period of his administration, which had covered twenty-eight years and that the hospital was now used largely to care for young Indian women during abnormal childbirth (Chapter 6).

A similar impressive comment was made to me by Dr. Romig, the superintendent of the government hospital for Eskimos and Indians at Anchorage, Alaska. He stated that in his thirty-six years among the Eskimos, he had never been able to arrive in time to see a normal birth by a primitive Eskimo woman. But conditions have changed materially with the new generation of Eskimo girls, born after their parents began to use foods of modern civilization. Many of them are carried to his hospital after they had been in labour for several days. One Eskimo woman who had married twice, her last husband being a white man, reported to Dr. Romig and myself that she had given birth to twenty-six children and that several of them had been born during the night and that she had not bothered to waken her husband, but had introduced him to the new baby in the morning.

Sherman,[10] who has made many important contributions to our knowledge of vitamin A, has shown in a recent communication that an amount of vitamin A sufficient to support normal growth and maintain every appearance of good health in animals, may still be insufficient to meet the added nutritive demands of successful reproduction and lactation. With the failure to reproduce successfully, there usually appears in early adult life an increased susceptibility to infection, and particularly a tendency to lung disease at an age corresponding to that at which pulmonary tuberculosis so often develops in young men and women. He states, further, that vitamin A must be supplied in liberal proportions not only during the growth period but during the adult period as well, if a good condition of nutrition and a high degree of health and vigor are to be maintained.

Hughes, Aubel and Lienhardt[11] have shown that a lack of vitamin A in the diets of pigs has resulted in extreme incoordination and spasms. They also emphasize that gilts bred prior to the onset of the nervous symptoms either aborted or farrowed dead pigs.

Hart and Gilbert[12] have shown that the symptoms most commonly seen in cattle having a vitamin A deficiency are the birth of dead or weak calves, with or without eye lesions. They report also a condition of newborn calves which simulates white scours, and the development of eye lesions in immature animals.

Hughes[13] has shown that swine did not reproduce when fed barley and salt, but did so when cod liver oil was added to this food.

Sure[14] has shown that a lack of vitamin A produces in females a disturbance in oestrus and ovulation, resulting in sterility. Further, he states, that resorption of the fetus may be produced by lack of vitamin A, even on a diet containing an abundance of vitamin E, which is known as the anti-sterility vitamin.

One of the most important contributions in this field has been made by Professor Fred Hale, of the Texas Agricultural Experiment Station, at College Station, Texas. He has shown that many physical deformities are readily produced by curtailing the amount of vitamin A in the ration of pigs. He produced fifty-nine pigs[15] that were born blind, every pig in each of six litters—where the mothers were deprived of vitamin A for several months before mating and for thirty days thereafter. In pigs, the eyeballs are formed in the first thirty days. He found, as have several others, that depriving pigs of vitamin A for a sufficient period produced severe nerve involvements including paralysis and spasms, so that the animals could not rise to their feet. He reported that one of these vitamin A deficient pigs that had previously farrowed a litter of ten pigs, all born without eyeballs, was given a single dose of cod liver oil two weeks before mating. She farrowed fourteen pigs which showed various combinations of eye defects, some had no eyes, some had one eye, and some had one large eye and one small eye, but all were blind.

In Fig. 117 I am able through Professor Hale's kindness, to show an eyeless pig and a normal eye of a pig (at the left) and (at the right) a pair of incomplete eyes from a pig born in the litter just mentioned. This one dose of vitamin A made possible the partial formation of optic nerves and eyeballs. A

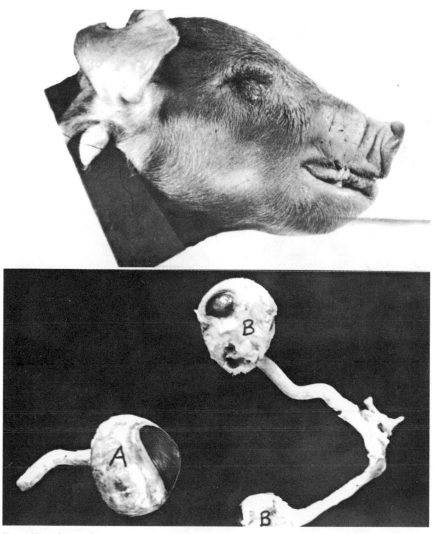

Fig. 117. Above, this pig was one of fifty-nine born without eyeballs and with other serious deformities due to lack of vitamin A in the mother's diet. Offspring of these blind pigs when normally fed had perfect eyes and no deformities. Below, A, at left shows normal eye of a pig at nine months. B, at right shows partial eyeballs and optic nerves produced in offspring when one dose of vitamin A was given two weeks before mating. (Courtesy of Professor Fred Hale.)

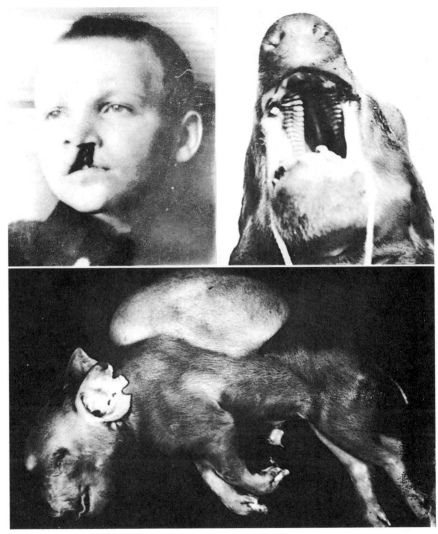

FIG. 118. Upper left: Boy has cleft palate, and harelip. Upper right: Pig has cleft palate, no eyes. Below, Pig has club feet, deformities of the ears, two tumors and no eyeballs due to lack of adequate vitamin A in the mother's diet. (Kindness of Professor Hale.)

typical eyeless pig is shown in Fig. 118 (lower). Note its deformed ears. Among the many physical injuries which develop in the pigs born to sows fed on a diet deficient in vitamin A are serious defects of the snout, dental arches, eyes and feet. This pig was born without eyeballs. It also had club feet and two tumors. In Fig. 118 (upper right) is shown a pig with cleft palate, and in Fig. 119 (upper right) one with double hairlip. In Fig. 118 (upper left) is shown a boy with cleft palate and defective eyes. One of the very important results of Professor Hale's investigations has been the production of pigs with normal eyes, born to parents both of whom had no eyeballs due to lack of vitamin A in their mother's diet. The problem clearly was not heredity. Two litters, one containing nine pigs and the other eight, which were born to mothers that had been deprived of vitamin A before mating and for thirty days thereafter, produced the following lesions: All had complete absence of eyeballs; some lacked development of the opening of the external ear; others had cleft palate, harelip, displaced kidneys, displaced ovaries, or displaced testes.

It is of interest that in October, 1935, Professor Hale reports that the Texas Agricultural Experiment Station was informed that a litter of fourteen pigs had been born blind in June, 1935, on a farm at Ralls, Texas. Of these, six pigs were raised and brought to the Station for further study. The farmer owning the pigs stated that no green feed was available on his farm from March, 1934, until May, 1935. It will be noted that this condition paralleled the experimental conditions at the station under which by restricting vitamin A before and immediately after gestation fifty-nine pigs were produced without eyeballs.

Professor Hale reports that in April, 1935, a litter of seven pigs were born blind at McGlean, Texas, which was suffering from drought conditions, similar to those at Ralls. The litter and dam were purchased by the Experimental Station. Matings were made between blind pigs. These were fed rations containing ample vitamin A, and normal pigs with normal eyeballs were produced. Even the mating of a blind son with his mother who had produced him when on deficient diet, produced only normal pigs when both had ample vitamin A. He states, "If an hereditary factor had been the cause of this congenital blindness, these matings would have produced some blind pigs, even if vitamin A were present in the ration."

The problem of congenital cleft palate has been very embarrassing to those parents whose children have been so afflicted. It is of interest that breeders of fancy dogs are frequently embarrassed by having this problem develop in their kennels or among litters born to parent stock obtained from their kennels.

In Fig. 119 (upper left) I have shown a water spaniel pup with cleft palate. This pup was not able to nurse because of the impossibility of producing suction without a palate. When fed artificially the milk was expelled through the nostrils. The mother had given birth to two previous litters all of which were dead at birth or died soon after. Her diet had been reinforced with mineral calcium phosphate in tablet form hoping to insure normal offspring. This is not nature's method.

I am informed by a veterinary that he has experienced trouble with harelip, cleft palate or serious facial deformities among dogs that are pets in homes where they are lavishly coddled and fed the things they like best. He stated that he has more trouble with head defects in bulldog pups than any other breed.

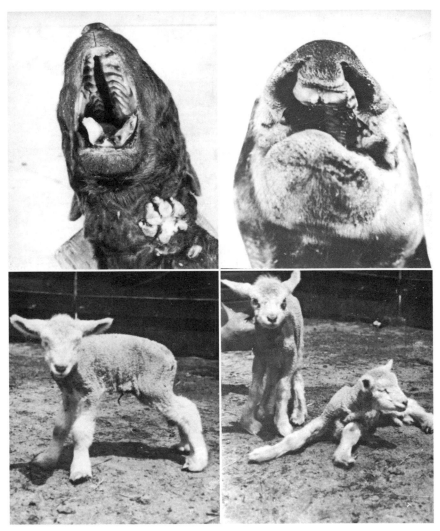

FIG. 119. Many young of modern domestic animals are born with deformities. At the upper left is seen a pup with cleft palate. In two previous litters all the pups were deformed and unable to live. At the upper right is one of Professor Hale's pigs with double harelip. Below two blind lambs and one with club foot.

There are few if any problems connected with modern degeneration on which so much light is thrown as that supplied by recent investigations on the problems of paternal responsibility for defects in the offspring. There are several reasons for this. Because the mother has the sole responsibility for the nourishment of the fetus during the formative period and she alone provides the handicaps incident to the process of birth, it is very natural that defects

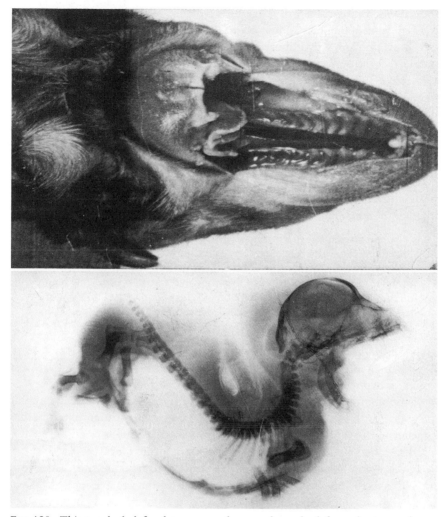

FIG. 120. This pup had cleft palate, as seen above, and grossly deformed spine, as shown below. It was one of two pups born in the same litter with the same defects and one of five pups born in four litters with these same defects. Five different mother dogs were involved but all pups were from the same father dog.

are practically all interpreted as being associated with these processes. This unfortunately, has been embarrassed further by the fact that since distortions in behavior do not appear until sometime after birth, normality was largely assumed to be present up to the time of their appearance, and therefore of necessity would be contributions from the child's environment. As such they would be subject naturally to treatment by applying influences to change the mental environment. Hence the entire problem of the role of the sex cells through controlling the architecture of the body including the brain has been largely overlooked. Very important light is thrown on this problem in the data provided on the pup shown in Fig. 120. This shows a dachshund pup with cleft palate and a very severe spinal deformity. This is not unlike deformities frequently seen, or unlike that of the pup shown in Fig. 119. The highly significant circumstance is the fact that these same deformities not only appeared also in another pup of this same litter but in one pup in each of three other litters about the same time. While four mothers were involved these four litters were all sired by one father. The paternal responsibility is clearly established.

At the right in Fig. 119 a lamb is shown with club feet and two lambs without eyeballs. I am told that in some of the sheep raising states quite a number of deformities occur in lambs at birth. One writer states:

> These deformities may maintain themselves in any number of ways. We have them two-headed, 5 and 6 legs, 2 tails, born without eyes, hermaphrodites, born with ribs on one side and any number of such deformities. A common deformity in sheep is under-shot and over-shot jaws. This simply means that the upper jaw extends farther to the front that the under jaw and the front teeth do not meet. This is called over-shot and the reverse is called under-shot.

It will be noted that a common deformity in sheep relates to an underdevelopment of either the upper or lower jaw which is one of the most common expressions of disturbed development in humans.

Some illustrations of the deformities that may occur in domestic animals are shown in Fig. 121. Above are seen two cows each with an extra foreleg attached to the shoulder; below, to the left is shown a double-faced calf which also had a cleft palate; to the right a cat with deformed legs.

In corresponding with Professor Hale, I inquired whether they had information as to the effect of vitamin A deficiency on the sire. He replied, "If we reduced the vitamin A content of the body of the sire, he would become sterile and, therefore, we could not try this procedure." The question arises as to what the effect would be of a less severe depletion of vitamin A of both parents.

It is a very easy matter to place the full responsibility on the mother, when defects develop in the children. These data indicate that either parent may contribute directly to certain of the defects of the children, due to defects in the germ plasm.

A practical case from my field studies includes a full-blooded Eskimo woman who was married twice, the second time to a white man, by whom she had several children. She had insisted on selecting and preparing the native foods for herself, though she prepared the white man's imported foods for him. With a total of twenty-six pregnancies she did not have any tooth

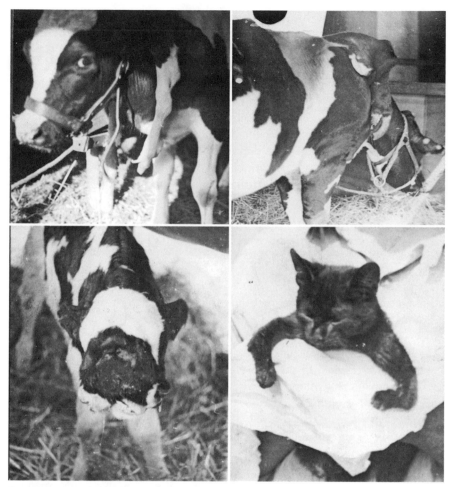

FIG. 121. Typical deformities in domestic animals. Above, two cows with an extra foreleg hanging from the shoulder. Below, left, double faced calf. Right, cat with deformed legs.

decay. He had rampant tooth decay, and a marked abnormality in the development of face and of the dental arches. Several of the children had incomplete development of the face and of the dental arches. One of the girls who was married had very narrow dental arches and nostrils and a typical boyish type of body build. Unlike her mother, this girl had a very severe experience in the birth of her only child and insisted that she would not take the risk of having another. Several daughters have narrow arches. The question arises whether the deficient nutrition of the father may have been the contributing factor in the injury of their children.

New light is being thrown on human problems by animal investigations. One study that is particularly instructive has been conducted by McKenzie and Berliner of the University of Missouri. (Bulletin No. 265.) The experimental animals used were sheep. Their studies indicated to them that they could predict the level of fertility of the sire by studies made on the seminal fluid. They found that the percentage of abnormal spermatozoa increased to 84 percent under unfavorable conditions and reduced to less than 15 percent under favorable conditions. When the unfavorable conditions characterized by these abnormal spermatozoa prevailed, the females did not conceive. High temperature proved to be an important controlling factor as indicated by variation in percentage of abnormal sperm. In one breed the average variation was from 2.5 percent in January to 22 percent defective in August; in another breed from 18 percent in January to 73 percent defective in August. They also found that the same result could be produced in the winter by keeping the sires in heated rooms or by applying heat externally. They further found that when the percentage of abnormal sperm was high, a condition of sterility was apparently established. In a personal communication from Professor McKenzie he states that their inference is that, with a high percentage of abnormal sperm, the ova either are not fertilized or that fertilization takes place and that prenatal death occurs in a certain number of the cases, and that there is an appreciable prenatal death loss in sheep, horses, cattle, and swine. I have referred to the data presented by Mall indicating that 15 percent of human conceptions in England are expelled as deformities in the second and third month of gestation. McKenzie also presents data relating to swine in which a sire that showed a high percentage of abnormal sperm was bred to two groups of sows of similar breed. One was maintained in a barn without access to pasture, the other received similar rations plus access to pasture. The group without pasture produced a high percentage of mummies, small litters, and abnormal pigs (open abdominal walls with viscera protruding and exposed spine in the region of the lumbar vertebrae). The second group on the same food with the addition of pasturage produced normally large-size litters without mummies. The following year this experiment was repeated reversing the groups of sows and using a similar high percentage of defective sperm in the same sire. The same results occurred, with the group maintained without access to pasture. This emphasizes the need for the vitamins and minerals that are provided in natural foods, particularly vitamin A and seems to relate to the studies of Hale in which the absence of vitamin A produced gross defects. These studies on domestic animals strongly emphasize the necessity that both parents shall have adequate nutrition before conception occurs and subsequently for the mother.

Until very recently there has been exceedingly little literature dealing with the factors contributing to the abnormal development of fetuses in either domestic animals or humans. Williams, who is one of the few students of this problem as it relates to domestic animals, in referring to this phase has commented that there is no treatise in the English language on teratology (development of monsters) in domestic animals.[16] He emphasizes that these defects are growing in numbers and economic importance. He refers to Burki's studies in Switzerland indicating that this difficulty has constantly and enormously increased in his territory. This veterinary has asked "Are our cows degenerating?" It is of interest that a type of deformity commonly recognized among veterinaries as a distortion of the head presenting a lack of development of the bones of the middle part of the face including the upper jaw is commonly called "bull-dog calf." This is particularly important in connection with the frequent human deficiency of lack of development in the middle third of the face. Williams emphasizes the common knowledge that Boston bull-dogs are not prolific and because of the difficulty of giving birth to their young, some veterinarians resort routinely to caesarian section. Fortunately, seriously deformed specimens are seldom born alive and usually do not continue to term. Williams states that Loje has observed ten grossly deformed calves of a particular type that were traced to the same sire; also a series of five with this deformity reported by Hutt were traced to one sire. Among the deformities in domestic animals cleft palate or absence of palate is very common. These studies on domestic animals strongly emphasize two facts; first, that deformities among these animals are very similar to those that develop in humans, and second, that the defects are largely related to the original germ cells and that the male may provide the defect quite as well as the female. Several of the primitive races have understood and provided against these mishaps.

Moench and Holt of the Cornell Medical School and New York Hospital[17] have made important studies on humans and have found a very high incidence of sterility when abnormal forms of spermatozoa reached 25 percent. Among the abnormal forms they found one particular family with a particular type of abnormal sperm reaching 12 percent. Their breeding record was decidedly bad and fetal malformations repeatedly occurred. In their group, in 63 sterile matings the men were normal 21 times and abnormal 37 times. They listed over 40 different abnormal or deformed types of sperm. They conclude:

1. In a normal semen the abnormal sperm heads do not exceed 19 to 20 percent.
2. When the sperm head abnormalities reach 20 to 23 percent, impaired fertility can be assumed.
3. When the sperm head abnormalities are above 25 percent, clinical sterility is usually present.

An important contribution to the question of the relation of the germ cells of the father to the type of defects that are prevalent in his family history has been made in recent studies conducted in Germany.[18]

> Two German surgeons concerned with enforcing the sterilization law in Berlin have taken advantage of their opportunities to make an important contribution to the study of fecundity.
>
> Several studies have been published previously, of the spermatozoa of normal men. This book offers a study of the spermatozoa of men who had been diagnosed as hereditarily defective. At the time of the operation, the upper part of the vas deferens was washed out, and the sperm thus obtained were studied in great detail, 20 different types of abnormality being distinguished.
>
> In their control studied, the normal man is found to produce 19 percent of morphologically defective sperm. By contrast, the chronic alcoholic patient produces 75 percent of defective sperm.
>
> Previously it has been assumed that as much as 25 percent or 30 percent of abnormal sperm were a good evidence of lowered fertility if not of sterility. But the fertility of these chronic alcoholics was not diminished, the authors claim.
>
> In cases of inherited mental defect, 62 percent of abnormal sperm were produced, accompanied by low fecundity, as is the case generally with the mentally defective male. On the other hand, in hereditary deafness, 62 percent and in hereditary blindness 75 percent of defective sperm appeared.
>
> Epilepsy and schizophrenia (dementia praecox) both supposed to be constitutional in origin, show less abnormality of spermatozoa (58 percent and 54 percent respectively) than blindness and deafness.

The fact that in the past almost the entire emphasis of change in physical, mental and moral qualities has been assigned to the forces of heredity, strongly emphasizes the lack of information regarding the nature of the forces at work and the points at which their influence constitute the determining factors. The data previously presented in this chapter dealing with the role of vitamins A and E throw valuable new light on this phase. It is important, however, that new data are available dealing with the factors which injure the germ cells and which Tredgold has spoken of as "poisoned germ cells."

In a personal communication received from Professor T. S. Sutton of the College of Agriculture, Ohio State University, he makes the following observation:

> For several years we have been interested in the study of the effects of vitamin A deficiency. Right now our main consideration is the effect of this deficiency on reproduction. We find that a diet low in vitamin A will cause reproductive failure, which seems to be caused chiefly by a degeneration of the germinal epithelium of the gonad. This is particularly true in the case of the male. I think we have rather convincing evidence that this is a direct

dietary damage to the gonad (ovary or testis), rather than a disruption of the endocrine balance which might result in sterility as appears to be the case in vitamin B deficiency.

The degenerative processes which occur in nerve tissues due to vitamin A deficiency have been studied by Professor Sutton and his associates.[19] They have been able to show detailed progressive degeneration within nerve fibers as a result of vitamin A deficiency.

In the light of the newer information it is quite clear why we may have any-one of the following distinct expressions in the reproductive process, namely, physical excellence of succeeding generations (such as is found among many of the primitive races as I have shown); complete reproductive failure or sterility or partial failure resulting in defectives of various types at the border-line between these two phases. It is the rapid and progressive increase in this last group which constitutes the progressive degeneration of our modern civilization.

One of the main problems in this study has to do with the relation of nutrition to the modification of the growth of the child, both in its formative period and in the stage of adolescence. I have shown that in many of these primitive racial stocks there occurs in the first generation after the displacement of native foods by imported foods a marked change in facial and dental arch forms. These changes happen most frequently in the later children in the families and come about notwithstanding the impact of heredity through all the previous generations of excellent physical development. Clinically, the evidence is abundant, that this change occurs in these primitive racial stocks regardless of color, geographic location, temperature, and climate. We are apparently dealing here with a factor which, while it may be related to the germ plasm and to the prenatal growth period, clearly involves other forces than those that are at work in the case of hereditary defectives. Since these changes have to do directly with disturbances in growth of the head, particularly of the face and of the dental arches, we are concerned with such evidence as may be available as to the nature of the forces that readily affect the anatomy of the skull.

The general architecture of the body is apparently determined primarily by the health of the two germ cells at the time of their union. This architectural design may not be completely fulfilled due to interference with nutritive processes both before and after birth. In this large problem of the relationship between physical design of the body and resistance or susceptibility to disease, we may have determining factors operating at different periods in prenatal and postnatal growth. The accumulating evidence strongly emphasizes that disease susceptibility is a widely variable factor and associated with certain types of developmental disturbances.

In a discussion of tuberculosis susceptibility before a meeting of specialists in that field, emphasis was placed upon the fact that other factors than the bacteria played controlling roles in the matter of susceptibility to tuberculosis.

Weisman has recently made an important contribution to the problem of physical development and susceptibility to tuberculosis. He has presented[20] statistical data indicating the type of chest deformity which predisposes an individual to tuberculosis. He states:

> In a study previously made on the shape of the normal and of the tuberculosis chest, it was found that the average normal chest was flat and wide and that the average tuberculous chest was deep and narrow. It was also shown that the deep chest was an underdeveloped, primitive type of chest, resembling an infant's chest in shape. Later studies on the shape of the chest and on environment showed that children from the poorer socio-economic environments had on the average a deeper chest, weighed less and were shorter than the children from the higher socio-economic levels. An investigation recently made on the incidence of tuberculosis in the various school districts in Minneapolis revealed that there is a very high incidence of tuberculosis among the children from the slums where the deep chest prevails. Ten times as many cases of tuberculosis were reported from a school district which is perhaps the poorest in the city as were reported from the best school districts.
>
> This study, which shows that there is a definite correlation between the deep chest and the positive reaction to tuberculin adds one more link to the chain of evidence supporting the contention that the deep chest is more or less associated with tuberculosis. It also helps to explain why there is such a high incidence of tuberculosis among the poor in the slum districts. The children in the slums are physically underdeveloped. They are not only shorter and lighter but they have on the average a deep, primitive, infantile type of chest, one that has not gone through the normal process of development. Even the new-born and infants are shorter and lighter and have a deeper chest than the average infant from a better environment.

It is important to note that Dr. Weisman associated the type of chest which predisposes the individual to tuberculosis, with a prenatal condition since he states "even the new-born and infants are shorter and lighter and have a deeper chest than an average infant from a better environment."

This work throws important light on why in the primitive groups the children born to parents who are living on the imported nutrition lower in vitamins and minerals than the native foods, not only showed a greatly increased incidence of tuberculosis over the children born to parents on the native diet but also proved to be those individuals who, in facial and dental arch form, presented positive evidence of prenatal injury. We also have a direct explanation for the observations that have been emphasized by Dr. George Draper, that physical form has a direct relationship to disease susceptibility of certain types, frequently spoken of as diatheses.

It is important in this connection to call to mind the statement made by some clinicians that tuberculosis patients with narrow nostrils tend to make a poor fight. These narrow nostrils are clearly related to prenatal injury resulting primarily from defective germ cells which determine the architecture, not heredity but intercepted heredity.

It is very easy to understand the effects of gross physical lesions such as the absence of eyeballs, harelip and cleft palate. These defects can readily be seen. The problem is very different, however, when we are dealing with disturbances of function due to minute anatomical lesions in either external or internal organs such as the brain. These latter will be discussed in the next chapter.

REFERENCES

[1] PRICE, W. A. *Dental Infections.* Cleveland, Penton, 1923.

[2] DRAPER, G. *Human Constitution.* Phila., Saunders, 1924.

[3] DRAPER, G. *Disease and the Man.* N.Y., Macmillan, 1930.

[4] WALD, G. Vitamin A in Eye Tissues. *J. Gen. Physiol.*, 18:905, 1935.

[5] MELLANBY, E. Vitamin A deficiency and deafness. *Biochem. J.* In press.

[6] MASON, K. E. Foetal death, prolonged gestation and difficult parturition in the rat as a result of vitamin A deficiency. *Am. J. Anat.*, 57:303, 1935.

[7] MEIGS, E. B. and CONVERSE, H. T. Some effects of different kinds of hay in the ration on the performance of dairy cows. *J. Dairy Sci.*, 16:317, 1933.

[8] BARRIE, M. M. Nutrition anterior pituitary deficiency. *Biochem. J.* In press.

[9] BACHARACH, A. L., ALLEHORNE, E., GLYNN, H. E. Investigations into the method of estimating vitamin E. 1. The influence of vitamin E deficiency on implantation. *Biochem. J.*, 21:2287, 1937.

[10] SHERMAN and MACLEOD. The relation of vitamin A to growth, reproduction and longevity. *J. Am. Chem. Soc.*, 47:1658, 1925.

[11] HUGHES, AUBEL and LIENHARDT. The importance of vitamins A and C in the ration for swine, concerning especially their effect on growth and reproduction. *Kansas Agric. Sta. Tech. Bull.*, No. 23, 1928.

[12] HART and GILBERT. Vitamin A deficiency as related to reproduction in range cattle. *Univ. of Calif. Agric. Exper. Sta. Bull.*, No. 560, 1933.

[13] HUGHES, E. H. Some effects of vitamin A deficient diet on reproduction of sows. *J. Agric. Res.*, 49:943, 1934.

[14] SURE, B. Dietary requirements for fertility and lactation; a dietary sterility associated with vitamin A deficiency. *J. Agric. Res.*, 37:87, 1928.

[15] HALE, F. The relation of maternal vitamin A deficiency to microphthalmia in pigs. *Texas S. J. Med.*, 33:228, 1937.

[16] WILLIAMS, W. L. The problem of teratology in clinical veterinary medicine. *Cornell Veterinarian*, 26:1, 1936.

[17] MOENCH, G. L. and HOLT, H. Sperm morphology in relation to fertility. *Am. J. Obst. and Gynec.*, 22:199, 1931.

[18] STIASNY, H. and GENERALES, K. Erbkranheit and Fertilitaet. Ferdinand Enke Verlag, Stuttgart, 1937. Review, *J. Heredity*, 29:9, 1938.

[19] SUTTON, T. S., SETTERFIELD, H. E. and KRAUSS, W. E. Nerve degeneration associated with avitaminosis A in the white rat. *Ohio Agric. Exper. Sta. Bull.*, No. 545, 1934.

[20] WEISMAN, S. A. Correlation of the positive reaction to tuberculin and the shape of the chest. *J.A.M.A.*, 109:1445, 1937.

Chapter 19

PHYSICAL, MENTAL AND MORAL DETERIORATION

A FTER one has lived among the primitive racial stocks in different parts of the world and studied them in their isolation, few impressions can be more vivid than that of the absence of prisons and asylums. Few, if any, of the problems which confront modern civilization are more serious and disturbing than the progressive increase in the percentage of individuals with unsocial traits and a lack of responsibility.

Laird[1] has emphasized some phases of this in an article entitled, "The Tail That Wags the Nation," in which he states: "The country's average level of general ability sinks lower with each generation. Should the ballot be restricted to citizens able to take care of themselves? One out of four cannot." He has illustrated the seriousness of this degeneration by presenting details as follows:

> Although we might cite any one of nearly two dozen states, we will first mention Vermont by name because that is the place studied by the late Dr. Pearce Bailey. "It would be," he wrote, "safe to assume that there are at least 30 defectives per 1000 in Vermont of the eight-year-old mentality type, and 300 per 1000 of backward or retarded persons, persons of distinctly inferior intelligence. In other words, nearly one-third of the whole population of that state is of a type to require some supervision."

From a broad view of the problem of modern degeneration it will be helpful to note the observations by Tredgold[2] in mental deficiency. He states:

> It is thus evident that the condition of mental deficiency, whilst presenting many interesting problems to the physician, the pathologist, and the psychologist, has also a much wider interest and importance. Since in Man the predominate feature is Mind, and since it is by its development and evolution that human progress has taken, and must take place, it is clear that the question of its disease, and particularly of its defect, is one of supreme importance to the statesman, the sociologist, the philosopher, and the whole community.

In connection with these investigations among primitive races it is interesting to note that the data are in complete harmony with the data which clinical pathologists, clinicians and anatomists have obtained in their study of the physical and structural characteristics of individuals who make up the

321

deficiency groups. In discussing the problem of the significance of the shape of the palate, Tredgold[2] states:

> Palate—The association of abnormalities of the palate with mental deficiency has long been recognized, and there is no doubt that it is one of the commonest malformations occurring in this condition. Many years ago Langdon Down drew attention to the subject, and more recently Clouston has recorded a large number of observations which show conclusively that, although deformed palates occur in the normal, they are far and away more frequent in neuropaths and the mentally defective. He states that deformed palates are present in 19 percent of the ordinary population, 33 percent of the insane, 55 percent of criminals, but in no less than 61 percent of idiots. Petersen, who has made a most exhaustive study of this question, and has compiled an elaborate classification of the various anomalies found palatal deformities present in no less than 82 percent of aments, (mental defectives), in 76 percent of epileptics, and in 80 percent of the insane.

Probably every city in the United States has made special provision for both mentally deficient groups and unsocial individuals, either in special schools or in special classes. In Cleveland, we have had a large school devoted to the problems of the so-called pre-delinquent boys, of whom nearly all have been before the courts and are assigned to this institution because they are not well enough adjusted to be kept in their normal school environment. In discussing the characteristics of these boys with the principal of that school, I asked him what the probabilities were that many of these boys would finally become involved in crime. His comment was, in effect, that they were virtually in the vestibule of a penal institute, when judged by the experience of previous boys from that school.

In approaching a study of this group, it is helpful to observe the experience of the well-equipped institutions organized for the correction of the abnormal trend which characterizes these boys. In this connection, there is a helpful report by the United States Dept. of Labor, Publication No. 203, which gives the result of tracing the after-careers of 621 boys who were in five of the best-known correctional institutions. It was found that 66 percent had been arrested and 58 percent convicted one or more times after having been paroled from the institution. It is apparent from data of this type that probably the forces that produce these abnormal expressions cause irreparable damage in the brain tissue. Practically all recent crime reports are recording an increase in juvenile crime. The Children's Bureau of the Dept. of Labor stated (Nov. 4, 1938): "that juvenile delinquency spurted during 1937 for the first time since 1930," but it cannot explain why until further study.

Reports to the bureau from 28 courts in 17 states and the District of Columbia showed that they handled 31,038 cases during 1937, an increase of 3,000 over 1936. The report showed that 44 percent of the cases involved children between 14 and 15 years old; 22 percent those between 12 and 13 years, and 10 percent those between 10 and 11. Boys' cases comprised 85 percent of the total.

As an approach to this problem I have made an examination of 189 boys in the Cleveland school for pre-delinquents. I gave particular attention to those physical signs of nutritional injury which seemed to be definitely assigned to the formative period of the child. We endeavored to obtain detailed information relative to the family history and to the birth of the child. We were fortunate in having the assistance of the officers, and of a nurse in the dental service of the Health Department of the Board of Education, a nurse who made visits to the homes of many of these boys to obtain the information directly from the mothers.

In this group of boys, there were twenty-nine for whom I had not sufficient details to include their cases in the studies. Of the 189 in the group, there were only three with sufficiently normal dental arches to be classified as normal. Accordingly, 98.4 percent proved to be individuals with more or less marked abnormality. Many of the faces were very badly deformed.

While often it will be difficult to place the responsibility entirely on either parent for the child's abnormal physical development, it is of interest to study the birth rank of these children. The average number of children in the families represented by these 160 children is 4.75. Of these, thirty-five, or 21.9 percent, are first children in the families represented; thirteen, or 9.1 percent, are only children; thirty-nine, or 24.4 percent, are last children; and thirty-six or 22.5 percent, are fifth children or later. Sixty-two, or 38.7 percent, are either the first or last child. It will be seen from these data that the first or last child, or even a late child in a large family, tended to have a distinctly poorer chance than the intermediate children in the families in which these studies were made. Statistical data relating the age of the mother and father to prenatal deficiency of their offspring reveal that abnormally young parents have a much higher percentage of defective children than do those in the most favorable child-bearing period of life. The group at the Cleveland school included only those boys who have been before the courts because of more or less serious phases of delinquency. If they are in a considerable part the products of a defective society, it seems quite unfair that they should be held entirely responsible for that delinquency, which has put them in this institution. If they are destined for a penal institute in which they will be held entirely responsible for that abnormality which resulted in their misdemeanor, as has been the procedure in the past, are they receiving just consideration? Society may be justified in protecting itself from their misdeeds by placing restrictions about them, but it does not seem that society is justified in shifting the entire responsibility to the affected individuals.

Recent studies of the mental capacity of felons brought before the Common Pleas Court in Cleveland have shown that of 3,197 convicted felons examined in the medical clinic only 42.3 percent were classified as normal. Fifty-five and nine-tenths percent were classed as defective delinquents and only 1.8 percent as insane. The outgrowth of this study has resulted in the drafting by the Cleveland Bar Association of a new criminal law for Ohio to be presented to the coming State Legislature. This bill provides for the creation of a new criminal class composed of what are called defective delinquents. This includes morons and others of abnormal mentality but not insane who commit felonies or misdemeanors. The purpose of this legislation is to afford special treatment for law violators falling within the new classification, making it possible to segregate delinquents in separate institutions. The Ohio law, like that of most other states, now recognizes only two types of criminals, sane and insane, and if not insane they must be punished.

It is proper that we should ask who is to blame for the abnormalities which render these young men incapable of making the necessary adaptation to our environment.

An important characteristic of the boys in the Cleveland school was their low intelligence. Practically all were recorded as retarded or mentally backward prior to their transfer to this institution.

It is important that we note the characteristics of groups that are similarly retarded, but who have not demonstrated sufficiently unsocial characters to have to be placed in the pre-delinquent groups. We shall recognize them as individuals who may never commit unsocial acts sufficient to get them into trouble, though they will doubtless continue in the group of mentally backward persons. Such a group is to be found in the Outwaithe School in Cleveland. The children in this school, which enrolls about one thousand students, were examined in order to ascertain whether there might be groups that are similarly afflicted physically. The school is distinctive because it has a very high percentage of children who are backward mentally. Many of these children have been concentrated there in order to bring them under the influence of special teachers. In an examination of a cross section of the children, almost all were found to have had distinct injury in the formative period, as evidenced by the changes in facial form. A preliminary survey of the backward children of this institution was made by having typical classes selected by an official of the school from ages ranging from eleven to seventeen. I examined the arches and made measurements of the head and face. With the assistance of the school nurse I obtained records of the other children in the families selected. This latter survey was supplemented by field work by the nurse. The intelligence quotients, as reported in the records, were also provided. In the twenty-nine individuals so studied, seven, or 25 percent were first children; fourteen, or 50 percent last children in the families. Only one individual was found with approximately normal dental arches, that is, approximately 3 percent of the individuals. Twenty-eight children, or 97 percent, had abnormality of one or both dental arches. These children were placed in this institution because they were backward mentally, although as a group they are comparable to the group studied in the Thomas A. Edison School, where the grouping was based on delinquent traits. A cursory examination was made by observing other pupils in this school in their classes and on the grounds. A large percentage of severe facial and dental arch deformities and a very high percentage with definite disturbances in facial growth were evident. These data are presented as applying to a group of individuals characterized by a disturbed mentality, to the extent that they were assigned to special classes for the mentally retarded. While the group constituting the school population at Outwaithe represented the relatively large group of pupils assigned to special classes for backward children and did not carry the stigmata of delinquency carried by those of the Thomas A. Edison School, both groups had many physical defects in common.

We are, accordingly, concerned with the relationship existing among various stages of mental backwardness, pre-delinquency and criminality. To throw light on this subject, I visited our State Penitentiary to observe the characteristics of facial and dental arch development of the individuals whose unsocial traits had brought them to this institution. I visited the dental clinic with the director, Dr. May, and saw the mouths of typical members of that colony as they were presented for oral examination. I asked the director what, if any, special features of the oral cavity he had observed to be characteristic of this group and different from those he had observed outside the institution in his private practice. He stated that he had noted continually that there was a tendency for the tongue to be too large for the mouth. This is a constant characteristic of another group of mentally injured, namely, the Mongoloid. This institution has a population of approximately four thousand individuals. A high percentage of them gave marked evidence of injury in the prenatal period as expressed in disturbances of facial form and the shape of the dental arches. In observing over half the population at work or exercise, I did not see one with a typically normal facial development. In Fig. 122 will be seen typical examples of this group. These show front and side views (see Hooton's recent book[3]).

Newspapers daily illustrated reports of crimes committed by young criminals show almost continually these evidences of prenatal injury. Note the two characters Bird and Nixon, Fig. 123.

It is important to emphasize the fact that the disturbances in the development of the head, face and brain may have a variety of expressions. In the more severe form characteristic of the Mongoloid group, as seen in Fig. 124

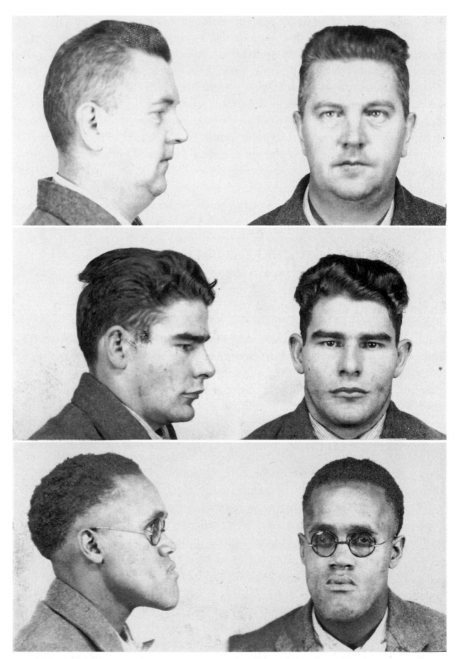

FIG. 122. Criminals. Were their unsocial traits related directly to incomplete brain organization associated with prenatal injury?

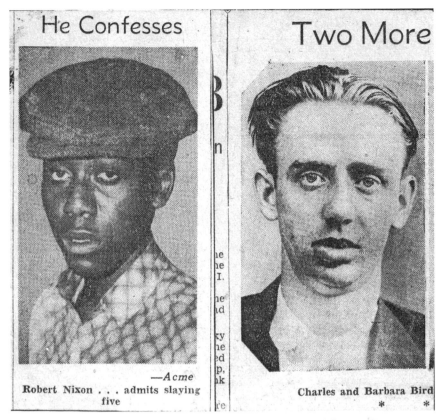

He Confesses

Two More

—Acme

Robert Nixon . . . admits slaying five

Charles and Barbara Bird
*   *

FIG. 123. Note the marked lack of normal facial development of these notorious young criminals. Nixon is only 18. These are typical samples seen frequently in the daily press.

the facial injury is typical and is associated with a mental disturbance which, in turn, has been shown to be associated with typical brain lesions. The individuals of that group, however, do not tend to be criminals. Indeed, their injury is too severe. As a group they are apt to be docile, tractable and happy. Indeed, in the mentally backward and criminal groups in their various stages, we find facial patterns typical of large numbers of individuals we see on the streets, who are in school or in business, and entirely capable of maintaining a respected and honorable position in society. Accordingly, it is not justified, and indeed would be entirely unfair, to associate their disturbed facial and dental arch development with traits that would be normally found in the grossly unsocial groups. We cannot by viewing the face evaluate the kind or extent of brain injury that is associated with prenatal malnutrition of that

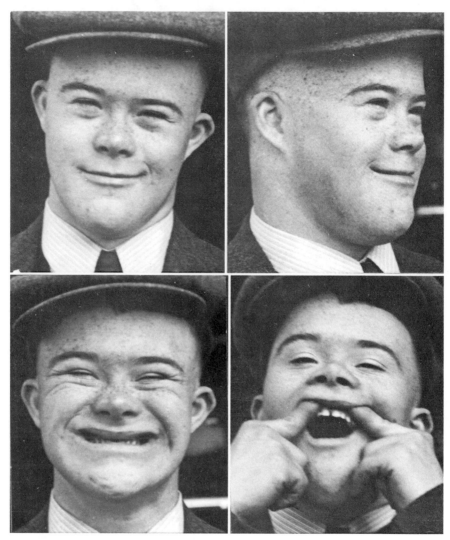

FIG. 124. This is a typical mongoloid defective. Note the marked lack of development of the middle third of the face and nose with the upper arch too small for the lower. Individuals of this type look alike and act alike and all have typical speech and behavior defects. These are now associated with definite defects in the brain. Nearly all are either a first or last child. A large percentage are born to mothers over forty years of age.

individual. Indeed, these various divergent facial patterns are accepted by our modern civilization as representative of the many varieties or patterns constituting a normal population. It is not until we see primitive groups living under a controlled natural environment that we see Nature's model and design of the human physiognomy.

We are concerned to know the percentage in any typical colony of our modern civilization that may be placed in the various classifications of normal, mildly backward mentally, severely backward mentally, unsocial, delinquent, criminal, idiots, epileptic and insane. Tredgold[2] reports two surveys in England and Wales which give figures on the proportion of the population that could be identified with definite lesions. It would be fortunate if a survey could be made in the United States that would indicate the extent of the increase in delinquents of various types, including racketeers and criminals. It would be very helpful if these data could be related to the degrees of prenatal injury. There are many phases of modern degeneration which lend themselves to study from the standpoint of the probable role of progressive decline in the efficiency of nutrition to the progressive increase in morbidity, mortality, mental deficiency and delinquency. This is discussed in the next chapter on Soil Depletion, Plant and Animal Deterioration.

From the point of view of this problem the differences between the modern white civilizations and many of the primitive groups is interesting. Criminal tendencies in isolated primitives are so slight that no prisons are required. I have referred to the Löetschental Valley in Switzerland, which, until recently, has been physically isolated from the process of modernization. For the two thousand inhabitants in that valley, there is no prison. In Uganda, Africa, the Ruanda tribes estimated to number 2.5 million, had no prisons.

Observation of Nature's normal facial patterns in the primitive racial stocks, establishes types within the limits of normality. The readers of this text by observing the individuals in any given families may see in how large a percentage of white families the progressive narrowing and lengthening of the face in the younger members of the family as compared with the older occurs. Further observations will enable one to recognize rapidly, even without experience and special training in anatomy, these evidences of prenatal injury.

I made a survey in the New England States, Quebec and Eastern Ontario, because the United States death rate from heart disease as reported by the American Heart Association was shown to be highest in Vermont and New Hampshire, followed closely by Massachusetts and New York. I first visited the New York State Hospital for tuberculosis patients at Raybrook, near Saranac. With the assistance of a member of the staff, I examined fifty young men and women in the wards. In that group, only three were found with normal facial and dental arch development. These three individuals were marble cutters who were suffering from silicosis. The forty-seven other individuals examined (94 percent) were found to have marked evidence of injury in the developmental period. At the state fair at Rutland, Vermont, to which residents came from various communities throughout the state, I was able to count, by observing and recording the individuals who passed, that in each 100 people, three out of four gave evidence of injury in the developmental period. Similar studies were made at the State Farm for delinquent boys and girls, almost all of whom had been before the courts. I found that a very high percentage, approximating 100 percent of those observed, had received injuries in the prenatal period. I then went to Quebec and studied groups of school children in the early teens. I observed groups in which a very high percentage gave marked evidence of prenatal injury. This seemed aggravated in districts where the farms had been abandoned, because the land was not producing as well as in the past. I studied Indians in two Indian Reservations, also, and there again found marked evidence of injury typical of our modernized communities. Similarly, a limestone district in Ontario was visited and critical observations were made of the facial form of the new generation in regions in which the fertility of the soil had been definitely depleted through exhaustion. These again showed evidence of prenatal injury through faulty nutrition. The prisoners in a jail were examined, and all of them except two habitual drunkards showed marked evidence of prenatal injury.

If space permitted, it would be interesting to include here a discussion and illustrations of the physical characteristics of the racketeers and criminals whose pictures are shown in our newspapers almost daily. It is rare that a normal face is depicted in this group.

As an approach to more detailed study of the available information regarding the processes that are involved in the production of facial deformities, it will be helpful to think of the face as constituting the floor of the anterior part of the brain. The pituitary body is situated on the underside of the brain just back of the eyes. It is the governing body for the activity of growth, and largely controls the functioning of several of the other glands of internal secretion. It is, as it were, the master of the ship. We are, accordingly, primarily concerned with the role that it plays, and the forces which control its own development and function. Its dependence upon vitamin E has been demonstrated by many workers. For example, Dr. M. M. O. Barrie[4] has reported that an inadequate amount of vitamin E produces marked disturbance in the growth of the offspring of rats. She states:

> The changes observed are similar in several ways to those produced by hypophysectomy (removal of pituitary gland). Marked degranulation of the anterior pituitary is found in both the abnormal young and the adult sterile animals. Lack of vitamin E therefore produces a virtual nutritional hypophysectomy in the young rat.

The work recently done in this field by Dr. Hector Mortimer and his associates in McGill University, Montreal, has included studies of skull development of rats. He has shown that the surgical removal of the pituitary body at the base of the brain in very young rats produces regularly a certain type of defect in skull development. This has been characterized by a lack of development forward of the muzzle or face, with a narrowing of the nose and dental arches. He found that by the addition of extracts made from the pituitary glands, which he had removed surgically, he entirely prevented the development of these defects, thereby establishing the relation of the injury to deficiencies of the hormones developed by that organ. Another approach to the problem on which he has expended much fruitful effort, has been in connection with the study of the skulls of individuals who are known to have disturbances in the functioning of the pituitary gland through the interference caused by tumors. Common illustrations are the cases of acromegaly or giantism. By associating these physical changes in bodily form with each x-ray, data obtained from skiagraphs, together with the history and the nature of the tumor, considerable information has been developed. Another important series of studies has included the correlation, by means of the x-rays, of the skulls of individuals suffering from certain types of physical and mental disturbances, with certain abnormalities in the skull as shown by the x-rays. By these various means Dr. Mortimer has been able to divide the various types of skull defects and developmental and growth defects into distinct classifications. With this yardstick he is able to classify individuals from their Roentgenograms. It is of interest that in his work, in association with Dr. G. Levine, Dr. A. W. Rowe and others at the Evans Memorial for Clinical Research and Neuro-Endocrine Research in Boston, important relationships have been established through the examination of over three thousand case histories. X-ray records of the skull are included in the studies. They report that independent and previous physiological investigations gave evidence at the time of the examination of disturbed pituitary function. Dr. Mortimer's excellent investigations seem to indicate clearly that facial and dental arch form are directly related to and controlled by the functioning of the pituitary body in the base of the brain. Dr. Barrie[4] reports that partial deficiency of vitamin E, as shown in the case of the female rat, results in the prolongation of gestation which may be continued as long as ten days beyond the normal period. The offspring under these conditions are abnormal. Further, animals deficient in vitamin E, occasionally give birth to a litter, but fail to lactate.

When we realize that one of the best sources of vitamin E is wheat germ, most of which is removed from white flour, usually along with four-fifths of the mineral, we see one cause of the tragedy that is overwhelming so many individuals in our modern civilization. In many individuals it may be wise to reinforce our modern white bread and starchy dietary with wheat germ, which can be obtained in package form from the manufacturers of flour. As this is put up in cans, all air is displaced with an inert gas when the cans are sealed. While in this way oxidation of the embryo which is very fragile, is prevented, as soon as the seal is broken, oxidation sets in and progresses rapidly, producing a product that is not comparable to the wheat embryo of freshly cracked whole wheat. My investigations indicate that Nature has put just the right amount of embryo in each grain of wheat to accompany that quantity of food. If the whole wheat is prepared and eaten promptly after grinding and exposing the embryo to oxidation, the effect desired by Nature is adequately provided.

It is important to emphasize in connection with the development of the deformities of the face that other skeletal deficiencies or abnormalities result from the same disturbing factors. One of these is the narrowing of the entire body, with a tendency to increase in height. This is shown in many of the family groups of modernized primitives. The effect of this narrowing of the body, which in girls results in the boyish type of figure due to the narrowing of the hips, introduces an entirely new and serious problem in the experience of our modern civilization when confronted with the problems of childbirth.

Among primitive races living in a primitive state, childbirth was a very simple and rapid process accompanied by little fear or apprehension; whereas, in the modernized descendants, even in the first and second generations of those individuals born to parents after they had adopted the foods of modern white civilizations, serious trouble was often experienced.

We have been considering the changes which take place in the skeletal growth as a result of the disturbances in the functioning of the pituitary body of the individual after birth, or of the mother during the prenatal period. We are also concerned with changes in the soft tissues, particularly the brain. I have presented data indicating that a very large percentage of mentally backward children have disturbances in facial development. The available data also indicate that a large percentage of those who are seriously injured in facial form have some disturbance in their mental or moral character. Whether there is relationship between the processes which develop these physical abnormalities in brain growth and mental efficiency, including emotional states and character traits, is now to be considered.

An important contribution has been made to this phase of the problem by Dr. James Papez, Professor of Anatomy at Cornell University,[5] who concludes his report:

> Is emotion a magic product, or is it a physiologic process which depends on an anatomic mechanism?...The evidence presented is...suggestive of such a mechanism as a unit within the larger architectural mosaic of the brain.

Research data have been presented which deal with the anatomical defects of the brain of individuals suffering from the typical mental and physical patterns of the so-called Mongolian idiot. In these cases the gyrus cinguli of the brain were found to be absent, which indicates the impossibility that these individuals function normally either physically or mentally.

Modern civilization has provided a large group of the defectives known as Mongolian idiots. They have very definite characteristics both physical and mental. Among the former, one of the most universal expressions is a vacant stare associated with a face that is markedly underdeveloped in the middle third, usually accompanied by narrow nostrils and a narrow upper dental arch.

One of the outstanding characteristics of the group is their inability to develop mentally beyond three to eight years of age. Because of the difficulty of building a character and intelligence level beyond infancy, these unfortunates are housed largely in state institutions for feebleminded. Since the physical picture is similar to that which occurs in a much less severe form in a large number of individuals in our modern civilization, it is important that we study this group in the light of the information that is available with regard to their physical, mental and moral characteristics, and in the light of such information as is available regarding their origin.

The surveys that have been made reveal the fact that nearly all of them are born to mothers more than forty years of age, and apparently at a period of very low efficiency in reproductive capacity. While most of the discussion and literature stress the importance of the age of the mother, some data are now available which throw responsibility also on the paternal side.

Korosi, as reported by Tredgold in *Mental Deficiency*, came to the conclusion as a result of the investigation of 24,000 unselected individuals that the children of fathers below twenty or above forty years of age are weaker than the children of fathers between these ages. Also, the children of mothers over forty years of age are weaker than those born to mothers below this age. Tredgold presents data connecting defective structures in the brain with certain phases of physical behavior and mental deficiencies. He quotes many authors whose data correspond with his own. Much of this material relates to accounts of incomplete prenatal development of nerve structures in the brain.

We are particularly interested in the origin and the nature of the brain lesions. Penrose,[6] in analyzing the relative etiologic importance of birth order and maternal age in Mongolism presents data obtained from an examination of 224 defectives in which the total number of children in all the families involved was 1,013. Accordingly, in these families approximately 20 percent were so affected. The average number of children per family was five and one-half.

He states:

> Mongolian imbeciles are very often born last in a long family. This fact, which was pointed out many years ago by Shuttleworth, has led clinicians to believe that Mongolism is to some extent a product of the exhaustion of maternal reproductive powers due to frequent child bearing.... The conclusion is widely accepted with the reservation that the affected child is not necessarily born at the end of the family. Several cases have been reported as first-born. There is, however, ample evidence that Mongolian imbeciles have a significantly later birth rank than normal children.

G. Ordahl[7] has reported on a study of ninety-one cases in which he found that fifty-six or 60 percent were the last born. The families averaged five children. He states that "uterine exhaustion is the most commonly advanced reason for Mongolism." Madge T. Macklin[8] says, "It is usually stated that it (Mongolism) occurs more frequently in the later pregnancies owing either to reproductive exhaustion or to too advanced age of the mother."

We are concerned at this point for evidence that will throw light on the relationship between the functioning of the pituitary body in the base of the brain and the development of this type of facial and mental deformity.

A striking case is that of a boy sixteen years of age who was a typical Mongolian idiot. He had two sisters who were much older than he. His mother was a partial invalid when he was born late in her life. We have no data relative to the details of the children who may have been lost. His father was living and well except for a railroad injury. This boy at the age of sixteen was infantile in many of his characteristics and developments. The genitals were those of a boy eight years old. The facial expression was that of the typical Mongolian idiot. By the Binet test he had a mentality of about four years. Roentgenograms of his hands showed that the epiphyseal bones had not united. He played on the floor with blocks and with rattles like a child. His interest was in children's activities. (Fig. 125.)

The outstanding physical characteristic was his maxillary arch which was so much smaller than the mandibular arch that it went entirely inside it. In order to give him a masticating surface, and with the hope of helping him both physically and mentally, since several cases had greatly benefited by such an operation, I determined to widen his arch by moving the maxillary bones apart about one-half inch. The position of his teeth before the moving of the bones is shown in Fig. 126. Roentgenograms showing the opening of the median suture with increase of pressure are also shown in Fig. 126. An important phase of this case was that the left nostril was entirely occluded, and probably had been all his life. A rhinologist spent half an hour trying to shrink the tissue with adrenalin and cocain sufficiently to get air or water through,

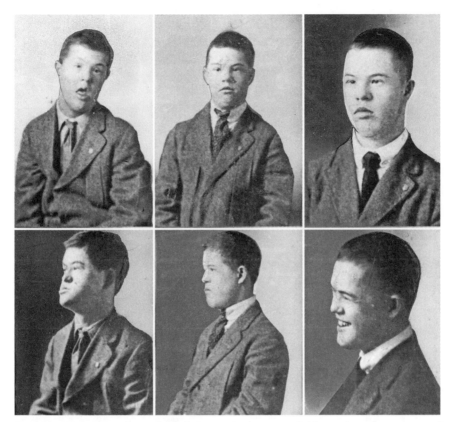

FIG. 125. These views show physical changes in the mongoloid type due to movement of maxillary bones to stimulate the pituitary gland in base of brain. Left, front and side view before, center, front and side view in thirty days. Right, front and side view six months after. Aged sixteen, infantile before, adolescent after operation.

and was not able to do so. The quantity of air that he was able to inhale through his right nostril was so scant that he continually breathed with his mouth open. At night he was forced to lie with something like his coat rolled into a hard ridge and placed under the back of his neck and his head pushed far back to a position that would open his mouth and retain it so, or he would awaken, strangling because of the closing of his mouth.

With the movement of the maxillary bones laterally, as shown progressively in Fig. 126, there was a very great change in his physical development and mentality. He grew three inches in about four months. His moustache started to grow immediately; and in twelve weeks' time the genitals developed from those of a child to those of a man, and with it a sense of modesty. His mental

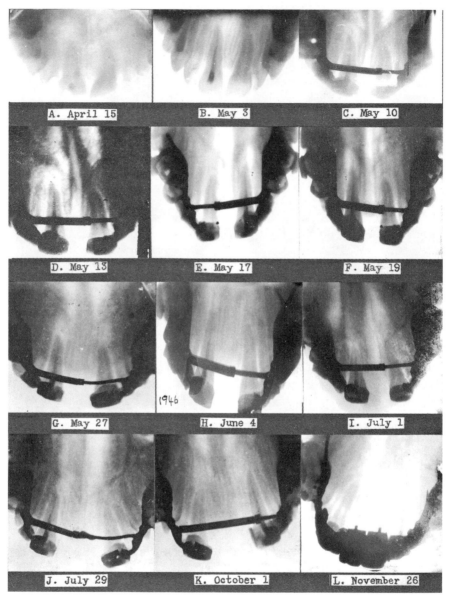

FIG. 126. These x-ray pictures show the position of the teeth before operation to move maxillary bones; and progressively, by the dates shown, the widening of the upper arch. In twelve weeks' time the boy passed through adolescence. New bone rapidly filled in the space between the separated bones. The space was retained with a fixed bridge carrying two additional teeth. His mother was nearly fifty when he was born.

change was even more marked. The space between the maxillary bones was widened about one-half inch in about thirty days. This lateral pressure on the maxillary bones was accomplished by rigid attachments to the teeth of the two sides of the upper arch. The outward movement of the maxillary bones (which form the roof of the mouth and sides of the nose) by pressure on the temporal bones produced a tension downward on the floor of the anterior part of the brain, thus stimulating the pituitary gland in the base of the brain. In a few weeks' time he passed through stages that usually take several years. At first, he got behind the door to frighten us; later, he put bent pins on chairs to see us jump when we sat down, and finally he became the cause of a policeman's coming to the office from where he was conducting traffic on the corner below to find who it was squirting water on him when his back was turned. He developed a great fondness for calling people over the telephone, wanted to borrow my automobile to take his mother for a drive, and with his arm caressingly about the shoulders of one of the secretaries, invited her to go with him to a dance. All this change developed in about twelve weeks.

A most remarkable event happened in connection with this procedure. He lived in another city, and so, while with me, stayed in a boarding house at a little distance from my office in order that he might have frequent, and almost constant attention. On his return to his home town, his efficiency had increased to such an extent that his mother could send him with the money to the grocery store with the order for the day's groceries, and he could bring back the right change and could tell when it was correct. He could also come alone to me ninety miles by railroad and make two changes of trains and the various transfers on the street cars of the city with accuracy and safety.

He wore an appliance in his mouth to keep the bones in position. This appliance became dislodged; the maxillary bones settled together; immediately, or in a day or two, he lapsed into his old condition of lethargy accompanied by an old trouble, which had frequently been distressing, namely, nausea, this sometimes lasting for twenty-four hours. With the readaptation of the separating appliance and the reconstruction of the retaining appliance, he returned rapidly to his improved condition.

During the period he was in my care, he had learned to read child stories and newspaper headings, and had spent much time doing so. The changes in his physical appearance are shown in Fig. 125, above, front view, and below, side view. The first picture at the left shows his appearance before the operation; the second, thirty days after; and the last, six months later. The opening produced in the upper arch in front of half an inch was filled by supplying two teeth on a restoration, which at the same time held the maxillary bones in their new position. In six months he had developed whiskers and moustache. The progressive changes in the position of the maxillary bones with the opening of the median suture are shown in Fig. 126, together with the mechanical appliance. In the last view, the restoration carrying the porcelain teeth to fill the space is shown.

A very important contribution to our knowledge of the cause of Mongolism has recently been published by Dr. Clemens E. Benda,[9] Clinical Director of the Wrentham State School, Wrentham, Massachusetts, in association with the Harvard Medical School of Boston. He and his group have approached the problem of Mongolism from two different angles; first, as to determine whether it is accidental, and second, whether it is a unit of symptoms which can be related to more essential alteration. Their studies including careful anatomical studies have been made on the basis of an examination of 125 Mongoloids. He states:

> Summarizing our investigations, the pituitary in mongoloids reveals a peculiar and definite pathology. On the basis of fourteen cases we feel justified in emphasizing that in mongolism definite failure of the pituitary development is to be found. Mongolism appears as a hypopituitarism of a specific type, in which the absence or deficiency of basophiles seems to be essential.

The evidence indicates that this severe type of facial and brain injury is related directly to a lowered reproductive capacity of the mother associated with age, since the majority are born to mothers beyond forty years of age, and to an inadequate nutrition of the mother, particularly in vitamin E since this vitamin plays so important a role in the nutrition of the pituitary body.

Important new data have been provided in an analysis of births in the United States in connection with the development of the Mongolian group. Bleyer[10] has reported a study of 2,822 cases. He reports that of the total births in the United States in 1934, of 1,095,939, there were 1,822 reported as Mongoloids. The average age of the mothers of these individuals was forty-one years. He reports data indicating that in the age group of mothers forty to forty-four the chances of the development of a Mongoloid would be seventy-five times as high as normal expectancy, and in the age forty-five to forty-nine the chances are 125 times normal expectancy. In a group of 1,942 Mongoloids, 1,100 or 57 percent were last children. These data are in keeping with those of several other investigators, and emphasize the problem of depleted reproductive capacity.

The interesting problems involved in the birth of identical twins throw light on the origin of both physical and mental characters. It is a matter of great significance in connection with these studies that anomalies which we can associate with parental deficient nutrition are reproduced in both twins. Important additional light has been thrown on this phase by a family of six pairs of fraternal twins born to the same parents. These are reported by Dr. William W. Greulich, of New Haven.[11] It is significant that nine of these individuals (one of the oldest pair is deceased, and the youngest twins are yet babes in arms) show marked narrowing of the nostrils and lack of development of the middle third of the face, narrowing of the face and tendency to be mouth-breathers. Further, the severity of this condition appears to be progressively more severe in the younger pairs of twins, sufficiently grown to show facial development. There is accordingly, evidence here of progressive lowering of reproductive efficiency, and the fact that both individuals are involved similarly has great significance, since they are fraternal twins arising from a single ovum. This seems clearly to relate this disturbance with a deficient germ plasm. Factors that are reproduced in identical twins would include both hereditary characters and those that are produced by a disturbance in environment resulting in an interference with normal hereditary processes. In a case of twins that are not identical, there is significance in the development of similar deformities which are likely to be of acquired origin rather than of hereditary origin. In Fig. 127 is seen a pair of twins. Note that they have similar disturbance in the development of the dental arches with the upper laterals depressed and the cuspids crowded outward in the arch.

A very important source of information which deals with the relation of disturbances of the physical development of the head and mentality is provided by a study of the members of the teen-age group who are classed as mentally backward. In an examination of a Cleveland school in a colored district that

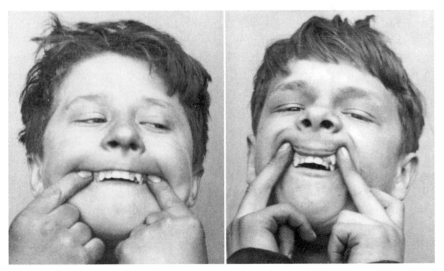

Fig. 127. These boys are twins, not identical. Note, however, both have same type of deformity of the dental arch, apparently due to the same cause.

has been set aside largely for boys and girls who are distinctly deficient in their ability to learn, it was disclosed that a very large percentage suffered from gross facial deformities when judged by these standards. Typical individuals in this group are shown in Fig. 128, one is white, lower left. It is clear that these boys were all physically injured in the formative period. Their clinical history indicates that the brain was involved in this disturbed development.

One of the problems involved in the development of the group of disturbances having physical and mental expressions, is associated with the sensitiveness of the body during the period of adolescence. Many students of degenerative problems have emphasized various phases of this large problem. Burt[12] commented: "It is almost as though crime were some contagious disease, to which the constitutionally susceptible were suddenly exposed at puberty, or to which puberty left them peculiarly prone." The age of adolescence is also the period of greatest susceptibility to dental caries. Data derived from chemical studies of the blood and saliva show that in this period of susceptibility to dental caries the supplies of minerals and vitamins are inadequate to meet Nature's demands, and the system borrows minerals from the skeleton to maintain vital processes. Lichtenstein and Brown[13] report data which reveal that educational quotients, like intelligence quotients, fall with increase in age during the years of developing puberty. They show that the educational quotient at nine years of age for the group studied was 100; at eleven years of age, 89; at twelve years, 83; and at thirteen years, 74. The changes in facial and dental arch form, which I have described at length in this volume, develop in this age period also, not as a result of faulty nutrition of the individual but as the result of distortions in the architectural design in the very early part of the formative period. Apparently, they are directly related to qualities in the germ plasm of one or both parents, which result from nutritional defects in the parent before the conception took place, or deficient nutrition of the mother in the early part of the formative period. Case records show that the first signs of delinquency generally make their appearance during these years. The age reported most frequently was that of thirteen.

One expression of the rate of the progressive degeneration that is taking place in the United States is the increase in delinquency and crime in young people between twelve and twenty years of age, as well as in crime in general. Edgar Hoover, Director of the Bureau of Investigation, has recently published data showing comparative figures for 1936 and 1937, during which time crimes in the United States increased from 1,333,526 to 1,415,816, an increase of six percent. This increase is occurring in spite of the rapid development of social organizations for improving the environment.

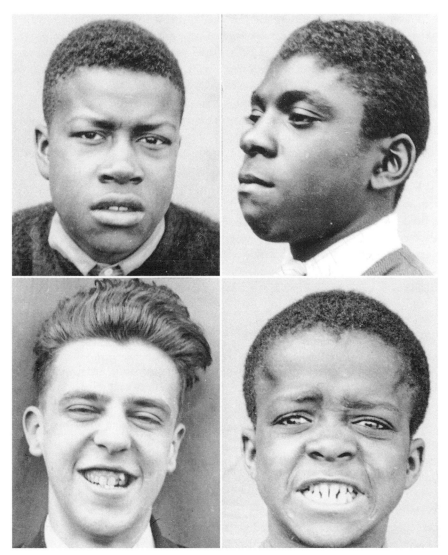

FIG. 128. These four boys are typical of a group of several hundred in a special school for backward children. Practically all showed some evidence of incomplete facial and dental arch development. The range of defects is wide. Blacks are similarly injured as whites. This is inhibited heredity.

Preventive measures among the unsocial group, who pass through the stages of predelinquency and crime, have been almost entirely confined to improvement in the social surroundings of the growing youth. While, no doubt, individuals with a low factor of safety are less likely to develop serious criminal tendencies under favorable environments, such factors as constitute a first-conditioning force, i.e., injury of the germ plasm, and deficient nutrition in the developmental period are not corrected by these efforts. These new data relating to the nature of the underlying causes strongly emphasize the need for beginning much earlier. Indeed, the preparation for the next generation should begin early in the life of the preceding generation.

Many investigators have emphasized the sensitiveness of the nervous system to disturbances in the formative period. Considerable data have been presented indicating that the tissues of the nervous system are the most easily affected of all the structures of the body. The extent of the injuries to the nervous system vary through a wide range.

Harris in his chapter on "Congenital Abnormalities of the Skeleton" in Blacker's[14] *Chances of Morbid Inheritance* has presented data indicating the sensitive period at which the ovum is most likely to be injured:

> Few normal human embryos have been subjected to careful study. The vast majority of human embryos examined have been abnormal, and it is their abnormality which has led to their abortion between the sixth and thirteenth weeks of embryonic life, a critical period associated with the development of the placenta, during which the death rate is probably in the neighborhood of at least 15 percent.

In tracing the development of the human embryo, he tells why the growth process is very different from that of the development of embryos of lower forms. He states regarding deformed ova: "Ova that survive the eighth week tend to live on to term, and are born as monsters." I have referred previously to a personal communication from Professor Shute, of the University of Western Ontario, which states that he had been impressed with the high percentage of deformities in aborted fetuses. This seems to be Nature's method of eliminating defective individuals. Harris says further:

> It is sometimes suggested that threatened abortions in early pregnancy should not be treated by rest and quiet, as it is quite possible that the uterus is attempting to rid itself of a pathological ovum which might become a monster in the future.

The available data emphasize strongly that a very small percentage of the total gross deformities ever develop to menace society. Harris quotes Mall:[15]

> He estimated from the records of 100,000 pregnancies that there were 80,572 normal births, 11,765 abortions of normal embryos and early mon-

sters, and 615 monsters born at term. Thus at term 1 child in 132 is born with some anatomical defect. For each such case appearing at term, 12 others died and were aborted during pregnancy.

These data deal with gross defects involving physical deficiencies in the infant and indicate that the defects that are produced in the formative period, which are less severe than the above, are not recognizable at birth and may not be until long afterwards. According to Harris, "During the fourth week of embryonic life the head, brain and spinal cord are most susceptible to adverse conditions." He traces the sensitive areas of the various structures through the various weeks in the embryonic history. The deformities of the face among the primitive races which I have illustrated extensively frequently are not revealed until the eruption of the permanent dentition and the development of the adult features. While it is true that many children show deformity in facial development even in babyhood and childhood, those individuals are usually much more seriously injured when the adult face is developed.

Bloom[16] has presented the anatomical and histological characteristics of a defective born to a mother fifty-one years of age, whose general health was reported as good. The infant's facial pattern was markedly divergent from normal and practically no brain tissues had been formed. This expression of an extreme injury was entirely beyond that with which we are concerned in the study of the mental and the moral cripples who constitute an increasing part of our society. This is presented to emphasize Nature's inexorable requirement that each parent shall be individually physically fit for the responsibility of producing the next generation. Several primitive races studied have realized this responsibility.

There are some phases of modern physical degeneration in which most of us take part with remarkable complacency. We would consider it a great misfortune and disgrace to burn up the furniture in our homes to provide warmth, if fuel were available for the collection. This is precisely what we are doing with our skeletons by a process of borrowing, simply because we fail to provide new body repairing material each day in the food. You are all familiar with the tragic misfortune that overtakes so many elderly people through the accident of a broken hip or other fractured bone. Statistics show that approximately 50 percent of fractured hips occurring in people beyond 65 years of age never unite. We look upon this as one of the inevitable consequences of advancing age. In Chapter 15, I have referred to the small boy whose leg was broken when he fell in a convulsion while walking across the kitchen floor. That bone did not break because the blow was hard but because the minerals had been borrowed from the inside by the blood stream in order to maintain an adequate amount of the minerals, chiefly calcium and phosphorus in the blood and body fluids. He had been borrowing from his skeleton for months because due to a lack of vitamins he could not absorb even the minerals that were present in the inadequate food that he was eating. The calcium and the phosphorus of the milk were in the skimmed milk that he was using but he needed the activators of the butter-fat in order to use the minerals. Simply replacing white bread with these activators and the normal minerals and vitamins of wheat immediately checked the convulsions.

We have many other expressions of this borrowing process. Much of what we have thought of as so-called pyorrhea in which the bone is progressively lost from around the teeth thus allowing them to loosen, constitutes one of the most common phases of the borrowing process. This tissue with its lowered defense rapidly becomes infected and we think of the process largely in terms of that infection. A part of the local process includes the deposit of so-called calculus and tartar about the teeth. These contain toxic substances which greatly irritate the flesh starting an inflammatory reaction. Many primitive peoples not only retain all of their teeth, many of them to an old age, but also have a healthy flesh supporting these teeth. This has occurred in spite of the fact that the primitives have not had dentists to remove the deposits and no means for doing so for themselves. Note particularly the teeth of the Eskimos. The teeth are often worn nearly to the gum line and yet the gum tissue has not receded. Many of these primitive groups were practically free from the affection which we have included in the general term of pyorrhea or gingivitis. Pyorrhea in the light of our newer knowledge is largely a nutritional problem. While nutrition alone often will not be adequate for correcting it, when established practically no treatment will be completely adequate without reinforcing the nutrition in so far as deficient nutrition has been a contributing factor. Nutrition plus the frequent removal of deposits, plus suitable medication will check and prevent pyorrhea but not correct the damage that has already been done. The elements that are chiefly needed in our nutrition are those that I have outlined as being particularly abundant in the menus as used by several of the primitive races. These are discussed in detail in Chapter 15.

Another important aspect of this problem of borrowing has to do with the progressive shrinking of the skeleton as evidenced by the shortening of the stature. I have measured many individuals who have lost from two to six inches in height in a decade or two. I have seen a few individuals who have lost as much as ten inches of their height by this process of borrowing from the skeleton. Our bodies need a certain amount of fresh minerals every day with which to manufacture blood. The days that these minerals are not provided in the foods they will be taken from our storage depots, the skeleton.

A particularly tragic phase of this problem of borrowing from the bone is seen in growing girls and is chiefly due to their ambition to avoid enlargement of their bodies to keep down their weight. The girls deprive themselves of body-building material at a time when their bodies are growing and are requiring considerable new minerals. Forming bone has a prior claim on minerals, which is sufficiently commanding to induce the individual to borrow from bones that are already formed to provide for the necessary lengthening and growth. By this process many of the bones of the body are softened, particularly the bones of the spine. Curvatures develop, one of the expressions of which may be round or stooped shoulders.

Among primitive races this type of girl, so commonly seen in our modern civilization, is absent. Probably not one of these girls has ever suspected the suffering and sorrow that is being stored up for future life as a result of this bad management at a critical time in her development. Fig. 134 illustrates one of the tragedies of this borrowing process. Practically all of these physical evidences of degeneration can be prevented and fortunately many of them can be relieved in large part with an adequate nutrition. Even ununited fractures often can be induced to unite by an adequate reinforcement of the nutrition. This is true not only for young people but for elderly people as well.

In addition to the problems growing out of physical injuries through lack of development before birth, which express themselves as facial and other deformities, there is increasing need for concern for physical handicaps entailed in underdevelopment of the hips. The difficulty encountered at childbirth in our modern civilization has been emphasized by Dr. Kathleen Vaughan[17] of London. In her book, *Safe Childbirth*, she states that faults of development more than race modify pelvic shape. In the Foreword to her book, Dr. Howard A. Kelly, Professor Emeritus of Gynaecological Surgery, Johns Hopkins University, says:

> Dr. Vaughan presents such an array of facts and data that the book must impress every reader. It is of vital importance that her conclusions be considered, for in my opinion our methods of bringing up our girls and the habits of our women with many of the customs of "civilized" life must be radically readjusted.

This important work should be made available for reference in the school libraries of the United States. Further data from it are presented in Chapter 21.

The great contrast in discomfort and length of time of the labor of modern mothers is to be contrasted with ease of childbirth among primitive mothers. Many workers among the primitive races have emphasized the vigorous health and excellence of the infant at birth. We have here, therefore, emphasis on the need in the interest of the infant that the mother shall have an easy and short labor. Both of these factors are directly influenced by the vitamin content of the mother's body as supplied by her nutrition and also by the physical development of her body if her mother at the time of gestation and prior to conception had adequate vitamins in her food to insure perfect germ cells.

The sensitivity of the brain to injury resulting from medication given the mother has been emphasized by Dr. Frederic Schreiber of Detroit. In his paper before the American Medical Association meeting in San Francisco, June, 1938, he was quoted as saying[18] that the analysis showed that 72 percent of the children had shown difficulty in breathing at the time of birth or in the first few days following birth. He concluded, therefore, that this difficulty in breathing was the cause of the brain damage.

Difficulty in breathing would lead to a shortage of oxygen. An insufficient supply of oxygen in the blood stream would have serious effects upon the tissues of the brain. In this connection, he cited evidence found in post-mortem examinations that deficiency of oxygen caused microscopic changes in the brain.

X-ray photographs of some of the children examined by Dr. Schreiber showed various degrees of brain atrophy.

The contribution of Dr. Schreiber also emphasizes strongly the susceptibility of the brain tissue to injuries which may handicap the individual throughout life.

REFERENCES

[1] LAIRD, D. The tail that wags the nation. *Rev. of Revs.*, 92:44, 1935.

[2] TREDGOLD, A. F. *Mental Deficiency (Amentia)*. Ed. 5. New York, William Wood, 1929.

[3] HOOTON, E. A. *Crime and the Man*. Cambridge, Harvard University Press, 1939.

[4] BARRIE, M. M. O. Nutritional anterior pituitary deficiency. *Biochem. J.* In press.

[5] PAPEZ, J. A proposed mechanism of emotion. *Arch. Neur. and Psychiat.*, 38:713, 1937.

[6] PENROSE, L. S. The relative aetiological importance of birth order and maternal age in Mongolism. *Proc. Roy. Soc. Lond.*, 115:431, 1934.

[7] ORDAHL, G. Birth rank of Mongolians: Mongolism, definite form of mental deficiency, found more frequently in the later birth ranks. *J. Hered.*, 18:429, 1927.

[8] MACKLIN, M. T. Primogeniture and developmental anomalies. *Human Biol.*, 1:382, 1929.

[9] BENDA, A. E. Studies in the endocrine pathology of mongoloid deficiency. *Proc. Am. A. Ment. Deficiency*, 43:151, 1938.

[10] BLEYER, A. Idiocy—the role of advancing maternal age. *Proc. Am. Assn. Ment. Defic.*, 61:

[11] GREULICH, W. W. The birth of six pairs of fraternal twins to the same parents. *J.A.M.A.*, 110:559, 1938.

[12] BURT, C. L. *The Young Delinquent.* London, University of London Press, 1925.

[13] LICHTENSTEIN, M. and BROWN, A. W. Intelligence and achievement of children in a delinquency area. *J. Juvenile Research*, 22:1, 1938.

[14] BLACKER, C. P. *Chances of Morbid Inheritance.* Baltimore, William Wood, 1934, Chapter 18.

[15] MALL, F. P. On the frequency of localized anomalies in human embryos and infants at birth. *Am. J. Anat.*, 22:49, 1917.

[16] BLOOM, D. D. Abnormalities encountered in dissection of the head and neck of an anencephalic monster. *J. Dent. Res.*, 16:226, 1937.

[17] VAUGHAN, K. *Safe Childbirth.* Baltimore, William Wood, 1937.

[18] SCHREIBER, F. Brain Damage at Childbirth. *Cleveland Press*, June 23, 1938.

Chapter 20

SOIL DEPLETION AND PLANT AND ANIMAL DETERIORATION

THE DATA available on the subject of soil depletion and animal deterioration are so voluminous that it would require a volume to present them adequately. When we realize the quantities of many of the minerals which must enter into the composition of the bodies of human beings and other animals, we appreciate the difficulty of providing in pasture and agricultural soils a concentration of these minerals sufficient to supply the needs for plant growth and food production.

If we think of growing plants and grasses in terms of average soil tilled to a depth of seven inches, we are dealing with a total of approximately two million pounds of soil per acre, of which two thousand pounds will be phosphorus in its various chemical forms, some of which will not be readily available for plants. If one-half of this phosphorus were present in an available form, there would be enough for only one hundred poor crops, utilizing ten pounds to the acre for the seed alone; or for forty good crops, taking twenty-five pounds per acre, assuming that the seed were to be removed from that land and not replaced. A sixty-bushel crop of wheat or corn per acre takes twenty-five to twenty-eight pounds of phosphorus in the seed. The soil is depleted of calcium similarly, though that mineral is not usually present in such limited amounts nor so rapidly taken away as is phosphorus. The leaves and stems of rapidly growing young plants and grasses are rich in calcium and phosphorus. As the plants ripen the phosphorus is transported in large amounts to the seed while most of the calcium remains in the leaves. A large part of the commerce of the world is concerned with the transportation of chemical elements as foods, chief of which are calcium and phosphorus. Whether the product of the soil is ultimately used as wheat for bread, milk and meat for foods, or wool and hides for clothing, every pound of these products that is shipped represents a depletion of soil for pasturage or for grain production.

If we think of one hundred good crops constituting the limit of capacity of the best soils, and one-fourth of that for a great deal of the acreage of the tillable soil, we are probably over-generous. This problem of depletion may seem to many people unimportant, either because there has been no consciousness that depletion has been taking place, or because they believe that replenishment is a simple matter.

In correspondence with government officials in practically every state of the United States I find that during the last fifty years there has been a reduction in capacity of the soil for productivity in many districts, amounting to from 25 to 50 percent. I am informed also that it would cost approximately fifty dollars per acre to replenish the supply of phosphorus.

Many people realize that farms they knew in their childhood have ceased to be productive because they have "run out." The movement of population to cities and towns is, in part, the result of the call of the social center and in part a consequence of the need of forsaking depleted soil. While there are many things that influence the movement from the farms, there is much to be learned from the government census reports which deal directly with farm acreage and values.

If we relate the levels of life of human and domestic animals to the problem of soil depletion, we find two important groups of data. First, there are those which relate to specific land areas, some small and some very large; and second, those which relate to civilizations and groups, both large and small that have passed out of existence or are rapidly deteriorating. A study of the skeletons of the past and present often discloses a progressive breakdown. For example, we may mention the important anthropological findings of Professor Hooton of Harvard, who, in his examinations of various pueblos of the Western Plains, especially at the Pecos Pueblo where the progressive burials have been uncovered, has brought to light the calendar of a civilization extending over a thousand years. These findings show that there has been over the period of years a progressive increase in skeletal deformities, including arthritis and dental caries, together with a reduction in stature, suggesting a direct relationship to progressive depletion of the soil.

In a recent magazine article, I have presented data[1] comparing the mineral content of different pasture grasses, and relating these to deficiencies in cattle. Unfortunately, space does not permit reviewing these data here in detail. They show that calcium varied from 0.17 percent for a dry pasture grass in Arizona to 1.9 percent in a Pennsylvania pasturage plant, to 2 percent in a British Columbia pasturage plant, a range of over tenfold. Similarly, phosphorus was shown to vary from 0.03 percent to 1.8 percent, a range of sixty fold. Neither pasture animals nor human beings can eat a sufficient amount of low mineral plant food to provide the total mineral requirements of ordinary metabolism. In cases of overload, such as pregnancy and lactation in adults, and rapid growth in children, the demand is increased greatly. For example, a high-milk-production cow from southern Texas on a certain low mineral pasture will run behind her normal requirements about 60 grams of phosphorus and 160 grams of potassium per day. In that district large numbers of cattle were unable at the time to maintain their own bodies, let alone reproduce or provide milk. Many cattle in the district developed loin disease. It was found that moving them to another plot of ground where the soil was not depleted provided recovery.

About thirty-seven billion dollars, or approximately 40 percent of the cash income of salaries and wages of the people in the United States, is used for the purchase of foods. When we add to this the expenditure of energy by the people living on the land, it represents a total, probably exceeding fifty billion dollars a year that is spent for the chemicals that are provided in the foods, a large amount of which, perhaps 50 percent, will have been expended for calcium and phosphorus, perhaps 25 percent for other chemicals, and 25 percent for special vitamin or activator carrying foods. Of this enormous transportation of minerals from the soil an exceedingly small proportion gets back to the tillable land in this country. Orr[2] states that "Consumption in the United Kingdom of livestock products mostly derived from grass lands has been estimated at about four hundred million pounds sterling per annum (*nearly two billion dollars*)." This includes dairy products, meats and hides. Never in the history of the world has there been such a large scale depletion of the soil by transportation away from the tilled and pasturage areas. Sickness in the United States has been calculated to cost nearly half as much as food, and is increasing.

An important discovery has been made with regard to the feeding of dairy cattle and other livestock: the nutritive value of young grass, when in a state of rapid growth, carries not only a very large quantity of minerals, but also digestible proteins in amounts that are approximately equivalent to those provided by the concentrated cereal cattle foods, such as linseed cake. It is observed also that not only do the milk products of such cows remain at a high level while the cows are on the rapidly growing young grass, particularly a rapidly growing young wheat grass or young rye grass, but the animals themselves are in better physical condition than when on grain concentrates. Further, that calves fed on the milk of those cows grow much more rapidly than they do when the cows are on other fodder and have a much higher resistance to disease. Grass, to provide these nutritional factors, must be grown on a very rich, well-balanced soil. A young plant, of necessity, produces a rapid depletion of soil. Minerals and other chemicals are removed and therefore there is need for adequate replacement.

In Chapter 18 I have reported investigations made by Professors Meigs and Converse at the Beltsville Experimental Station, in which they have shown that feeding cattle on a grade of dried hay that was low in chlorophyll resulted in the development of dead or blind calves, and further that when the milk of these cows was fed to three normal calves they died in fifty-seven, sixty-two and seventy-one days respectively. These calves had been fed on whole milk until twenty days of age. They show that the main deficiency in this ration was vitamin A.

Since mammals require milk in infancy and since it is the most efficient single food known, I have made a special study of milk and its products. The role of the vitamins and other activating substances in foods is quite as important and essential as that of minerals. These activating substances, in general, can be divided into two groups, those that are water-soluble and those that are fat-soluble, the former being much more readily obtained in most communities, than the latter. Since the fat-soluble and also the water-soluble vitamins are essential for mineral utilization and particularly since the fat-soluble activators are so frequently found to be inadequately supplied in diet and are usually more difficult to obtain, a special effort has been made to determine the level of these in dairy products in many different places for different seasons of the year. To accomplish this, I have obtained each year since 1927 samples of cream and butter, mostly butter, for analysis for their activator content. The work has rapidly extended so that for the eleventh year we are receiving now (1939) samples from several hundred places distributed throughout the world, usually once or twice a month throughout the year. Methods used for these studies are both biologic and chemical. These data are used in connection with morbidity and mortality statistics for the same districts.

The progressive changing of the levels of life is shown by the morbidity and mortality statistics of the various areas of the United States and Canada. The American Heart Association publishes, from time to time, very important data relative to the number of deaths from heart disease in the various states of the Union. It is of interest to note that the highest mortality levels that are obtained are found in those states, in general, that have been longest occupied by modern civilizations, namely, the Atlantic States, the New England States, the Great Lakes States and the Pacific States. Their data published in their booklet *Heart Disease Mortality Statistics* and based on the United States Registration area reveal that the death rate per 100,000 population was 123 in 1900. The data sent me in November 1937 from the United States Census Bureau, Department of Commerce, in Washington, report the death rate from heart disease per 100,000 for 1934 as 239.9, in other words an increase of 86.9 percent in thirty-four years. Figures provided by the Bureau of Census for England and Wales show the death rate per 100,000 to be 269.3; and for Scotland, 232. While the average figure for the United States Registration area of 224 deaths per 100,000 seems very high, it is exceedingly important to note that the New England States were much higher, leading the entire country. Massachusetts reported 307.3; New Hampshire, 323.1; Vermont, 310.8; New York, 302.1; Maine, 297.5. The rate of increase in the decade of 1921 to 1930 was 51.3 percent for Delaware; 52 percent for Connecticut, 51 percent for Pennsylvania, 59.4 percent for Missouri, 60.0 percent for Washington; 55 percent for Wisconsin; 64 percent for Louisiana; 71 percent for Florida; 63 percent for South Carolina; 81 percent for Montana; 61 percent for Kentucky; and 51.9 percent for North Carolina. Such rates of increase as these are cause for alarm.

Sir Arnold Theiler, who spent a quarter of a decade studying the problems of nutritional deficiency diseases among pasture animals in South Africa, has discussed at length the reduction of phosphorus in available quantities for plant development as constituting, by far, the most important mineral deficiency. He reported data obtained from many countries through the world, indicating that the deterioration of cattle and sheep can be directly traced to an inadequate amount of phosphorus in the soil. He states, in discussing the relation of this problem to the conditions as they found in Australia, that:[3]

> Amongst the Australian data the figures showing depletion of phosphorus as a result of sale of products off the farm without adequate replacement by manuring, are interesting. Thus Richardson estimates that it would take two million tons of superphosphate to replace the phosphorus removed in the form of milk, mutton and wool. In the "ranching stage" of the development of a country the fact is often forgotten that the balance of Nature is frequently disturbed to the detriment of generations to come.

It is important to keep in mind that morbidity and mortality data for many diseases follow a relatively regular course from year to year, with large increases in the late winter and spring and a marked decrease in summer and early autumn. The rise and fall of the level of morbidity with the changing season produces curves that are exceedingly regular for the same place from year to year. The distribution, however, is distinctly different for different latitudes and altitudes. It is further of special importance to note that the curves for the Southern Hemisphere, with its opposite seasons, are in reverse of those of the Northern Hemisphere, and have very similar levels for the same seasonal periods. I have obtained the figures for the levels of morbidity for several diseases in several countries, including the United States and Canada. I find that the distribution of the rise and fall in morbidity and mortality does not follow the sunshine curve but does follow the curve of vegetable growth. Accordingly, I have made studies by dividing the United States and Canada into sixteen districts, four from East to West and four from North to South. I have plotted by months the levels of mortality for heart disease and pneumonia in these various districts, from figures obtained from the governments of these two countries. Similarly, I have plotted curves for the vitamin content found in butter and cream samples obtained from these sixteen districts. When these are arranged in accordance with the levels by months they are found, in each case, to be opposite to the mortality from heart disease and pneumonia. It is also important to note that while these curves show a higher midsummer level of vitamins in dairy products in the northern tier of districts, the period of high level is shorter than in the more southern division. Two peaks tend to appear in the summer cycle of curves for the vitamins, one representing the spring period of active growth and the other, the fall period. These peaks are closer together in the north than in the south.

A particularly important phase of this study is the finding of a lower level of vitamins throughout the year in those districts which correspond with the areas of the United States and Canada that have been longest settled, and consequently most depleted by agriculture. A similar study has been made based on the data published in a report by Tisdall, Brown and Kelley,[4] of Toronto. Their figures for children's diseases which included chicken pox, measles, nephritis, scarlet fever, hemorrhage of newborn, tetany and retropharyngeal abscess were arranged according to the incidence for each month. All of these diseases show a relatively high incidence during February and March, rising in December and January, falling during April and May, reaching a very low level in midsummer and then making a rapid increase during the autumn. These are opposite to the vitamin levels found in the dairy products of Ontario for the same months.

In Chapter 3, I discussed data obtained during two summers in the Löetschental and other Swiss valleys. The Löetschental Valley has been isolated from contact with surrounding civilizations by its unique physical environment. For twelve hundred years during which time a written history of the valley has been kept, the people have maintained a high level of physical excellence providing practically all their food, shelter and clothing from the products raised in the valley. Cattle and goats provided milk, milk products and meat. The stock was carefully sheltered during the inclement weather and great care was used to carry back to the soil all of the enrichment. This, of course, is a process that is efficiently carried out in many parts of the world today. In this manner extensive depletion of the minerals required for food for animals and human beings may be prevented. Their practice is in striking contrast to that in many of the agricultural districts of the United States in which the minerals are systematically shipped from the land to the cities, there to be dissipated to the ocean through the sewerage system. Among many primitive races there is some attempt to preserve the fertility of the soil. For example, in Africa, many of the tribes that depend in part on agriculture, cleared off only a few acres in the heart of a forest and cropped this land for a limited number of years, usually less than ten. Great care was taken to prevent the loss of the humus both through drenching rains and wind erosion. The decaying vegetation and lighter soil that might be dislodged by the water were caught in the entanglement of roots and shrubbery surrounding the agricultural patch. The surrounding trees protect the soil from wind erosion. Care was taken not to form gullies, furrows and grooves that could carry currents of water and thus float away the valuable humus from the soil. This again is in contrast to conditions in other parts of the world, particularly in the United States. Sears[5] has stated that "Bare ground left by the plow will have as much soil washed off in ten years as the unbroken prairie will lose in four thousand. Even so, soil in the prairie will be forming as fast as, or faster than it is lost."

In Nature's program, minerals are loaned temporarily to the plants and animals and their return to the soil is essential. To quote again from Sears:

> What is lent by earth has been used by countless generations of plants and animals now dead and will be required by countless others in the future. In the case of an element such as phosphorus, so limited is the supply that if it were not constantly being returned to the soil, a single century would be sufficient to produce a disastrous reduction in the amount of life.

The history of preceding civilizations and cultures of mankind indicate the imbalances that have developed when minerals have been permanently transferred from the soil. There are only a few localities in the world where great civilizations have continued to exist through long periods and these have very distinct characteristics. It required only a few centuries, and in some profligated systems a few decades to produce so serious a mineral depletion of the soil that progressive plant and animal deterioration resulted. In such instances, regular and adequate replenishment was not taking place.

The replenishment may be made, as in the case of the prairie with its plant and animal life, through a replacement in the soil of borrowed minerals, a program carried out efficiently by a few intelligent civilizations. The balance of the cultures have largely failed at this point. Another procedure for the replenishing of the depleted soils is by the annual spring overflow of great water systems which float enrichment from the highlands of the watersheds to the lower plains of the great waterways. This is illustrated by the history of the Nile which has carried its generous blanket of fertilizing humus and rich soil from the high interior of Africa northward over its long course through Sudan and Egypt to the Mediterranean, and thus made it possible for the borders of the Nile to sustain a population of greater density than that of either China or India. The salvation of Egypt has been the fact that the source of the Nile has been beyond the reach of modernizing influences that could destroy Nature's vast stores of these replenishing soil products. Where human beings have deforested vast mountainsides at the sources of the great waterways, this whole problem has been changed.

A similar situation has occurred in China. Her two great rivers, the Yangtze and the Yellow River, having their sources in the isolated vastness of the Himalayas in Tibet, have through the centuries provided the replenishment needed for supporting the vast population of the plains of these great waterways. Together with this natural replenishment the Chinese have been exceedingly efficient in returning to the soil the minerals borrowed by the plant and animal life. Their efficiency as agriculturists has exceeded that of the residents of most parts of the populated world.

The story in Europe and America has been vastly different in many districts. The beds of roots of trees and grasses that hold the moisture and induce precipitation have been rudely broken up. An important function of the plant and tree roots is the entanglement of dead plant life. Vegetation holds back moisture at the time of melting snows and rainy seasons so efficiently that disastrous floods are prevented and a continuing flow of water maintained over an extended period. Under the pressure of population more and more of the highlands have been denuded for agriculture; the forests have often been ruthlessly burned down, frequently with the destruction of very valuable timber. The ashes from these great conflagrations provided fertilizer for a few good crops, but these chemicals were dissipated rapidly in the swift flow of the water in which they were soluble, with the result that vast areas that Nature had taken millenniums to forest have been denuded and the soil washed away in a few decades. These mountainsides have become a great menace instead of a great storehouse of plant food material for the plains country of the streams. Loss of timber which was needed greatly for commerce and manufacture has been another disastrous result. The heavy rains of the spring now find little impediment and rush madly toward the lower levels to carry with them not the rich vegetable matter of the previous era, but clay and rocks which in a mighty rush spread over the vast plains of the lowlands. This material is not good soil with which to replenish and fertilize the river bottoms. On the contrary, it often covers the plains country with a layer of silt many feet deep making it impossible to utilize the fertile soil underneath.

We have only to look over the departed civilizations of historic times to see the wreckage and devastation caused by these processes. The rise and fall in succession of such cultures as those of Greece, Rome, North Africa, Spain, and many districts of Europe, have followed the pattern which we are carving so rapidly with the rise and fall of the modernized culture in the United States.

The complacency with which the masses of the people as well as the politicians view our trend is not unlike the drifting of a merry party in the rapids above a great cataract. There seems to be no appropriate sense of impending doom.

An outstanding example of our profligate handling of soil and watersheds may be seen in our recent experiences in the Mississippi Basin. The Ohio River draining the western slopes of the Allegheny Mountains has gone on rampages almost annually for a decade carrying with it great damage to property and loss of life. Other branches of the Mississippi, particularly the Missouri, draining the eastern slopes of the Rocky Mountains have gone out of control so that vast areas are flooded with silt. There is now a concerted effort to stem this series of cataclysms by building dykes along the great waterways to raise the banks and dams in the higher regions of the watershed to hold back the floods. These artificial lakes become settling pools for the silt and soon lose their efficiency by being filled with the debris that they are holding back from the lower levels. An effort is also being made to reforest which is purposeful, but when we consider the millenniums of time that Nature has required to build the tanglewood of plant life, shrubbery and trees over the rocks and through the gullies to act as great defenses for holding back the water, these modern programs offer very little assurance for early relief.

Another very destructive force is the wind. When surfaces are denuded either at high or low altitudes the wind starts carving up the soil and starts it on the march across the country. We call the demonstrations dust storms. When we travel through our Western States, it is not uncommon to see buildings and trees partially buried in these rolling dunes of drifting sand. When we were traveling across the desert of Peru in 1937, we saw in many places mountain-like dunes rolling slowly across the country, frequently so completely blocking former traffic routes that long detours were necessary. When we were flying over eastern Australia in search of groups of primitive Aborigines, we saw great forests gradually being engulfed with these marching billows of sand so that most of the trees were covered to their tips.

Few people will realize that it is estimated that only about 45 percent of the land surface of the United States is now available for agricultural purposes and grazing. This includes vast areas that are rapidly approaching the limit of utility.

In one of my trips to the Western States I visited a large ranch of some fifty thousand acres. I asked the rancher whether he was conscious of a depletion in the soil of the ranch in its ability to carry pasture cattle. He said that it was very greatly depleted, that whereas formerly the cows on the ranch were able to produce from ninety-three to ninety-five healthy calves per hundred cows annually, nearly all of sufficiently high physical quality to be available for reproductive purposes, now he was getting only forty to forty-four calves per hundred cows annually and usually only ten or eleven of these were physically fit for reproductive purposes. He stated also that he was able to raise as many calves for restocking the ranch on the plant food produced on the fifty acres to which he was applying a high fertilization program as on the rest of the fifty-thousand-acre ranch. Of late most of the calves for the ranch had to be imported from other states.

In a city in the vicinity I inquired of the director of public health what the death rate was among their children up to one year of age. He stated that the figures were progressively increasing in spite of the fact that they were giving free hospitalization and free prenatal and postnatal care for all mothers who could not afford to pay for the service. This death rate had more than doubled in fifty years. I asked how he interpreted the increasing mortality rate among the infants and mothers. His comment was in effect that they could not explain the cause, but that they knew that the mothers of this last generation were far less fit physically for reproduction than their mothers or grandmothers had been.

To many uninformed people the answer will seem simple. Those who are responsible for these programs, recognize the difficulty in replenishing the exhausted minerals and food elements in adequate quantity. I have been informed by the director of the department of agriculture of the state of Ohio that it would cost fifty dollars per acre to restore the phosphorus alone that has been exhausted during the last fifty to one hundred years. He stated that the problem is still further complicated by the fact that the farmer cannot go to a bank and borrow money to buy this fertilizer. If, however, he buys adjoining acreage to double his own, he can then borrow twice as much money as he can on his own farm. But this is not all of the difficulty. Recent data indicate that if sufficient phosphorus in a form easily available for plant use were supplied to the land at once, it would kill the plant life; it must be provided in a form in which by a process of weathering it is made slowly available for plant utilization. Phosphorus is only one of the minerals that is readily taken from the soil. Other minerals also are difficult to provide. I have been able practically to double the weight and size of beets in five weeks by the addition of a tablespoonful of ferric ammonium citrate to each square foot of garden soil.

An important commentary on soil depletion is provided by the large number of farms that have been abandoned in many districts throughout the United States. The severe industrial depression which has thrown large numbers of shop and mill workers out of employment, has induced a considerable number of these to return to the land for subsistence. As one drives through farming districts that once were very fertile many farms are seen apparently abandoned insofar as tillage is concerned.

In my studies on the relation of the physiognomy of the people of various districts to the soil, I have found a difference in the facial type of the last generation of young adults when compared with that of their parents. The new generation has inherited depleted soil. In many communities three generations of adults are available for study. The yardstick for these comparisons has been developed in the preceding chapters. It will be of interest for the readers to apply this yardstick to their own brothers and sisters in comparison with the parents and particularly their grandparents. The most serious problem confronting the coming generations is this nearly unsurmountable handicap of depletion of the quality of the foods because of the depletion of the minerals of the soil.

REFERENCES

[1] PRICE, W. A. New light on the control of dental caries and the degenerative diseases. *J. Am. Dent. Assn.*, 18:1889, 1931.

[2] ORR, J. B. The composition of the pastures. London, H. M. Stationery Office. E.M.B., 18, 1929.

[3] THEILER, A. and GREEN, H. Aphosphoris in ruminants. *Nutrition Absts. and Rev.*, 1:359, 1932.

[4] TISDALL, BROWN and KELLEY. The age, sex and seasonal incidence of certain diseases in children. *Am. J. Dis. Child.*, 39:163, 1930.

[5] SEARS, P. B. *Deserts on the March.* Norman, University of Oklahoma Press, 1935.

Chapter 21

PRACTICAL APPLICATION OF PRIMITIVE WISDOM

IF THE observations and deductions presented in the foregoing chapters are exerting as controlling an influence on individual and national character as seems to be indicated, the problem of the outlook for our modern civilization is changed in many important aspects. One of the most urgent changes in our viewpoint should be to look upon the assortment of physical, mental and moral distortions as due, in considerable part, to nutritional disturbances in one or both parents which modify the development of the child, rather than to accepted factors in the inheritance. The evidence indicates that these parental disturbances of nutritional origin may affect the germ plasm, thus modifying the architecture, or may prevent the mother from building a complete fetal structure, including the brain. In other words, these data indicate that instead of dealing entirely with hereditary factors, we are dealing in part with distortions due to inhibitions of normal hereditary processes. This changes the prospects for the offspring of succeeding generations. Atavism will still have plenty to her credit even if she must give up her claim to distortions of individual characteristics.

Jacobson[1] has summarized the determining factors in individuality and personality when he says "The Jekyll-Hydes of our common life are ethnic hybrids." Most current interpretations are fatalistic and leave practically no escape from our succession of modern physical, mental and moral cripples. Jacobson says of our modern young people:

> Very much of the strange behavior of our young people to-day is simply due to their lack of ethnical anchorage; they are bewildered hybrids, unable to believe sincerely in anything, and disowned by their own ancestral manes. To turn these neurotic hybrids loose in the world by the million, with no background, no heritage, no code, is as bad as imposing illegitimacy; their behavior, instead of expressing easily, naturally and spontaneously a long-used credo, will be determined by fears and senseless taboos. How can character be built upon such foundations?
>
> There is a ludicrous as well as a pathetic side to the situation presented by a Greek puzzled by his predominantly German children, or by the German woman unable to understand her predominantly Spanish progeny. It is a foolish case over again of hen hatching ducklings, of wolf fostering foundlings.

If our modern degeneration were largely the result of incompatible racial stocks as indicated by these premises, the outlook would be gloomy in the extreme. Those who find themselves depressed by this current interpretation of controlling forces would do well to recall the experiments on pigs referred to in Chapters 17 and 18, in which a large colony all born blind and maimed because of maternal nutritional deficiency—from deficient vitamin A—were able to beget offspring with normal eyes and normal bodies when they themselves had normal nutrition.

Much emphasis has been placed on the incompatibility of certain racial bloods. According to Jacobson,[1]

> Aside from the effects of environment, it may safely be assumed that when two strains of blood will not mix well a kind of "molecular insult" occurs which the biologists may someday be able to detect beforehand, just as blood is now tested and matched for transfusion.

It is fortunate that there is a new explanation for the distressing old doctrine which holds that geniuses cannot be born unless there is an abundant crop of defectives. In this connection Jacobson says,

> The genius tends to be a product of mixed ethnic and nervously peculiar stock—stock so peculiar that it exhibits an unusual amount of badness. The human family pays dearly for its geniuses. Just as nature in general is prodigal in wasting individuals for the development of a type, or species, so do we here find much human wastage apparently for a similar purpose. One may think of the insane and the defectives as so many individuals wasted in order that a few geniuses may be developed. It would seem, that in order to produce one genius there must be battalions of criminals, weaklings and lunatics. Nietzsche must have had biologic implications of this sort in mind when he spoke of the masses as merely "fertilizers" for the genius. This is why the genius has been compared to the lily on the dunghill. He absorbs all the energy of his family group, leaving the fertilizing mass depleted.

Our recent data on the primitive races indicate that this theory is not true, since in a single generation various types and degrees of physical, mental or moral crippling may occur in spite of their purity of blood and all that inheritance could accomplish as a reinforcement through the ages.

The extent to which the general public has taken for granted that there is a direct relationship between mental excellence and mental deficiency is illustrated by the commonly heard expression "great wits and fools are near akin" which expresses tersely the attitude of a modern school of psychiatry. This doctrine is not supported by controlled data from scientifically organized investigations. One of the principal exponents quoted is Maudsley who stated "it is not exaggeration to say that there is hardly ever a man of genius who has not insanity or nervous disorder of some form in his family." Many reviews of the lives of great men have been published in support of this doctrine. Havelock Ellis, however, one of the leading psychologists and psychiatrists of our day, has shown that the percentage of cases substantiating this doctrine is less than 2 percent and less than half that proportion found in the population at large, which in a tested group he found to be 4.2 percent. East of Harvard in discussing this problem states, after reviewing the evidence pro and con: "Thus it is seen that where one collates the work of the most competent investigators on the possibility of relation between insanity and genius the conclusion is unavoidable that none exists."

Those who still believe in the old fatalistic doctrines may answer the questions why the last child is affected seriously much more often than would be expected through chance; or why the most severe defectives are born after mothers have exceeded forty years of age; and still further why our defectives are found chiefly among the later members of large families. These facts are not explainable by Mendel's laws of heredity.

Professor J. C. Brash, of the University of Birmingham, in his monograph[2] discusses the current theories in detail. He emphasizes the role of heredity as the controlling factor in the origin of divergencies. However, all of the distortions of the face and jaws which he presents as being related to heredity can be duplicated, as I have shown, in the disturbances appearing in the first and second generation after primitive racial stocks have adopted the foods of our modern civilizations in displacement of their native foods. He emphasizes the importance of an adequate diet during the growth period of the child, and also the fact that malocclusion is not a direct manifestation of rickets. Hellman has emphasized the importance of childhood diseases. The disturbances which we are studying here, however, are not related to these influences.

Two of the outstanding advances in laboratory and clinical approach to this problem of the relation of the structure of the brain to its function as expressed in mentality and behavior have been the work of Tredgold in England, referred to in Chapter 19, and the "Waverly Researches in the Pathology of the Feeble-Minded," in Massachusetts. Tredgold recognizes two sources of brain injury, "germinal blight" and "arrest" and puts particular stress on the former as being pathological and not spontaneous, and related to the germ of either or both parents due to poisoning of the germ cell. The "arrest" problems have to do with intra-uterine environmental disturbances.

The Waverly group have made very detailed anatomical studies, both gross and microscopic, of brains of mental defectives and related these data to the clinical characteristics of the individuals both mental and physical when living. They have reported in detail two groups of studies of ten individuals each. In their summary of the second group they state:[3]

> The provisional conclusions drawn from the second series and the combined first and second series are much in agreement with the original conclusions drawn from the first series which were as follows: First that measurable brain can be correlated with testable mind in the low and high orders with fairly positive results. That is the small simple brains represented the low intellects or idiots and the most complex brain patterns corresponded to the high grade, moronic and subnormal types of feeble-mindedness.

The lessons from the primitive races demonstrate certain procedures that should be adopted for checking the progressive degeneration of our modernized cultures. If, as now seems indicated, mal-development with its production of physical, mental and moral cripples is the result of forces that could have been reduced or prevented, by what program shall we proceed to accomplish this reduction or prevention?

I have presumed in this discussion that the primitive races are able to provide us with valuable information. In the first place, the primitive peoples have carried out programs that will produce physically excellent babies. This they have achieved by a system of carefully planned nutritional programs for mothers-to-be. It is important to note that they begin this process of special feeding long before conception takes place, not leaving it, as is so generally done, until after the mother-to-be knows she is pregnant. In some instances special foods are given the fathers-to-be, as well as the mothers-to-be. Those groups of primitive racial stocks who live by the sea and have access to animal life from the sea, have depended largely upon certain types of animal life and animal products. Specifically, the Eskimos, the people of the South Sea Islands, the residents of the islands north of Australia, the Gaelics in the Outer Hebrides, and the coastal Peruvian Indians have depended upon these products for their reinforcement. Fish eggs have been used as part of this program in all of these groups. The cattle tribes of Africa, the Swiss in isolated high Alpine valleys, and the tribes living in the higher altitudes of Asia, including northern India, have depended upon a very high quality of dairy products. Among the primitive Masai in certain districts of Africa, the girls were required to wait for marriage until the time of the year when the cows were on the rapidly growing young grass and to use the milk from these cows for a certain number of months before they could be married. In several agricultural tribes in Africa the girls were fed on special foods for six months before marriage. The need for this type of program is abundantly borne out by recent experimental work on animals, such as I have reported in Chapters 17, 18 and 19.

Another important feature of the control of excellence of child life among the primitive races has been the systematic spacing of children by control of pregnancies. The interval between children ranged from two and a half to four years. For most of the tribes in Africa this was accomplished by the plural-wife system. The wife with the youngest child was protected.

The original Maori culture of New Zealand accomplished the same end by birth control and definite planning. In one of the Fiji Island tribes the minimum spacing was four years.

These practices are in strong contrast with either the haphazard, entirely unorganized programs of individuals in much of our modern civilization, or the organized over-crowding of pregnancies also current. The question arises immediately: what can be done in the light of the data that I have presented in this volume to improve the condition of our modern civilization? A first requisite and perhaps by far the most important is that of providing information indicating why our present haphazard or over-crowded programs of pregnancies are entirely inadequate. This should include, particularly, the education of the high-school-age groups, both girls and boys.

In the matter of instruction of boys and girls it is of interest that several of the primitive races have very definite programs. In some, childbirth clinics supervised by the midwife are held for the growing girls. With several of these tribes, however, the ease with which childbirth is accomplished is so great that it is looked upon as quite an insignificant experience. Among the ancient Peruvians, particularly the Chimu culture, definite programs were carried out for teaching the various procedures in industry, home-building and home management. This was accomplished by reproducing in pottery form, as on practical water jugs, the various incidents to be demonstrated. The matter of childbirth was reproduced in detail in pottery form so that it was common knowledge for all young people from earliest observation to the time the practical problems arose. Many of the problems related directly were similarly illustrated in pottery forms.

It is not sufficient that information shall be available through maternal health clinics to young married couples. If pigs need several months of special feeding in order that the mothers-to-be may be prepared for adequate carrying forward of all of the inheritance factors in a high state of perfection, surely human mothers-to-be deserve as much consideration. It is shown that it is not adequate that sufficient vitamin A be present to give the appearance of good health. If highly efficient reproduction is to be accomplished there must be a greater quantity than this. There is no good reason why we, with our modern system of transportation, cannot provide an adequate quantity of the special foods for preparing women for pregnancy quite as efficiently as the primitive races who often had to go long distances without other transportation than human carriers.

The primitive care of a newborn infant has been a matter of severe criticism by modernists especially those who have gone among them to enlighten them in modern ways of child rearing. It is common practice among many primitive tribes to wrap the newborn infant in an absorbent moss, which is changed daily. A newborn infant, however, does not begin having regular all over baths for a few weeks after birth. While this method is orthodox among the primitives it is greatly deplored as a grossly cruel and ignoble treatment by most moderns. Dr. William Forest Patrick of Portland, Oregon was deeply concerned over the regularly occurring rash that develops on newborn infants shortly after they are first washed and groomed. He had a suspicion that Nature had a way of taking care of this. In 1931 he left the original oily varnish on several babies for two weeks without the ordinary washing and greasing. He found them completely free from the skin irritation and infection which accompanies modern treatment. This method was adopted by the Multanomah County Hospital of Oregon which now reports that in 1,916 cases of unwashed, unanointed babies only two cases of pyodermia occurred. They record that each day the clothing was changed and buttocks washed with warm water. Beyond this the infants were not handled. Dr. Patrick states that within twelve hours after birth by Nature's method the infant's skin is clear, and Nature's protective film has entirely disappeared. In my observations of the infant's care among primitive races I have been continually impressed with the great infrequency with which we ever hear a primitive child cry or express any discomfort from the treatment it receives. Of course, when hungry they make their wants known. The primitive mother is usually very prompt, if possible, to feed her child.

Among the important applications that can be made of the wisdom of the primitive races is one related to methods for the prevention of those physical defects which occur in the formative period and which result in physical, mental and moral crippling. When I visited the native Fijian Museum at Suva, I found the director well-informed with regard to the practices of the natives in the matter of producing healthy normal children. He provided me with a shell of a species of spider crab which the natives use for feeding the mothers so that the children will be physically excellent and bright mentally, clearly indicating that they were conscious that the mother's food influenced both the physical and mental capacity of the child. The care with which expectant mothers were treated was unique in many of the Pacific Islands. For example, in one group we were informed that the mother told the chief immediately when she became pregnant. The chief called a feast in celebration and in honor of the new member that would come to join their colony. At this

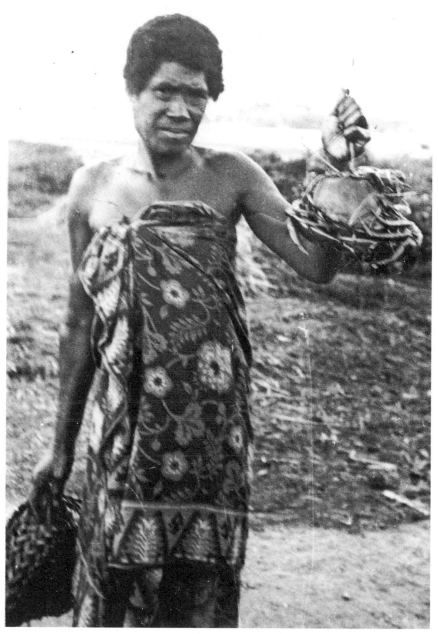

FIG. 129. This Fiji woman has come a long distance to gather special foods needed for the production of a healthy child. These and many primitive people have understood the necessity for special foods before marriage, during gestation, during the nursing period and for rebuilding before the next pregnancy.

feast the members of the colony pledged themselves to adopt the child if its own parents should die. At this feast the chief appointed one or two young men to be responsible for going to the sea from day to day to secure the special sea foods that expectant mothers need to nourish the child. Recent studies on the vitamin content of crabs have shown that they are among the richest sources available. We have then for modern mothers the message from these primitives to use the sea foods liberally, both during the preparatory period in anticipation of pregnancy and during that entire period. In Fig. 129 will be seen a woman of one of the Fiji Islands who had gone several miles to the sea to get this particular type of lobster-crab which she believed, and which her tribal custom had demonstrated, was particularly efficient for producing a highly perfect infant.

For the Indians of the far North this reinforcement was accomplished by supplying special feedings of organs of animals. Among the Indians in the moose country near the Arctic Circle a larger percentage of the children were born in June than in any other month. This was accomplished, I was told, by both parents eating liberally of the thyroid glands of the male moose as they came down from the high mountain areas for the mating season, at which time the large protuberances carrying the thyroids under the throat were greatly enlarged.

Among the Eskimos I found fish eggs were eaten by the childbearing women, and the milt of the male salmon by the fathers for the purpose of reinforcing reproductive efficiency.

The coastal Indians in Peru ate the so-called angelote egg, an organ of the male fish of an ovoviviparous species. These organs were used by the fathers-to-be and the fish eggs by the mothers-to-be.

In Africa I found many tribes gathering certain plants from swamps and marshes and streams, particularly the water hyacinth. These plants were dried and burned for their ashes which were put into the foods of mothers and growing children. A species of water hyacinth is shown in Fig. 130. The woman shown in Fig. 130, with an enormous goiter, had come down from a nine-thousand-foot level in the mountains above Lake Edward. Here all the drinking water was snow water which did not carry iodine. She had come down from the high area to the six-thousand-foot level to gather the water hyacinth and other plants to obtain the ashes from these and other iodine carrying plants to carry back to her children to prevent, as she explained, the formation of "big neck," such as she had. The people living at the six-thousand-foot level also use the ashes of these plants.

Among many of the tribes in Africa there were not only special nutritional programs for the women before pregnancy, but also during the gestation period, and again during the nursing period.

As an illustration of the remarkable wisdom of these primitive tribes, I found them using for the nursing period two cereals with unusual properties. One was a red millet which was not only high in carotin but had a calcium content of five to ten times that of most other cereals. They used also for nursing mothers in several tribes in Africa, a cereal called by them linga–linga. This proved to be the same cereal under the name of quinua that the Indians of Peru use liberally, particularly the nursing mothers. The botanical name is quinoa. This cereal has the remarkable property of being not only rich in minerals, but a powerful stimulant to the flow of milk. I have found no record of the use of similar cereals among either the English or American peoples. In Chapter 14, I presented data indicating that the Peruvians, who were descendants of the old Chimu culture on the coast of Peru, used fish eggs liberally during the developmental period of girls in order that they might perfect their physical preparation for the later responsibility of motherhood. These fish eggs were an important part of the nutrition of the women during their reproductive period. They were available both at the coast market of Peru and as dried fish eggs in the highland markets, whence they were obtained by the women in the high Sierras to reinforce their fertility and efficiency for childbearing. A chemical analysis of the dried fish eggs that I brought to my laboratory from Alaska as well as of samples brought from

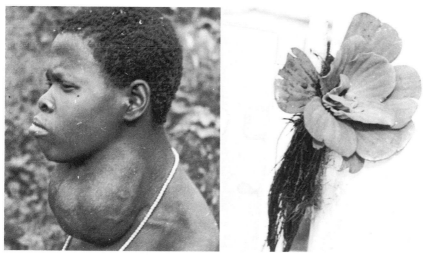

FIG. 130. This African woman with goiter has come down from the 9000-foot level in the mountains in Belgian Congo near the source of the Nile to a 6000-foot level to gather special plants for burning to carry the ashes up to her family to prevent goiter in her children. Right, a Nile plant, a water hyacinth burned for its ashes.

other places has revealed them to be a very rich source of body-building minerals and vitamins. Here again, I have found no record of their use in our modern civilization for reinforcing physical development and maternal efficiency for reproduction. As I have noted in Chapter 15 special nutrition was provided for the fathers by tribes in the Amazon jungle, as well as by the coastal tribes.

Professor Drummond, a British bio-chemist, in discussing the question of the modern decline in fertility, before the Royal Society of Medicine[4] suggested that the decline in the birth rate in European countries, during the last fifty years, was due, largely, to the change in national diets which resulted from the removal of vitamins B and E from grains when the embryo or germ was removed in the milling process. He called attention to the fact that the decline in the birth rate corresponded directly with the time when the change was made in the milling process so that refined flour was made available instead of the entire grain product.

Of the many problems on which the experience of the primitive races can throw light, probably none is more pressing than practical procedures for improving child life. Since this has been shown to be largely dependent upon the architectural design, as determined by the health of the parental germ cells and by the prenatal environment of the child, the program that is to be successful must begin early enough to obviate these various disturbing forces. The normal determining factors that are of hereditary origin may be interrupted in a given generation but need not become fixed characteristics in the future generations. This question of parental nutrition, accordingly, constitutes a fundamental determining factor in the health and physical perfection of the offspring.

One of the frequent problems brought to my attention has to do with the responsibility of young men and women in the matter of the danger of transmitting their personal deformities to their offspring. Many, indeed, with great reluctance and sense of personal loss decline marriage because of this fear, a fear growing out of the current teaching that their children will be marked as they have been.

On the presumption that all mentally crippled individuals will be in danger of transmitting these qualities to their offspring there is a strong movement continually in operation toward segregating such individuals or incapacitating them by sterilization. Several primitive racial stocks have produced large populations without criminals and defectives by means of an adequate nutritional program which provided normal development and function. May it not be that even our defectives, when they have resulted from poisoning of germ cells or interference with an adequate normal intrauterine environment, may be able to build a society with a high incidence of perfection, that will progressively return toward Nature's ideal of human beings with normal physical, mental and moral qualities?

Because of its interpretation of the individual's responsibility for his mental and moral qualities, society has not only undertaken to protect itself from the acts of so-called unsocial individuals but has proceeded to treat them as though they were responsible for the injury that society has done to them. Does it not seem inevitable that this apparently false attitude will change if it be demonstrated that they are the result of a program of inadequate nutrition for the parents.

As we have seen, the children born in many of the families of primitive racial stocks after the parents have adopted our modernized dietary, may have marked changes in the facial and dental arch forms. In our modernized white civilization this change occurs so frequently that in a considerable percentage of the families there is seen a progressive narrowing of the dental arches in the succeeding children of the same family. Since the position of the permanent teeth which erupt at from seven to twelve years of age, can be determined by x-rays early in child life, this procedure provides an opportunity to anticipate deformities that will make their appearance with the eruption of the permanent teeth.

In Fig. 131, may be seen the x-rays of the upper arches of three children. Even under conditions causing the permanent teeth to develop irregularly the deciduous dental arch will not show the deformity that will be expressed later in the permanent dental arch. The abnormal placement of the developing permanent teeth, however, will show the deformity that is later to be produced in the face even though the deciduous arch is normal in design. Both deciduous and permanent teeth can be seen at the same time. In Fig. 131 it will be seen that there is a progressive deformity revealed in the position of the permanent teeth in these three children. (Most severe in the youngest.) This narrowing of the curve made by the permanent teeth is a condition characteristic of a large number of individuals, occurring in at least 25 percent of the families throughout the United States; in some districts the percentage will reach 50 to 75 percent.

Another striking illustration of this progressive injury in the younger members of the family, detected early by the x-rays, is shown in Fig. 132. Note the breadth of the arch of the permanent teeth of the oldest child (to the left), and the marked narrowing of the arch of the two younger children (to the right).

While the application of orthodontic procedures for the improvement of the facial form and arrangement of the teeth will make a vast improvement in facial expression, that procedure will not modify disturbances in other parts of the body, such as the abnormal underdevelopment of the hips and pelvic

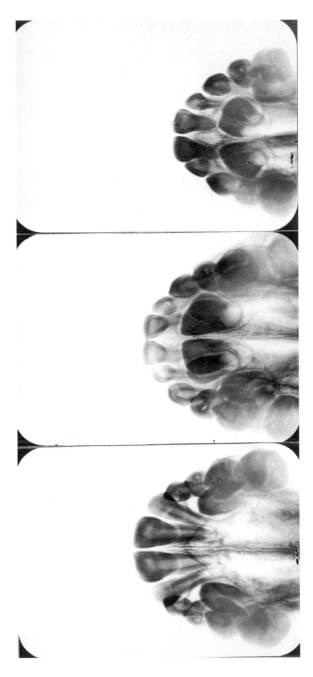

FIG. 131. X-rays of teeth of three children in one family show in the teeth and upper arch a progressive injury in the younger children as indicated by the progressive narrowing of the placement of the tooth buds of the upper permanent teeth. Note the narrowing curve of the arch.

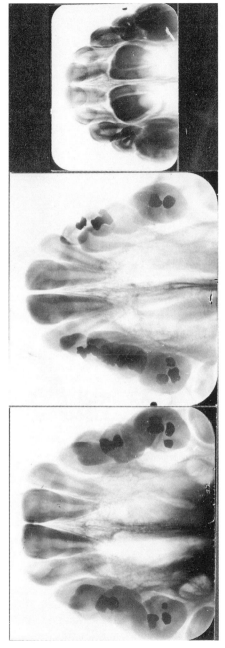

FIG. 132. These x-rays illustrate the progressive injury in the two younger children in this family. Note the progressive narrowing of the permanent arch illustrated by the lapping of the laterals over the centrals in the youngest, and decreasing distance between the cuspids.

bones. If an improvement in nutrition for the mothers-to-be is adequately provided in accordance with the procedures of the primitives, it should be possible to prevent this progressive lowering of the capacity of our modern women to produce physically fit children.

Fig. 133 is another illustration. The oldest child, ten years of age, is shown at the upper left. She has a marked underdevelopment of the width of the face and dental arches. The nostrils are abnormally narrow and she tends to be a mouth-breather. She is very nervous and is becoming stooped. In the lower

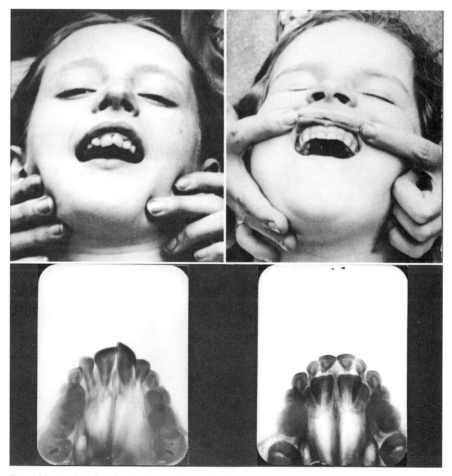

FIG. 133. In this family the first child to the left was most injured in the formative period as shown in the form of the face and dental arches above and x-rays below. The first child required fifty-three hours of labor and the second three hours, preceded by special nutrition of the mother.

left photograph, is shown an x-ray of the narrowed upper arch. At the right is shown her younger sister, six years of age. It will be seen that the proportions of her face are much more normal and that she breathes with complete ease through her nose. She has none of the nervous trouble of her older sister. In the x-rays, below, at the right, it will be seen that her permanent arch, as indicated by the positions of the permanent teeth, although not so far advanced as that of her sister, has good design. The history of these pregnancies is of interest. The duration of labor for the first child was fifty-three hours and for the second three hours. Following the birth of the first child the mother was a partial invalid for several months. Following that of the second child the experience of childbirth made but slight impression on the strength and health of the mother. During the first pregnancy no special effort was made to reinforce the nutrition of the mother. During the second pregnancy the selection of foods was made on the basis of nutrition of the successful primitives. This included the use of milk, green vegetables, sea foods, organs of animals and the reinforcement of the fat-soluble vitamins by very high-vitamin butter and high-vitamin natural cod liver oil. It is a usual experience that the difficulties of labor are greatly decreased and the strength and vitality of the child enhanced where the mother has adequately reinforced nutrition along these lines during the formative period of the child.

The problem of maternal responsibility with regard to the physical capacity of their offspring to reproduce a healthy new generation comprises one of the most serious problems confronting modern degenerating society. In a previous chapter I have discussed the difficulty that zoological garden directors have had in rearing members of the cat family in captivity. It has been a very general experience until the modern system of feeding animal organs was instituted, that unless the mothers-to-be had themselves been born in the jungle the lack of development of the pelvic arch would frequently prevent normal birth of their young. In the Cleveland Zoo a very valuable tigress, that had been born in captivity, found it impossible to give birth to her young. Although a Caesarian operation was performed, she lost her life. The young also died. One of the veterinaries told me that the pelvic arch was entirely too small to allow the young to pass through the birth canal. Studies of the facial bones of this animal showed marked abnormality in development.

The result of disturbance in the growth of the bones of the head and of the development of general body design is quite regularly a narrowing of the entire body, and often there is a definite lengthening. Statistics have been published relative to the increase in the height of girls in colleges during the last few decades. This is probably a bad rather than a good sign as actually it is an expression of this change in the shape of the body. I am informed by gynecologists that narrowing of the pelvic arch is one of the factors that is contributing to the increased difficulties that are encountered in childbirth by our modern generation.

A typical case illustrating the relationship between the lack of pelvic development and deformity of the face, is presented in Fig. 134. This girl presented a very marked underdevelopment of the lower third of the face which produced the appearance of protrusion of her upper teeth so that it was quite difficult or impossible for her to cover them with her lips. An operation to improve her appearance consisted in removing the first bicuspid on each side above and then moving the bone carrying the anterior teeth backward with appliances, the width of the two removed teeth. This changed the relationship of the teeth as shown in the two upper views in Fig. 134. The operation greatly improved her facial appearance and she lost the inferiority complex which had prevented her from mingling with young people. When she went to the hospital for her first child, there was special concern because of her weak heart, and every effort was made to obtain a normal birth rather than one by Caesarian section. This proved impossible and the Caesarian operation was done. Great difficulty was experienced in saving the life of the mother and child. Her boyish figure, of which she had been so proud, and which had been a part of her serious deformity, during her formative period had nearly resulted in her undoing. She nursed her baby for some time but the overdraft of reproduction on her frail body was so great that she aged rapidly, her back weakened and she stooped forward as shown in Fig. 134, lower right. In the view at the lower left, it will be seen that the teeth remained in their new position. A point to keep in mind is that her physical deficiency was probably directly caused by an inadequate nutrition of her mother during the intrauterine development and prior to conception. It is, of course, possible that the father also contributed a poisoned germ cell that constituted a disturbance in the architectural design of the offspring. In this connection, it is important to have in mind the tragic influence of a program of deliberate starvation of mothers-to-be in order that the bones of the baby may be soft and thus provide an easy birth. Some literature has been published indicating the foods that would be efficient in accomplishing this. This means almost certain wreckage or handicapping of the child's life.

Information from many sources may suggest that the expectant mother needs more calcium and more vitamin D. She may go to the pharmacy with a prescription or on her own initiative obtain calcium tablets and so-called vitamin D as a synthetic preparation. We are concerned here with data which will throw light on the comparative value of the treatment the modern mother will thus give herself with that that the primitive mother would provide.

Dr. Wayne Brehm who is associated with two Columbus, Ohio, hospitals has recently published the results[5] of a study of the effect of the treatment received in 540 obstetrical cases divided into six groups of ninety individuals

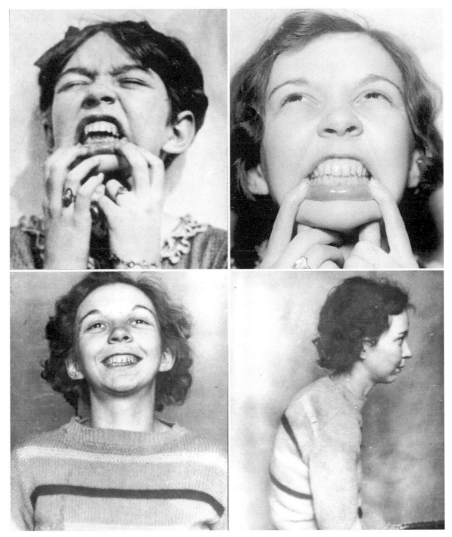

FIG. 134. This girl suffered with a serious deformity of her face. She also had very contracted pelvic arch. The facial deformity was improved as shown. She nearly lost her life with the birth of her first baby which was removed by Caesarian operation. Note her badly deformed back from the overload of reproduction.

each, on the basis on which their nutrition was reinforced in order to study the comparative effects of the different treatments. The reinforcement of the diet consisted in Group 1 of taking calcium and synthetic vitamin D as viosterol; Group 2, calcium alone; Group 3, viosterol alone; Group 4, calcium and cod liver oil; Group 5, cod liver oil alone and Group 6, no reinforcement. For those receiving the calcium and viosterol there was extensive calcification in the placentae, marked closure of the fontanelle (the normal opening in the top of the infant skull) and marked calcification in the kidneys. For those receiving calcium alone there was no placental calcification, slight closure of the fontanelle and no calcification of the kidneys. Group 3 receiving viosterol had moderate to marked placental calcification, moderate closure of the fontanelle and no calcification of the kidneys. Those receiving cod liver oil alone had very slight placental calcification, slight fontanelle closure and no calcification in the kidneys. Those receiving no reinforcement had very slight placental calcification, normal fontanelle closures and no calcification of the kidneys. The effect on the mother was a prolonging of labor in Group 1 and at birth the fetal heads were less moulded not being able to adjust their shape to the shape of the birth tube. These infants had a general appearance of ossification or postmaturity. This strongly emphasizes the great desirability of using Nature's natural foods instead of modern synthetic substitutes.

It is a matter of great importance that the most serious disturbances in reproduction and childbirth are occurring in the most civilized parts of the world. In Chapter 19 I have referred to the important work of Dr. Kathleen Vaughan entitled "Safe Childbirth." She has not only had wide experience among several tribes in India and in the British Hospitals but has collected a large quantity of information regarding the experience of many races throughout the world. Her data strongly emphasize the necessity that the growing girl shall be allowed to have an active outdoor life not only until the completion of the building of her body at about fourteen years of age, but through the child-bearing period. In practically all countries a restricted sedentary indoor life greatly increases the complications associated with childbirth. She quotes Whitridge Williams to the effect that: "At the onset of pregnancy the (males) are 125 to 100 (females), and he adds that sex is determined in the germ cells, primarily or immediately after their union, and is immutable by the time segmentation of the ovum begins." Notwithstanding this advantage, prenatal and infant mortality reduces the proportion of boys to a level below that of girls. Dr. Vaughan in her reference to the data on the annual report of the chief medical officer, the Minister of Health, states as follows:

> Our infant mortality returns show that over half the number of infants dying before they are a year old die before they have lived a month (and 6,744 of them before they are twenty-four hours old), strongly suggesting that their vitality was impaired by the process of birth. The figures of those who did not survive one month are 20,060, and of these *more than half are males. So we lose over ten thousand boys every year under a month old!* (Public Health Report, No. 55, British). Hear what Dr. Peter McKinley has to say on the subject. "The death rate of infants in the period immediately subse-

quent to birth is nine times as high as that which occurs later in the first years of life." He shows how the difficulty experienced by the mothers during parturition leads to the death of infants at and just after birth, and says in this connection, "Infant deaths under a month are significantly associated with the death rates of mothers in childbearing." He quotes Netherland statistics showing that of stillbirths due to difficulty during birth, male stillbirths predominate, and says, "These figures might be taken in support of the view that the greater size of the male head is a cause of some greater difficulty in labour than there is with a female birth." Here, indeed, in civilized childbirth is the laboratory where the sex of the population is finally determined—the actual births of boys and girls are nearly equal in number, but the small ones slip through; the larger children are the ones who are killed during birth, or so damaged that life is heavily handicapped, and we are left with an enormous surplus female population. This destruction of male infants, which goes on day by day and year by year, puts the consequences of the Great War into the shade. Our surplus female population (now reaching over one and a half million in excess of the male) is directly due to it. We have no need of Pharaoh's midwives to kill our boys off at birth (Exodus i. 16). Civilization does it unaided, for all civilized races as they pass their zenith and are on the downgrade have eventually had to face the same problem, the outnumbering of men by women, and most of them have met it as the East does to-day by female infanticide. A more intelligent policy would be to prevent the males dying at birth. We see that difficult childbirth leads to a high maternal mortality, but it is also the cause of a high infant mortality falling most heavily upon the male infants, and it is also responsible for the production of mental defectives in ever-increasing numbers.

Dr. Vaughan's work places emphasis on the necessity that the human body be properly built, especially that of the mother-to-be. She shows clearly that the shape of the pelvis is determined by the method of life and the nutrition. In all primitive tribes living an outdoor life childbirth is easy and labor is of short duration. She shows that this is associated with a round pelvis and that the distortion of the pelvis to a flattened or kidney shape, even to a small degree, greatly reduces the capacity and therefore the ease with which the infant head may pass through the birth canal. In Dr. Vaughan's wide experience she has observed two ways by which a rough estimate of the pelvic shape and capacity may be anticipated: first, by the gait of the individual, because the angle of the hips is determined by the shape of the pelvis; and second, by the teeth and jaws. She has recognized an association between facial and dental arch deformities and deformed pelvis.

During my investigations in eastern Australia I was informed that the birth rate among the whites had declined over a large area and to such an extent that many families had no children and many women could produce only one child. The diets used in that district were very largely refined white-flour products, sugar, polished rice, vegetable fats, canned goods and a limited amount of meat. The alarm regarding the declining birth rate in Australia has recently been a matter of discussion by the New South Wales legislature as indicated by an Associated Press dispatch from Sydney, Australia, dated August 1, 1938: "A 'stork derby' with sweepstakes prizes was proposed in the New South Wales Legislature today to boost Australia's falling birth rate."

A report just received from the Bureau of Home Economics, Department of Agriculture, Washington, presents figures for the average amount of the various foods used in different income groups in different parts of the United States. These showed that in general about one-third of the income up to $2500 was spent for food per family; further, that the total flour equivalent ranged from 0.39 to 0.50 pound per capita per day. These quantities will furnish about 829 to 1063 calories per day, per capita. It will be seen at once that this provides a large number of the calories required for growing children and sedentary adults per day. With this number of calories derived from refined flour products there is no adequate provision for a normal amount of such body-building materials as minerals and vitamins. These have been removed, largely, in the milling process, and are largely denied to our modern civilization insofar as the cereal foods are concerned. This includes vitamin E, so essential for the functioning of the pituitary gland, the master governor of the body.

One of the most important lessons we may learn from the primitive cultures is the detail of their procedures for preventing dental caries. Since I have devoted an entire chapter (Chapter 16) to this I will make only a brief comment here. Simply stated, the practical application of the primitive wisdom for accomplishing this would involve returning to the use of natural foods which provide the entire assortment of body-building and repairing food factors. This means the recognition of the fact that all forms of animal life are the product of the food environments that have produced them. Therefore, we cannot distort and rob the foods without serious injury. Nature has put these foods up in packages containing the combinations of minerals and other factors that are essential for nourishing the various organs. Some of the simpler animal forms are able to synthesize in their bodies some of the food elements which we humans also require, but cannot create ourselves. Our modern process of robbing the natural foods for convenience or gain completely thwarts Nature's inviolable program. I have shown how the robbing of the wheat in the making of white flour reduced the minerals and other chemicals in the grains, so as to make them sources of energy without normal body-building and repairing qualities. Our appetites have been distorted so that hunger appeals only for energy with no conscious need for body-building and repairing chemicals.

A first requisite for the control of tooth decay is to have provided an adequate intake of the body-building and repairing factors by the time the hunger appeal for energy has been satisfied. A sufficient variety of foods must be used to supply the body's demand for those elements which it needs in large quantities, that is, calcium and phosphorus, and the other elements which it needs in smaller quantities, though just as imperatively. One of the serious human deficiencies is the inability to synthesize certain of the activators which include the known vitamins. This makes necessary the reinforcement of the nutrition with definite amounts of special foods to supply these organic catalysts, especially the fat-soluble activators, including the known vitamins, which are particularly difficult to provide in adequate quantities. I have shown that the primitive races studied were dependent upon one of three sources for some of these fat-soluble factors, namely, sea foods, organs of animals or dairy products. These are all of animal origin. I have indicated in Chapter 16 the nutritional programs that have proved in clinical testing adequate for providing the body with nutrition that will not only prevent tooth decay, but check it when it is active. The stress periods of life, namely, active growth in children and motherhood, do not constitute overloads among most of the primitive races because the factor of safety provided by them in the selection of foods is sufficiently high to protect them against all stresses. I have indicated the type of nutrition that is especially needed for these stress periods in our modern civilization. Also, that it is not necessary to adopt the foods of any particular racial stock, but only to make our nutrition adequate in all its nutritive factors to the primitive nutritions. Tooth decay is not only unnecessary, but an indication of our divergence from Nature's fundamental laws of life and health. (See Chapter 16 for primitive menus.)

The responsibility of our modern processed foods of commerce as contributing factors in the cause of tooth decay is strikingly demonstrated by the rapid development of tooth decay among the growing children on the Pacific Islands during the time trader ships made calls for dried copra when its price was high for several months. This was paid for in 90 percent white flour and refined sugar and not over 10 percent in cloth and clothing. When the price of copra reduced from $400 a ton to $4 a ton, the trader ships stopped calling and tooth decay stopped when the people went back to their native diet. I saw many such individuals with teeth with open cavities in which the tooth decay had ceased to be active.

In undertaking to make practical application of primitive wisdom to our modern problems, the field is so broad that only a limited number of items may be included. It is important to emphasize the difference between the procedures used in the preparation of boys and girls for life in many of the primitive groups, and in our modern social organization. Few people will realize the remarkable training given the primitive children, with the fathers and mothers as tutors. To illustrate, among the Indians of the far North in Canada near the Arctic Circle, the girls rather than the boys select a companion for life. This is done with the help of her parents. Before a boy is considered worthy of consideration he must demonstrate that he can build the winter cabin, provide the firewood for maintaining the home of the parents, and all of the provisions of wild game, during the trial period of several weeks. After an adequate demonstration of bravery as well as of skill, in which the boy must kill a grizzly bear, he is accepted into the home for a period of trial marriage. The girl has the privilege of making her choice by trial, but when the choice is made there is complete faithfulness on the part of both. Girls are prepared for life's duties by being taught to make clothing, prepare food, care for children and assist in the maintenance of the home. I have seldom, if ever, seen such happy people as these forest Indians of the far North.

In Chapter 10, in discussing the Australian Aborigines, I have similarly described the preparation of boys for the responsibility of manhood. No modern college graduate has to win his spurs under more exacting examinations and tests than do those boys.

In Africa several specialties call for special training. The medicine men spend several years under the training of a tutor. Each boy must provide a specified number of cattle per year which are eaten by the group.

Probably the most indelible impression that is left by my investigations among primitive races, is that which came from examining 1,276 skulls of the people who had been buried hundreds of years ago along the Pacific Coast of Peru and in the high Andean Plateau, without finding a single skull with the typical marked narrowing of the face and dental arches, that afflicts a considerable proportion not only of the residents in modernized districts in Peru, but in most of the United States and many communities of Europe today. I know of no problem so important to our modern civilization as the finding of the reason for this, and the elimination of the cause of error. Perhaps few will recognize the significance of this important point. This may be the reason why the prospect is not encouraging.

One of the important lessons we should learn from the primitive races is that of the need for maintaining a balance between soil productivity, plant growth and human babies. Even in a country with so low a fertility as found in the greater part of Australia, the Aborigines for a very long period were able to maintain this balance. Their system of birth control was very efficient and exacting.

A survey made by a committee appointed by the League of Nations indicates the need per capita of approximately one-half acre of land for wheat, two acres for dairy products, and ten acres for beef producing pasture for the supply of meat. When we realize that Ohio has been occupied by our modern civilization for only one hundred fifty years and that it is estimated that during that time approximately half of the topsoil has been lost through water and wind erosion we realize that Nature's accumulated vegetable enrichment has been greatly reduced in this area within a short time from this one source alone. In Chapter 20 I have shown that there is only enough phosphorus in the top seven inches of agricultural land for approximately fifty crops of high-yield wheat or one hundred crops of moderate-yield. Other grains make similar drafts upon the land. I have given data indicating a relationship between progressive soil depletion and progressive increase in heart disease.

It is apparent that the present and past one or two generations have taken more than their share of the minerals that were available in the soil in most of the United States, and have done so without returning them. Thus, they have handicapped, to a serious extent, the succeeding generations, since it is so difficult to replenish the minerals, and since it is practically impossible to accumulate another layer of topsoil, in less than a period of many hundreds of years. This constitutes, accordingly, one of the serious dilemmas, since human beings are dependent upon soil for their animal and plant foods, for body-building. The minerals are in turn dependent upon the nutritive factors in the soil for establishing their quality. The vitamin and protein content of plants has been shown to be directly related to availability of soil minerals and other nutriments. A program that does not include maintaining this balance between population and soil productivity must inevitably lead to disastrous degeneration. Over-population means strife and wars. The history of the rise and fall of many of the past civilizations has recorded a progressive rise, while civilizations were using the accumulated nutrition in the topsoil, forest, shrubbery and grass, followed by a progressive decline, while the same civilizations were reaping the results of the destruction of these essential ultimate sources of life. Their cycle of rise and degeneration are strikingly duplicated in our present American culture.

Various therapeutic measures in use today have come to us from primitive peoples. One of the greatest scourges of the world is malaria fever. Everywhere it has been fought successfully with quinine. Indeed, many parts of the world would not have been tenantable for whites without it. Yet few people realize that quinine was the gift of the ancient Peruvian Indians.

In Chapter 15 I presented data regarding the treatment used by several primitive races for preventing and correcting serious disturbances in the digestive tract. This consisted in the use of clay or aluminum silicate which modern science has learned has the important quality of being able to adsorb and thus collect toxic substances and other products. Important new light is now thrown on the probable role of this substance in the primitive diet and its possible application in our modern problems of sensitization reactions or allergies. In the first volume of my work on "Dental Infections," I presented data relating toxic sensitization reactions to dental infections. These were shown in both animals and human beings. I discussed the relation of these reactions to histamine and emphasized their similarity to the effect produced by inoculation with histamine. An important new chapter has recently. been added to this problem by the work of Dr. C. F. Code for which he has received an award by the American Association for the Advancement of Science. He reported his findings before the Association meeting at Richmond, Virginia, in December, 1938. Dr. Code has apparently discovered that histamine is the actual product responsible for the symptoms of the various allergies. Its excess accumulation in the blood is the actual cause of the symptoms whether expressed as asthma, hay fever or skin eruptions such as produced by pollens, various foods, dust and other sensitizing agents. He has shown that the eosinophils, a type of white blood cell, are the source of excess histamine in the blood. It is accordingly indicated that the primitive treatment by the use of kaolin, aluminum silicate, as an adsorbent was used directly for controlling such symptoms. It is now further indicated that this treatment can be helpful for the prevention of modern allergies. Previous investigations have shown that histamine is produced in the alimentary tract as a putrefaction product of proteins by the action of certain micro-organisms of the colon group.

Modern science boasts the discovery of vitamin C, lack of which took its toll of thousands of the white mariners through hundreds of years with scurvy. The first recorded cure of that disease was made by the Indians in Canada when the British soldiers were dying in large numbers. The Indians taught them to use a tea made from the steeped tips of the shoots of the spruce. When I was among the Indians of the far north I asked a chief why the Indians did not get scurvy. He then proceeded, as I have related in Chapter 15, to explain to me how the Indians prevented scurvy by the use of special organs in the animals. While it is true that we have come to associate the absence of vitamin C as the causative factor in scurvy, we do not know how many other affections may be due to its absence in adequate quantity in our foods. Almost weekly, new diseases are being associated with vitamin deficiencies in our modern dietaries.

One of our modern tendencies is to select the foods we like, particularly those that satisfy our hunger without our having to eat much, and, another is to think in terms of the few known vitamins and their effects. The primitive tendency seems to have been to provide an adequate factor of safety for all emergencies by the selection of a sufficient variety and quantity of the various natural foods to prevent entirely most of our modern affections. Their success demonstrates that their program is superior to ours. An important advance in modern international relationships provides for exchange of professorships and, thus, interchanges of wisdom. We have shown a most laudable and sympathetic interest in carrying our culture to the remnants of these primitive races. Would it not be fortunate to accept in exchange lessons from their inherited knowledge? It may be not only our greatest opportunity, but our best hope for stemming the tide of our progressive breakdown and also for our return to harmony with Nature's laws, since life in its fullness is Nature obeyed.

As I have sojourned among members of primitive racial stocks in several parts of the world, I have been deeply impressed with their fine personalities, and strong characters. I have never felt the slightest fear in being among them; I have never found that my trust in them was misplaced. As soon as they had learned that I was visiting them in their interest, their kindness and devotion was very remarkable. Fundamentally they are spiritual and have a devout reverence for an all-powerful, all-pervading power which not only protects and provides for them, but accepts them as a part of that great encompassing soul if they obey Nature's laws.

Ernest Thompson Seton has beautifully expressed the spirit of the Indian in the opening paragraph of his little book *The Gospel of the Red Man*:

> The culture and civilization of the White man are essentially material; his measure of success is, "How much property have I acquired for myself?" The culture of the Red man is fundamentally spiritual; his measure of success is, "How much service have I rendered to my people?"
>
> The civilization of the White man is a failure; it is visibly crumbling around us. It has failed at every crucial test. No one who measures things by results can question this fundamental statement.

The faith of the primitive in the all-pervading power of which he is a part includes a belief in immortality. He lives in communion with the great unseen Spirit, of which he is a part, always in humility and reverence. Elizabeth Odell in the following lines seems to express the spirit of the primitives,

> Flat outstretched upon a mound
> Of earth I lie; I press my ear
> Against its surface and I hear
> Far off and deep, the measured sound
> Of heart that beats within the ground.
> And with it pounds in harmony
> The swift, familiar heart in me.
> They pulse as one, together swell,
> Together fall; I cannot tell
> My sound from earth's, for I am part
> Of rhythmic, universal heart.

REFERENCES

[1] JACOBSON, A. C. *Genius (Some Revaluations)*. New York, Greenburg, 1926.

[2] BRASH, J. C. The etiology of irregularity and malocclusion of the teeth. *Dental Board of United Kingdom*, London, 1930.

[3] Waverly researches in the pathology of the feeble-minded (Research series, cases XI to XX). *Mem. Am. Acad. Arts & Sci.*, 14:131, 1921.

[4] DRUMMOND, J. C. The medical aspects of decline of population. *J.A.M.A.*, 110:908, 1938.

[5] BREHM, W. Potential dangers of viosterol during pregnancy with observations of calcification of placentae. *Ohio S. M. J.*, 33:990, 1937.

Chapter 22

A NEW VITAMIN-LIKE ACTIVATOR

THE SERIOUSNESS of the dental caries problem in relation to both human progress and the dilemma of modern physical degeneration emphasizes the need of a bird's-eye view of the problems involved in restoring to man his original immunity.

For the entire period of human life on the earth, say one million years, some human skeletons have been preserved in burials. A study of these remains reveals that there has been more dental caries in the last hundred years than at any time previously and probably more than during any thousand-year period of his history. This situation suggests, if it does not demand, that we analyze critically the changes in man's environment and his interference with it.

As to our present knowledge of the problem, we find it evaluated in the recently published summary made by the Research Commission of the American Dental Association. Two hundred thirty-seven investigators and observers present their best judgment and experience in 276 pages. In this detailed report, we see that there is no recognized theory regarding the etiology of dental caries and no accepted program for the control of the disease. So far as progress is concerned, there is much evidence that, in general, the situation is getting worse from decade to decade.

While outstanding progress has been made in the knowledge of disease in general—knowledge that places great emphasis on the role of nutrition in modern degeneration—that splendid progress has revealed the nature and role of many of its new factors, especially vitamins. It is profoundly significant, however, that no single vitamin or combination of vitamins has completely solved the riddle of dental caries or pointed the way to a determination of its etiology. This suggests our ignorance as regards any specific substance for use in controlling dental caries. There must be some food substance that is not adequately provided in modern nutrition, perhaps owing to some fundamental change in quality, preparation or selection of the substance. To judge from the skeletal remains, people of the past obtained a substance that modern generations do not have. The present report will present evidence of a heretofore not generally recognized activating substance. It is not one of the recognized vitamins, but is a substance which belongs in the fat-soluble group.

The data to be presented will indicate that: (a) it plays an essential role in the maximum utilization of body-building minerals and tissue components; (b) its presence can be demonstrated readily in the butterfat of milk of mammals, the eggs of fishes and the organs and fats of animals; (c) it has been found in highest concentration in the milk of several species, varying with the nutrition of the animal; and (d) it is synthesized by the mammary glands and plays an important role in infant growth and also in reproduction.

Experimental Data

In 1926, Yoder[1] published a report on the "Relation Between Peroxidation and Antirachitic Vitamins," including a chemical procedure for determining antirachitic potency. When vitamin D was separated from vitamin A, its role included the functions of activated ergosterol, which came to be known as vitamin D. While Yoder's peroxidation method was early used as a chemical test for vitamin D, it was later found that it measured a nutritional factor much broader than its antirachitic function.

In my early reports on the vitamin content of dairy products,[2] I used this test as a measure of the vitamin D content. My data revealed that the nutritional factor it represented included aids to mineral utilization, as well as potency for dental caries immunity. I have accordingly used this method for testing the value of foods, particularly dairy products, for potency in controlling dental caries, and of associated health factors.

In my early report[3] on the levels of this activating substance in butter as measured by the chemical test reported by Yoder, I expressed the values as vitamin D; but, as my studies progressed, it was revealed clearly that the qualities which I was concerned with in butter were not comparable to vitamin D as represented by ergosterol that had been exposed to ultraviolet radiation. Since butter contained definite nutritional qualities not provided in irradiated ergosterol in addition to its antirachitic properties, I accordingly dropped the term vitamin D, as expressed in Yoder's test, and, for want of a better means of identification, used in my records the term activator X.

Since an acceptable chemical test for vitamin A that depended on the action of antimony trichloride in chloroform solution had been developed by Carr and Price,[4] I made an extensive number of studies of the vitamin A and activator X content of a large series of butter samples obtained from many states and provinces and from different countries throughout the world. These studies were related to two other important studies; namely, sunshine curves and mortality data from various districts. These studies, which have now been in progress since 1928, include an analysis of more than 20,000 samples of dairy products. In order to establish wide application of the data, samples were received every two to four weeks from several different parts of the world over a period of several years. These included samples from districts of the United States, northwestern Canada, Australia, Brazil and New Zealand.

It was quickly disclosed that neither total hours of sunshine nor temperature was the chief controlling factor. The factor most potent was found to be the pasture fodder of the dairy animals. Rapidly growing grass, green or rapidly dried, was most efficient. It was disclosed that these periods of growth were directly related to the rains and harvest, and, for the southern states, there were two distinct peaks in the vitamin and activator curves, one in the spring and the other in the autumn. In general, in moving northward through the United States and through the Canadian provinces, these two peaks came closer together and the total for the maximum rise was much higher in the northern dairy districts than in the southern. By obtaining samples over a very wide range, curves for vitamin A and activator X, as shown combined in Figure 135, were made for the products analyzed from various provinces of the United States and Canada. The total area was divided into sixteen divisions, each representing several thousand square miles.

A study of the data of the health departments of all these districts regarding mortality for heart disease and pneumonia disclosed that the curves were always found to be lowest when the vitamin content of the dairy products was highest. This study is well illustrated in Figure 135, which shows vitamin and sunshine curves for the various latitudes and the mortality curves by months for heart disease and pneumonia combined.

Many facts are revealed in this extensive study. Note, for example, how much higher the vitamin curves are for the north than for the regions farther south; also, how much lower the vitamin curves are in the eastern states and far west where the soil has been tilled the longest.

Simultaneously, dairy products were obtained for analysis from several countries in the southern hemisphere, chiefly, Australia, New Zealand, and Brazil. These again showed the distinct seasonal variation in vitamin A and activator X content of the dairy products, which were, similarly, in the opposite phase for heart disease and pneumonia. The curves, however, for the southern hemisphere were in the phase opposite to those of the northern hemisphere, but were parallel with the seasons.

As these data were developed, preliminary reports were made from time to time in current scientific journals. These reports are summarized in the bibliography. While it is clearly not possible to review the steps of progress in detail in this communication, certain essential facts are presented briefly, with illustrations. I have been deeply indebted to national, state and provincial officials, also to individuals in the United States, Canada, Australia and New Zealand, for continuous cooperation extending over several years. This assistance

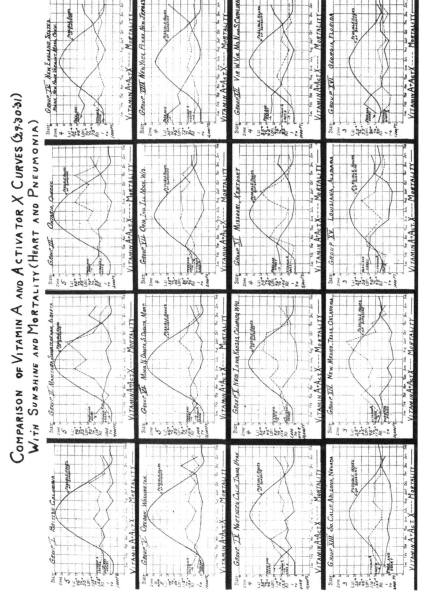

FIG. 135. Relation by months of possible hours of sunshine to each level of vitamin A, and activator X, and mortality rates for heart disease and pneumonia. This chart covers 16 areas of the United States and Canada in their geographic relationships. Mortality is the phase opposite to the vitamin A and activator X levels.

has made it possible to develop curves showing comparative values from month to month and from year to year.

In the early part of this work, progress was slow in the differentiation of those activating substances that were identified as vitamins and given alphabetical numbers. Little was known of their nutritional properties. It was early discovered in the history of mineral utilization that one of the most striking manifestations was involved in rickets; and since the therapeutic use of ergosterol that had been exposed to ultraviolet radiation resulted in rapid healing of rickets, being comparable to exposure of the individual to sunlight or suitable artificial radiation, that substance was given the identifying name of vitamin D and was assumed to have the total responsibility for mineral utilization in bone and tooth formation and maintenance. The substance was given the name of viosterol in the United States. It did not prove efficient, however, in the control of dental caries.

Much progress has been made in recent years in identifying four different vitamin D factors, of which viosterol or irradiated ergosterol is vitamin D^2. Vitamin D^3 is produced by the irradiation of a form of cholesterol. It is now recognized that activated ergosterol D^2 does not represent the factors essential for the utilization of calcium and phosphorus by the human body. Available data indicate that it is not a product of animal bodies. We accordingly are concerned with data that will relate to mineral metabolism in general and dental caries in particular.

I have found in these studies that, in the control of dental caries, while the consumption of whole butter is an aid in mineral metabolism, greater potency may be obtained by melting a high-vitamin butter and allowing it to crystallize for twenty-four hours at a temperature of about 70 degrees. It is then centrifuged, and, under the process, it separates into an oil that is limpid at that temperature, with a solid crystalline layer below. This oil is much higher in the activating factor than the whole butter. It is this substance that I shall refer to in this communication, unless otherwise explained, as a source of activator X.

There are many expressions of disturbed mineral metabolism in both the soft and the hard tissues of the body. Those of the skeleton are most easily demonstrated. Rickets in young children and animals is easily demonstrated by the roentgen rays and the progress in its healing is readily measured by this means.

Rats are used largely for testing the efficiency of various treatments for rickets. The effect of administration of activator X on rickets is striking.

In Figure 136 will be seen the roentgenographic appearance of the forelegs and the tails of two rats on the same deficiency diet; namely, Steenbock 2965. It will immediately be seen that all of the bones of No. 1 are very transparent and the carpal bones have not formed. The junction of the epiphyses and the diaphyses of the bones, especially of the tail, is shown to be characterized by a zone of separation. In rat No. 2, there is a marked density of the bones, seen as an area of opacity to the roentgen rays, and the carpal bones are well formed. The head of the humerus and the epiphyseal zones of provisional growth of the tail are well calcified, with only a line of separation between them and the diaphyses. This rat received, as an addition to the deficient diet, 2 percent of the diet as a butter oil concentrate obtained from a high-vitamin butter. Clinically, this condition constitutes healed rickets. The quantity of this butter used would constitute only about one-half ounce for a child eating 2 pounds of food per day. This is a very small quantity for a growing child. To the right in Figure 136 will be seen the mineral levels in the blood serum of these two rats. The calcium for rat No. 1 is at 6.26 mg. per hundred cubic centimeters, and in rat No. 2, it is 8.4. The inorganic phosphorus in rat No. 1 is at 1.93 mg. per hundred cubic centimeters and in rat No. 2, it is 2.5 mg. We see at once that this clinical condition in these two rats is attended by marked correction of the blood chemical levels.

The product that was administered to rat No. 2 is a normal constituent of a normal milk, Nature's only complete diet for mammalian infants and by far the most important single item of food for growing human beings in all periods of stress.

I shall use as illustration of a case profiting by the use of this dietary factor, the case of a boy 4 years of age (Fig. 93, page 270), brought to me with a fracture. He was in a cast. Rampant tooth decay was present. The diet had consisted of white bread and skimmed milk, which had been the source of his nutrition for an extended period owing to the poverty of the family at the time of the depression. He had been suffering from convulsions, which had been increasing in severity over a period of eight months. His leg had been broken when he had fallen to the floor in one of his convulsions three months before receiving the reinforced diet. The minister who brought him to me had been called to the home to baptize the boy for burial because he was considered so near death.

The only treatment given was a change in diet from skimmed milk and white bread to whole milk and a gruel made of freshly ground whole wheat. Over this gruel was poured about a dessert spoonful of butter oil from a sample of butter that had been produced when the cows were eating rapidly growing green wheat. After his first meal, the boy slept his first night without a convulsion. He was fed five times the next day on the same diet, and had no convulsions. Recovery was very rapid.

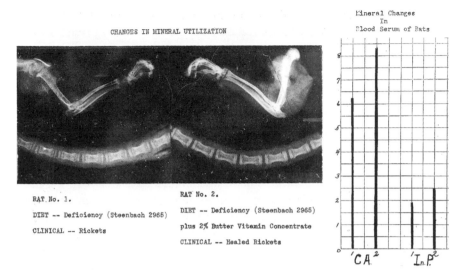

CHANGES IN MINERAL UTILIZATION

Mineral Changes
In
Blood Serum of Rats

RAT. No. 1.

DIET -- Deficiency (Steenbach 2965)

CLINICAL -- Rickets

RAT No. 2.

DIET -- Deficiency (Steenbach 2965)

plus 2% Butter Vitamin Concentrate

CLINICAL -- Healed Rickets

FIG. 136. Treatment of rickets in rats by adding 2 percent of butter oil concentrate containing activator X to deficiency diet. Healing of rickets in the carpal and tail bones of rat No. 2 and improvement in blood minerals are marked.

Figure 93 shows the broken leg before and after the use of the reinforced diet for one month. The x-ray film shows the healed fracture. The patient had been taken out of the cast the day before. The x-ray film of the broken femur shows clearly the healing of the fracture. The photograph is indicative of the excellent physical condition of the child. Without operation on his teeth, dental caries was controlled. He grew to be an athletic young man, active in sports, particularly baseball.

During the severe industrial depression, rampant caries developed in a great number of cases in the families of mill workers. Children in these families provided excellent clinical material. A typical result of work done for these families is shown in a study of an experimental group of twenty-seven mission children selected on the basis of rampant dental caries. At the beginning of the test, in the average chemical analysis of all of the saliva specimens of the group, the inorganic phosphorus had passed from the powdered bone in an amount of 2.4 percent of the total inorganic phosphorus of the saliva. In two months, this condition changed to a movement toward the powdered bone averaging 3.42 percent of inorganic phosphorus for the entire group; in four months, to 8.13 percent; in five months, to 11.36 percent, and in seven months, to 11.75 percent.

Since these children were all from poor homes, many of the families being on relief, one extra good meal a day at midday was provided for the entire group at the mission. This was preceded by administration to each child of one teaspoonful of a mixture containing a high-vitamin butter oil obtained by centrifuging the butter at 70 degrees from a twenty-four-hour crystallization of the melted butter. This butter was selected on the basis of its high content of activator X. It was mixed with equal parts of a high-vitamin, natural cod liver oil. The clinical effect was apparent complete control of dental caries for the entire group, as shown in the x-ray films. In many of these cases, the open cavities were left without fillings; and, in all such cases, the exposed dentin took on a hard glassy finish. There were many other evidences of betterment.

One of the boys, who was so weak at the beginning of the test that it was considered questionable whether it was safe for him to walk the two blocks from his home to the mission for the one reinforced meal a day, in six weeks was able to play basketball. He was dashing about as a star player, and there was no evidence of undue fatigue on his part in this strenuous game.

Under the stress of the industrial depression, the family dietary for the children in this mission group was very deficient. During the experiment, the home meals were not changed, nor was the home care of the teeth. The preliminary studies of each child included complete x-ray examination of all the teeth, chemical analyses of the saliva, a careful plotting of the position, size and depth of all cavities, a record of the height and weight and a record of school grades, including deportment. It is important to note that the home diet which had been responsible for the tooth decay, was exceedingly low in body-building and repair material and high in sweets and refined starches. It usually consisted of a highly sweetened coffee and white bread, vegetable fat, pancakes made of a white flour and eaten with syrup and doughnuts fried in vegetable fat.

The diet provided these children in the supplemental meal was as follows: About 4 ounces of tomato juice or orange juice and a teaspoonful of a mixture of equal parts of a very high-vitamin, natural cod liver oil and an especially high-vitamin butter oil was given at the beginning of the meal. The child then received a bowl containing approximately a pint of a very rich vegetable and meat stew, made largely from bone marrow and fine cuts of tender meat. The meat was usually broiled separately to retain its juice and then chopped very fine and added to the bone-marrow meat soup, which always contained finely chopped vegetables and plenty of very yellow carrots. The next course consisted of cooked fruit, with very little sweetening, and rolls made from freshly ground whole wheat and spread with high-vitamin butter. The wheat for the rolls was ground fresh every day in a motor-driven coffee mill. Each child was given also 2 glasses of fresh whole milk. The menu was varied from day to day by substituting for the meat stew fish chowder or organs of animals. From time to time, food similar to that eaten by the children was placed in a 2-quart jar and brought to my laboratory, where chemical analysis showed that these meals provided approximately 1.48 gm. of calcium and 1.28 gm. of phosphorus in a single helping of each course. Since many of the children took "seconds," their intake of these minerals was much higher. Since the accepted figures for the requirements of the body for calcium and phosphorus are 0.68 gm. of calcium and 1.32 gm. of phosphorus, it is obvious that this one meal a day, plus the other two meals at home, provided a factor of safety. Clinically, this program completely controlled the dental caries of each member of the group, as determined by x-ray and explorer examination.

It is important to note with regard to the effect of the special nutritional program on this group of mission children that two different teachers came to me to inquire as to what had been done to make a particular child change from one of the poorest in the class in capacity to learn to one of the best. Dental caries is only one of the many expressions of our modern deficient nutrition.

An example of the change produced in the structure of the teeth as a result of the reinforced nutrition in this mission group is illustrated in Figure 97, page 259, which shows three first permanent molars in which caries apparently had decalcified the dentin to the vicinity of the pulp chamber, causing exposure. The pulps were still vital. It will be noted at the left, in Figure 97, that each of the three molars apparently had an exposure of the pulp. In the views to the right, a progressive filling in of the pulp chambers can be noted from a deposition of secondary dentin, making a roof over the pulp and thereby providing a protection which enabled the pulp to remain vital and useful for an extended period. This is frequently experienced as a result of reinforcing the diet with high-vitamin and high-activator butter, together with reducing the carbohydrate intake to a normal level as supplied by natural foods and by increasing the foods that provide body-building and tooth-forming minerals. The condition that is found in the tooth is one in which the minerals cease to be taken in minute amounts from the tooth structure and, owing to the change in the saliva, the minerals in ionic form pass from the saliva bathing the tooth cavity into the demineralized dentin, in many cases a hard and even glassy surface resulting.

It is important to keep in mind that silver nitrate will not penetrate appreciably into tooth enamel after the tooth has been erupted for a year or more, in a normal mouth with normal saliva and high immunity to dental caries, though it will penetrate an appreciable distance in a recently extracted tooth in the same mouth. This experiment is easily made with impacted third molars, in which silver nitrate will often penetrate a millimeter into the enamel.

An excellent illustration of the rescue of a large number of apparently doomed teeth in the same mouth is shown in Figure 137. The patient, a girl aged 14, had lost all four of the first permanent molars and the diagnosis made by her local dentist indicated the necessity of removing all of the erupted teeth and the construction of two artificial dentures. Studies indicated that she had forty-two open cavities in twenty-four teeth in addition to fillings. The patient was placed on a reinforced diet including approximately one-half teaspoonful of a mixture of a high-vitamin A and high-activator X butter oil mixed with equal parts of a very high-vitamin, natural cod liver oil taken in capsules three times a day. She was on this regimen for about seven months, with the result that there was very little evidence of extension of the caries, notwithstanding that no fillings were placed, with the exception of two or three temporary ones. The condition of these teeth before the dietary change is shown in the two upper rows of Figure 137.

Because of the extreme severity and extent of the dental operations needed, restoration was not undertaken locally, but the patient was sent to Cleveland from a southern state; also for the management and care of her case. The operative program was completed by my associate Dr. Richard Spayde. The roots of three of the straight-rooted teeth with extensive pulp exposure were filled. Another tooth had had its roots filled before the patient came to me. The lower two rows of teeth show them as restored.

This girl, at 15, had all her teeth, with the exception of the four first permanent molars, extracted earlier in life. The teeth have been well restored with good masticating surfaces and the appearance of the patient is excellent. She is so enthusiastic that she wishes to give lectures on nutrition to aid others with their dental problems. Important light is thrown on this case by both the chemical analysis of the saliva and the bacterial count. The inorganic phosphorus of the saliva, shaken with powdered bone, was changed from +19.1 to −29.5. The bacterial count change for L. acidophilous was from 680,000 to none.

This form of nutritional control of dental caries is so satisfactory that I can recommend it with confidence as adequate to control well over 95 percent of dental caries, in the hands of painstaking, efficient and informed dentists.

During the years that these investigations on the nature and source of this special activating substance in butter, which I have called activator X, have been in progress, no reports have been noted from other workers of its discovery until the last few years. Then Schantz, Elvehjem and Hart[5] reported the comparative nutritive value of butterfat and certain vegetable oils. Their data were summarized in Dairy Council Digest, March 1940, as follows:

> A series of feeding experiments on rats showed differences in the nutritive value of common fats. The rats which received butterfat grew better than the rats fed vegetable oils, were better in appearance, and had better reproductive capacity. Apparently butterfat contains a substance not present in the other fats tested, which is essential for the growth and health of young

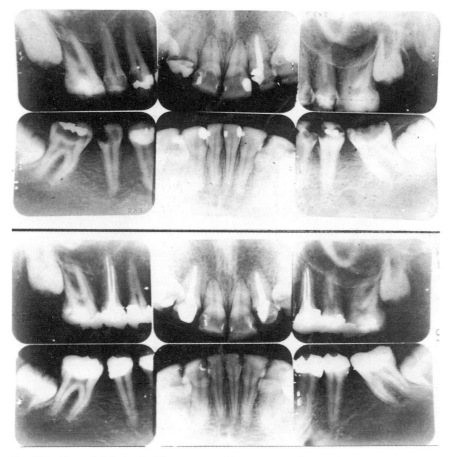

FIG. 137. Case of girl who had forty-two cavities in twenty-four teeth. With the diet rein-forced with activator X, the pulp chambers built in secondary dentin and all the teeth were saved. Full dentures had been recommended.

animals. This difference is not due to vitamins A, D, or E, but to a difference in the chemical constitution of the fats. These findings are significant to the knowledge of nutrition because they indicate additional reasons why milk fat has superior value for human diets.

Hart emphasizes the importance of these findings. He says:

Milk is indispensable for the best nutrition of children and serves as a con-centrated protective source of nutritional essentials for all ages. This being true, dairying must continue as a part of our agriculture if our standards of living are to be maintained. A people without milk and in general the means to make a better milk, must suffer from high infant mortality, poor child nutrition, and forego the liberal use of a product so nearly complete in all nutritional factors. Milk is the one food with a liberal concentration of all the nutrients, except a small number of minerals, that can claim the distinction of protecting against deficiency diets. It can be improved by better feeding. But the mammary gland in its distinctive synthetic capacity and as a concentrator elaborates a commercial and readily available product for which there is no equally effective substitute.

Hart and his group later reported additional data under the title "Rations for the Study of the Relative Nutritive Value of Fats and Oils," *Science* (Dec. 3, 1943), which he summarized as follows: "It is apparent that lactose has an as yet unknown effect on intestinal conditions which is counteracted by butter but not by corn oil."

December 1943, he reported further studies in the *Journal of Nutrition*, under the title, "Further Studies on the Comparative Value of Butterfat, Vegetable Oils, and Oleomargarines," which he summarized as follows:

1. With lactose as the sole carbohydrate in the diet, rats showed superior growth when fed butterfat or lard as compared to corn oil, coconut oil, cottonseed oil, soybean oil, peanut oil, olive oil and hydrogenated cottonseed oil.
2. With a mixture of carbohydrates composed of sucrose, starch, dextrose, dextrin, and lactose in the diet, the average growth response of the animals fed vegetable oils was equal to that of the animals fed butterfat and lard. The growth rate on this ration was more rapid than when all of the carbohydrate present was lactose.
3. Properly fortified oleomargarine fats had growth potential equal to butterfat over a period of 6 weeks when the above mixture of carbohydrates was incorporated in the rations.
4. Properly fortified oleomargarines did not give growth equal to butterfat when lactose was the sole carbohydrate in the diet. On such a regime rats fed butterfat grew slightly better than rats fed oleomargarines of animal origin, but decidedly better than rats fed oleomargarines of vegetable origin.

Another group of workers using calves as the experimental animals has recently reported a similar superiority of butterfat in feeding trials. T. W. Gullickson, F. C. Fountaine and J. B. Fitch;[6] of the Division of Dairy Husbandry, University of Minnesota, used animal and vegetable fats with skimmed milk, with the following results:

Feeding tests were conducted to compare the feeding value of the following fats and oils for calves: butterfat, lard, tallow, coconut oil, peanut oil, corn oil, cottonseed oil, and soybean oil....In average daily gain in weight as well as in general well-being, the calves fed butterfat excelled those in all other groups. Following closely were those receiving lard and tallow. Corn oil, cottonseed oil and soybean oil were the least satisfactory....They appeared unthrifty, listless and emaciated. Some calves in these groups died and others were saved only by changing to whole milk.

We are concerned to note the probable relationship between the factor that has been disclosed by the Wisconsin and Minnesota groups and my activator X and vitamin A. Table I shows the relation of activator X and vitamin A to butterfat structure as reported by the Wisconsin Group, which shows the comparative readings in six spaced samples of butter produced by the same cows. This herd was fed in Deaf Smith County of northwest Texas near Hereford. The samples were obtained about ten days apart, beginning with February and extending through to April. In March, the fodder was reinforced with green alfalfa hay.

TABLE 1. RELATION OF ACTIVATOR X TO
VITAMIN A AND BUTTERFAT STRUCTURE*

1942 Date	Saponification Number	Iodine Number	A	Vitamins Int. Units	Activator X
2/23	188.0	25.0	0.10	95	0.1
3/4	185.5	31.9	2.2	2,000	18.0
3/16	190.0	32.0	2.2	2,000	18.0
4/2	225.0	33.0	4.5	4,300	32.0
4/8	223.0	33.0	5.5	5,200	32.0
4/13	234.0	35.0	5.5	5,200	26.0

*Data on six ten-day samples of cream from same herd, near Hereford, Texas, showing marked increase in both nutritional factor reported by Wisconsin group and activator X factor, strongly indicating that they are the same.

It will be noted that all of the factors, namely the saponification number, iodine number, vitamin A and activator X, progressed through a wide range and are in general parallel. The addition of the green pasture also produced a marked change in the color of the butterfat. The first two samples of butter, when separated from the cream, were as white as lard. A very slight tint was showing in the third sample, which increased progressively to a brilliant golden yellow through the next three samples. The relation of the changes in these four factors to each other and to the green pasture addition to their fodder is shown graphically in Figure 138, which also shows a change in the color of the butter as photographed on panchromatic plates. It will be noted that the evidence is very striking in that the factor which I have been studying and referring to as activator X is possibly the same factor that has recently been observed and reported by both the Wisconsin and the Minnesota groups.

It is important that we observe the effect of the administration of the activator X factor to patients suffering with rampant dental caries on the incidence of caries, the change in chemical analysis of the saliva and *L. acidophilous growth*. I have previously reported that in the inorganic phosphorous of the saliva, as determined by an adaptation of the Kuttner and Cohen[7] technic for

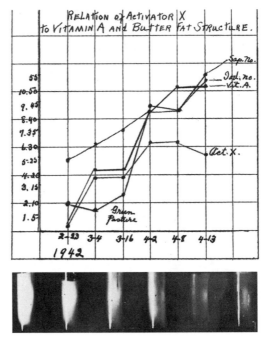

FIG. 138. Above: Four butter factors, saponification number, iodine number, vitamin A and activator X graphically shown. There was a rapid rise of all when green pasturage was added. Below: Difference in natural color of butters.

blood, in which the proteins of the saliva are precipitated by sodium acid molybdate and trichloracetic acid, there is a marked change in the behavior of the phosphate ions of the saliva when it is shaken with powdered bone or powdered tooth substance. In the mouths of susceptible individuals, the inorganic phosphorous is increased by transfer of the phosphate ions from the powdered bone or tooth chips, whereas, in normal saliva of patients with immunity to dental caries, the movement is from the saliva to the negative absorbent; namely, powdered bone or tooth chips. This is graphically shown in Figure 139 for a group of six typical cases.

In this group, the saliva, before the treatment began, gained 11.5 percent in inorganic phosphorus; whereas, after treatment, the saliva lost 13.9 percent of its inorganic phosphorus. The change in nutrition included an increase in the activator X and vitamin A content as concentrated from a high-vitamin butter and a reduction in carbohydrates; also an increase in mineral-providing foods. Before the change in nutrition, when the tooth decay was considered active, *L. acidophilous* averaged, for the group, 323,000 colonies per cubic centimeter of saliva, and, after treatment, averaged 15,000. These data are typical of many hundreds of clinical cases in which dental caries has been reduced apparently to zero, as indicated by both x-ray and instrumental examination.

We human beings of modern civilization are at a great disadvantage in the selection of foods in that we seem to have lost a sixth sense by which we would recognize a specific need for special food. Many of the primitive races and most animals retain the capacity to satisfy the body needs by choosing the foods that will provide minerals and vitamins. This is well illustrated in one of my experiments with chickens.

Three brooders, each carrying twenty-five chickens, 3 days old, were provided with a diet of grain. No opportunity was given the chicks to supplement the diet, as chickens in the open or birds in the wild can supplement theirs by picking up green food and insects. In order to provide an additional source of food, each brooder was supplied with a measured quantity of butter selected on the basis of its vitamin A and activator X content.

Brooder No. 1 had a butter that was high in both vitamin A and activator X; brooder No. 2, a butter high in vitamin A and low in activator X, and brooder No. 3, a butter low in vitamin A and activator X. It was observed that the chicks in brooder No. 1 developed much better than those in either of the two other brooders even though the vitamin A content was high in both brooder No. 1 and brooder No. 2. An important part of the experiment was observation of the effect of these diets on the chemical content of the blood. On the eighth day, a sufficient number of chickens were killed for blood tests

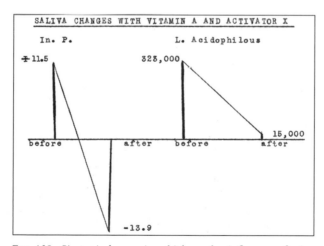

FIG. 139. Six typical cases in which, under influence of reinforced diet, inorganic phosphorus factor changed from average of +11.1 to −13.9 and *L. acidophilous* count fell from 323,000 to 15,000.

BLOOD CHANGES IN CHICKS WITH THREE GRADES OF BUTTER.

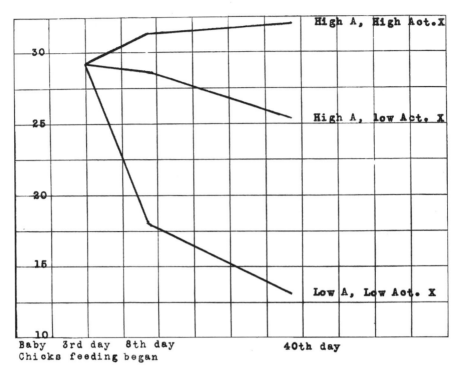

FIG. 140. Changes in blood of chicks depending on vitamin A and activator X content. The product of serum calcium and serum inorganic phosphorus went up when both were used and fell to a low level when butter with low vitamin A and activator X content was used.

to determine the level of the product of serum calcium and serum inorganic phosphorus (CaXP).

A product of 40 is considered normal for most species. At the beginning of the test, this factor stood at 29.7. On the eighth day, for the chickens receiving the butter high in both vitamin A and activator X, this factor had increased to 31.2; for the chicks in brooder No. 2, receiving the butter high in vitamin A and low in activator X, it decreased to 28.8, and for those in brooder No. 3, receiving the butter low in both vitamin A and activator X, it had fallen to 17.8. On the twentieth day, this progressive change was even more marked, being at 32 for the chicks receiving butter high in both vitamin A and activator X and at 25 for those receiving butter high in vitamin A and low in activator X. For those receiving butter low in both vitamin A and activator X, this product of serum calcium and serum inorganic phosphorus had fallen to 13. This result is strikingly illustrated in Figure 140.

The significance of these data is very great since they throw an important light on the lowering of the level of defense for many of our modern degenerative processes, including dental caries.

An important observation was made with regard to the behavior of the chicks in these three groups, particularly as to the amount of the butter they consumed and the effect on their general health. It was noted that the chicks in pen No. 1 ate much more butter than those in either pen No. 2 or pen No. 3. This suggested the desirability of making an observation of the ability of the chickens to select from three samples of food the one that was highest in vitamin A and activator X. Accordingly, a new group of forty chickens was started in a large brooder. The same deficient diet was used and three containers supplying the same three grades of butter were placed in the large brooder, fresh each day. The butter was weighed before and after each feeding and the containers were shifted to different parts of the brooder so that the same grade of butter was not in the same place twice in succession. This was repeated for fifty-seven days, when it was found that the chickens selected and ate about two and one-half times as much of the high activator X butter as of the low. I could not distinguish between these butters, nor could any member of my staff. This clearly indicated an ability on the part of the chicks to select the best food.

An important modification of this chick experiment related to the capacity of this butter vitamin and activator to maintain life. The same three grades of butter were used and the chicks were on McCollum's deficiency diet 3142. When 28 percent of the chicks had died in the pen with the low vitamin A and low activator X butter, only 16 percent had died in the group receiving butter high in vitamin A and low in activator X, and none had died in the pen with the butter high in both vitamin A and activator X. When 72 percent of the chicks were dead in group 3, 53 percent were dead in group 2, and only 24 percent in group 1.

It has generally been assumed that cod liver oil is an adequate source of the fat-soluble vitamins, but that this is not true for human beings, animals or birds is readily illustrated by the following experiment in which turkeys were used that were afflicted with weak legs. Three groups of turkeys were used. Those in pen No. 1 were controls; those in pen No. 2 received cod liver oil in addition to the stock food on which they were being fed, and those in pen No. 3 received in addition to foods mentioned butter high in vitamin A and activator X. After a seven-day period, the controls had gained only 8.3 percent in weight and those in pen No. 2, on cod liver oil as an addition to the stock food, had gained 16.7 percent; while those in pen No. 3, receiving in addition the high-vitamin-A and activator X butter, gained 37.5 percent in weight, more than twice the gain of those in pen No. 2 and more than four times that of the controls in pen No. 1. The difference in their appearance and condition is shown in Figure 141. We are concerned to note the changes in the blood. The calcium and phosphorus increase is shown graphically at the right in Figure 141. The calcium increased 2 mg. in groups 2 and 3, the phosphorus, 1 mg. in group 3.

Space does not permit a detailed presentation of my experimental studies showing the direct relationships among the soil, chemical content, the plants produced by the soil and the effect of those foods on human beings and animals.[8]

Interpretation of these data in relation to current thought regarding the etiology and control of dental caries requires strong emphasis on the need for a broader view than is involved in the interpretation that dental caries is purely a local problem in the mouth and solely due to the presence and activity of aciduric organisms propagated by favorable pabulum supplied in the food and chiefly by sugar. It is also strongly indicated that we must not think of dental caries in terms of oral hygiene, as important as that process is.

My studies of fourteen primitive racial stocks in various parts of the world, selected on the basis of their unique physical environment, have in accordance with the accumulated wisdom of the racial stock, people are relatively free from dental caries. This was true notwithstanding the fact that almost no effort was made at oral hygiene. At their point of contact with the foods of modern civilization, they rapidly lost their immunity, in large part because of the high-sugar and refined starch content, which provided pabulum. However, many other expressions of degeneration appeared besides dental caries. The percentages of teeth attacked by dental caries in these groups, the more isolated as compared with the modernized, are shown in Table 2.

TABLE 2. PERCENTAGE OF TEETH ATTACKED BY
CARIES IN PRIMITIVE AND MODERNIZED GROUPS

	PRIMITIVE	MODERNIZED
Swiss	4.60	29.8
Gaelics	1.20	30.0
Eskimos	0.09	13.0
Northern Indians	0.16	21.5
Seminole Indians	4.00	40.0
Melanesians	0.38	29.0
Polynesians	0.32	21.9
Africans	0.20	6.8
Australian Aborigines	0.00	70.9
New Zealand Maori	0.01	55.3
Malays	0.09	20.6
Coastal Peruvians	0.04	40.0+
High Andes Indians	0.00	40.0+
Amazon Jungle Indians	0.00	40.0+

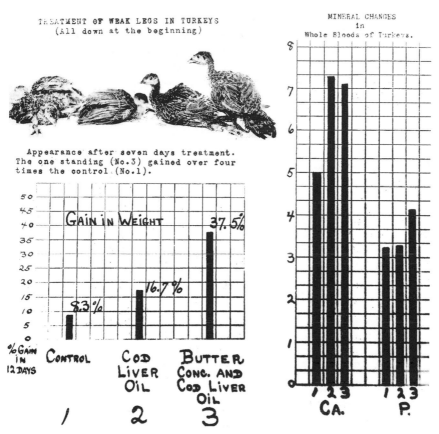

FIG. 141. Young turkeys which, when fed on stock food, rapidly developed weak legs. They recovered much more rapidly with activator X and cod liver oil than with cod liver oil alone, as shown in the photograph. The gain in weight was twice as great in seven days as were the gains in the cod liver oil group and four times as great as that of the control group. The graph shows the changes in amounts of calcium and phosphorus.

On the basis of the chemical analysis of the foods, it was disclosed as shown in previous chapters that the primitive diets of these various groups in various environments all indicated a high content of minerals and vitamins, including activator X. I have reported these data in several communications.[9]

Table 1 and Figure 138, above, show the chemical characteristics of butters produced in Deaf Smith County, Texas. Much publicity has been given to the observation that dental caries had a much lower incidence in the town of Hereford than in most other districts in the United States. It is of special interest that during the years that I have been obtaining butter samples from various parts of the United States and Canada and several other countries, I have been making a special study of the dairy products in the immediate district of northwest Texas and eastern New Mexico in the adjoining counties of Curry, New Mexico and Deaf Smith County, Texas. On the basis of the samples of butter received from these counties and analyzed, during 14 years, when I had butter shipped to Cleveland because of its very high content of activator X and vitamin A to use in my experimental groups of human beings and animals I found its use highly effective in the control of human dental caries, when accompanied by an adequately adjusted food intake. During these years, it has been found that the high level of activator X and vitamin A was directly associated with the specially favorable pasturage, chiefly wheat grass and other cereal grasses and alfalfa in a lush green state of growth. The cows were pastured on this wheat grass during the fall, winter and spring until time for the wheat plants to stalk. The winter wheat was usually sown in August.

In the immediate districts in which the especially high-vitamin butter was produced by this pasturage, it has now been shown that the butter content is directly related to the soil. Excavations to trace the wheat roots show that they pass down 6 feet or more through 3 feet of top soil, varying in depth, into a caliche soil which is very rich in calcium. This caliche consists of glacial pebbles cemented together with calcium carbonate. All of the plants growing on these areas that have this soil foundation are particularly rich in minerals and vitamins.

I have obtained samples of wheat from thirteen districts surrounding Hereford for chemical analysis. It is of interest that while these samples all show a relatively high level of thiamine, vitamin B^1, there is still a marked variation which is not related directly to the protein, calcium or phosphorus content.

Farm stock produced in this area has a much higher market value and a greater capacity for reproduction than the stock in most states. The capacity of most of our states for supporting domestic animals has progressively decreased until, in many districts, the capacity of the farms has gone down to about 50 percent. When animal life degenerates because of inadequate food, human beings react similarly. The data disclose a physical basis for our modern physical degeneration including dental caries.

Summary

1. Data have been presented revealing a wide range of nutritive factors, one of which has not been generally recognized and to which, for want of an accepted identification, I have referred to as activator X. This is found in the food fats of animal origin and is particularly high in butterfat when dairy animals are eating lush green pasturage directly or rapidly cured and stored for stall-feeding.

2. Data have been presented indicating that this factor, activator X, plays an important role in such vital processes as the control of dental caries and the healing of fractured bones.
3. It has been shown that dairy products in Hereford vicinity may vary through a range of fiftyfold in a few weeks' time in the vitamin A and activator X content, the range depending directly on the fodder. There is a sharp rise at the time that the green pasturage is added to the ration of the cows.
4. This factor, which I have discovered in my investigations of butterfats, gives strong evidence of being the same factor that has recently been announced by the Dairy Department of the University of Wisconsin and of the University of Minnesota, which they identify by determining the saponification number and iodine number and by animal feeding.
5. The addition of butter high in activator X to the diets of human beings suffering from tooth decay causes a marked change in the chemical constituents of the saliva and the growth of *L. acidophilous*.
6. Data have been prated indicating that chickens have the ability to recognize and select butters high in activator X and that this prolongs their lives.
7. Turkeys are shown to grow much more rapidly when this factor is available in their food than when cod liver oil alone is used, and its addition to their diet prevents and cures weak legs.
8. Clinically, the use of butter high in activator X, in conjunction with a favorable selection of natural foods, as shown through a period of seventeen years, is highly effective in the control of dental caries.
9. Primitive races controlled dental caries with diets high in body-building factors which included activator X.

REFERENCES

[1] YODER, L. Relation between peroxidation and anti–rachitic vitamins. *J. Bio1. Chem.*, 70:297, October 1926.
[2] PRICE, W. A. Seasonal variations in butter-fat vitamins and their relation to seasonal morbidity, including dental caries and disturbed calcification. *J.A.D.A.*, 17:850–873, May 1930.
[3] *Idem*: Calcium and phosphorus utilization in health and disease. 1. Role of activators for calcium and phosphorus metabolism. *Domin. D. J.*, 41:315, October 1929. 2. The nature and source of calcium and phosphorus activators. *Ibid.*, 41:351, November 1929.
[4] CARR, F. H., and Price, E. A. Colour reactions attributed to vitamin A. *Bochem. J.*, 20:497–501, 1926.

[5] SCHANTZ, E. J., ELVEHJEM, C. A., and HART, E. B. The comparative nutritive value of butterfat and certain vegetable oils. *J. Dairy Sc.*, 23:181, 1940.

[6] GULLICKSON, T. W., FOUNTAINE, F. C., and FITCH, J. B. Various oils and fats as substitutes for butterfat in the ration of young calves. *J. Dairy Sc.*, 25:2, February 1942.

[7] KUTTNER, T., and COHEN, H. Microcolorimetric studies. 1. Molybdic acid, stannous chloride reagent. *J. Biol. Chem.*, 75:517, November 1927.

[8] PRICE, W. A. Control of dental caries and some associated degenerative processes through reinforcement of the diet with special activators. *J.A.D.A.*, 19:1339, August 1932.

[9] *Idem*: *Nutrition and Physical Degeneration*. Comparison of primitive and modern diets and their effects. New York, Paul Hoeber, Inc. (Medical Book Department of Harper and Brothers), 1939.

Chapter 23

FOOD IS FABRICATED SOIL FERTILITY

BY WILLIAM A. ALBRECHT
UNIVERSITY OF MISSOURI, COLUMBIA

INTRODUCTION

In chapter 20 I have discussed briefly Soil Depletion and Plant and Animal Deterioration. Dr. Albrecht has made new and important contributions to this field. He has graciously consented to my presenting here a condensed summary which he has provided. This address was given before the regional A.A.A. conference at Durham, N.H., June 1944. In referring to that address Dr. Henry Bailey Stevens, Director General Extension Service, University of New Hampshire, made these comments:

> "Sometimes a powerful thought, like a flash of lightning, throws a great area from darkness into sudden light. Such an illumination was experienced by those of us who heard the two addresses by Dr. Wm. A. Albrecht. I confess that I am not sure yet how far or along what strange paths this message will take us. Apparently we can no longer think of foods as having a fixed value; for such value varies according to the soil content. . . . It would seem that nutrition is a much more profound science than has been generally recognized and that in studies heretofore its surface has perhaps only been scratched." *Extension Bulletin 66.* General Extension Service, University of New Hampshire, Durham, N H

Dr. Albrecht has published many research reports and is greatly aiding by his contributions, in the large problem of human rehabilitation.

DR. PRICE

Food is fabricated soil fertility. It is food that must win the war and write the peace. Consequently the questions as to who will win the war and how indelibly the peace will be written will be answered by the reserves of soil fertility and the efficiency with which they can be mobilized for both the present and the post-conflict eras.

National consciousness has recently taken consideration of the great losses by erosion from the body of the surface soil. We have also come to give more than passive attention to malnutrition on a national scale. Not yet, however, have we recognized soil fertility as the food-producing forces within the soil that reveal national and international patterns of weakness or strength.

Soil fertility, in the last analysis, must not only be mobilized to win the war, but must also be preserved as the standing army opposing starvation for the maintenance of peace.

What is soil fertility? In simplest words it is some dozen chemical elements in mineral and rock combinations in the earth's crust that are being slowly broken out of these and hustled off to the sea. Enjoying a temporary rest stop enroute, they are a part of the soil and serve their essential roles in nourishing all the different life forms. They are the soil's contribution—from a large mass of nonessentials—to the germinating seeds that empowers the growing plants to use sunshine energy in the synthesis of atmospheric elements and rainfall into the many crops for our support. The atmospheric and rainfall elements are carbon, hydrogen, oxygen and nitrogen, so common everywhere.

It is soil fertility that constitutes the five percent that is plant ash. It is the handful of dust that makes up the corresponding percentage in the human body. Yet it is the controlling force that determines whether Nature in her fabricating activities shall construct merely the woody framework with leaf surfaces catching sunshine and with root surfaces absorbing little more than water or whether inside of that woody shell there shall be synthesized the innumerable life-sustaining compounds.

Soil fertility determines whether plants are foods of only fuel and fattening values, or of body service in growth and reproduction. Because the soil comes in for only a small percentage of our bodies, we are not generally aware of the fact that this five percent can predetermine the fabrication of the other ninety-five percent into something more than mere fuel.

History Records Changing Politics Rather than Declining Soil Fertility

Realization is now dawning that a global war is premised on a global struggle for soil fertility as food. Historic events in connection with the war have been too readily interpreted in terms of armies and politics and not premised on mobilized soil fertility. Gafsa, merely a city in North Africa, was rejuvenated for phosphorus-starved German soils. Naura, a little island speck in the Pacific, is a similar nutritional savior to the Japanese. Hitler's move eastward was a hope looking to the Russian fertility reserves. The hoverings of his battleship, Graf Spee, around Montevideo, and his persistence in Argentina were designs on that last of the world's rich store of less exploited soil fertility to be had in the form of corn, wheat and beef much more than they were maneuverings for political or naval advantage. Some of these historic material events serve to remind us that "an empty stomach knows no laws" and that man is in no unreal sense, an animal that becomes a social and political being only after he has consumed some of the products of the soil. . . .

Geographic divisions to give us an East and a West, and a North and a South for the eastern half of the country, are commonly interpreted as separations according to differences in modes of livelihood, social customs, or political affiliations. Differences in rainfall and temperature are readily acknowledged. But that these weather the basic rock to make soils so different that they control differences in vegetation, animals, and humans, by control of their nutrition is not so readily granted. That "we are as we eat" and that we eat according to the soil fertility, are truths that will not so generally and readily be accepted. Acceptances are seemingly to come not by deduction but rather through disaster.

Patterns of Nourishment Are Premised on the Pattern of Soil Fertility

We have been speaking about vegetation by names of crop species and by tonnage yields per acre. We have not considered plants for their chemical composition and nutritive value according to the fertility in the soil producing them. This failure has left us in confusion about crops and has put plant varieties into competition with—rather than in support of—one another. Now that the subject of nutrition is on most every tongue, we are about ready for the report that vegetation as a deliverer of essential food products of its own synthesis is limited by the soil fertility.

Proteinaceousness and high mineral contents, as distinct nutritive values, are more common in crops from soil formed in regions of lower rainfall and of less leaching as for example the "Midlands" or the midwestern part of the United States. "Hard" wheat, so-called because of its high protein content needed for milling the "patent" flour for "light" bread, is commonly ascribed to regions of lower annual rainfalls. "Soft" wheat is similarly ascribed to the regions of higher rainfalls. The high calcium content of the other liberal mineral reserves, and the pronounced activities of nitrogen within the less-leached soil, however, are the causes when experimental trials supplying the soil with these fertility items in high rainfall regions can make hard wheat where soft wheat is common. The proteinaceous vegetation and the synthesis by it of many unknowns which, like proteins, help to remove hidden hungers and encourage fecundity of both man and animal are common in the prairie regions marked by the moderate rainfalls. It is the soil fertility, rather than the low precipitation, that gives the Midwest or those areas bordering along approximately the 97th meridian these distinctions: (a) its selection by the bison in thundering herds on the "buffalo grass"; (b) the wheat which taken as a whole rather than as a refined flour is truly the "staff of life"; (c) animals on range nourishing themselves so well that they reproduce regularly; and (d) the more able-bodied selections for the military service of whom seven out of ten are chosen in contrast to seven rejected out of ten, in one of the southern states where the soils are more exhausted of their fertility.

Protein production, whether by plant, animal or man, makes demands on the soil giving elements. Body growth among forms of higher life is a matter of soil fertility and not only one of photosynthesis. It calls for more than rainfall, fresh air and sunshine.

The heavier rainfall and forest vegetation of the Eastern United States mark off the soils that have been leached of much fertility. Higher temperatures in the southern areas have made more severe the fertility-reducing effects of the rainfall. Consequently, vegetation there is not such an effective synthesizer of proteins. Neither is it a significant provider of calcium, phosphorus, magnesium, or the other soil-given, foetus-building nutrients. Annual production as tonnage per acre is large, particularly in contrast to the sparsity of that on the western prairies. The East's production is highly carbonaceous, however, as the forests, the cotton and the sugar cane can testify. The carbonaceous nature is contributed by air, water and sunlight more than by the soil. Fuel and fattening values are more prominent than are aids to growth and production.

Here is a basic principle that cannot be disregarded. It has signal value as we face nutritional problems on a national scale. It is of course, true that soil under higher rainfalls and temperatures still supply some fertility for the plant production. Potassium however, dominates that limited supply to give prominence to photosynthesis of carbonaceous products. The insufficient provision of calcium and of all requisite elements usually associated with calcium does not permit the synthesis, by internal performances of plants, of the proteins and many other compounds of equal nutritive value. The national problem is largely one of mobilizing the calcium and other fertility elements for growing protein and not wholly of redistributing proteins under federal controls. The soil fertility pattern on the map delineates the various areas of particular success or particular trouble in nutrition. It marks out the areas where, by particular soil treatments, the starving plants can be given relief.

The Fertility Pattern of Europe Is a Mirror Pattern of Our Own

The more concentrated populations in the United States are in the East and on the soils of lower fertility. For these people, Horace Greeley spoke good advice when he said "Go West young man." It was well that they trekked to the semi-humid midwest where the hard wheat grows on the chernozem soils, and where the bread basket and the meat basket are well-laden and carried by the same provider, viz, the soil. It was that move that spelled our recent era of prosperity.

In Europe the situation is similar but the direction of travel was reversed and the time period has been longer. It is Western Europe that represents the concentrated populations on soils of lower fertility under heavier rainfall. Peoples there reached over into the Pioneer United States for soil fertility by trading for it the marked "made in Germany." More recently the hard wheat belt on the Russian chernozem soils has been the fertility goal under the Hitlerite move eastward. Soil fertility is thus the cause of no small import in the world wars.

Calcium and Phosphorus Are Prominent in the Soil Fertility Pattern as It Determines the Pattern of Nutrition of Plants and Animals

Life behaviors are more closely linked with soils as the basis of nutrition than is commonly recognized. The depletion of soil calcium through leaching and cropping and the almost universal deficiency of soil phosphorus, connect readily with animals when bones are the chief body depositories for these two elements. In the forest, the annual drop of leaves and their decay to pass their nutrient elements through the cycle of growth, and decay again, are almost a requisite for tree maintenance. Is it any wonder then that dropped antlers and other skeletal forms are eaten by the animals to prohibit their accumulation while their calcium and phosphorus stay in the animal cycle? Deer in their browse will select trees given fertilizers in preference to those untreated. Pine tree seedlings along the highway as transplantings from fertilized nursery soils are taken by the deer when the same tree species in the adjoining forests go untouched. Wild animals truly "know their medicines" when they take plants on particular levels of soil fertility.

The distribution of wild animals, the present pattern or distribution of domestic animals, and the concentrations of animal diseases, can be visualized as super-impositions on the soil fertility pattern as it furnishes nutrition. We have been prone to believe these patterns of animal behaviors wholly according to climate. We have forgotten that the eastern forest areas gave the Pilgrims limited game among which a few turkeys were sufficient to establish a national tradition of Thanksgiving. It was on the fertile prairies of the Midwest, however, that the bison were so numerous that only their pelts were commonly taken.

Distribution of domestic animals today reveals a similar pattern, but more by freedom from "disease"—more properly freedom from malnutrition—and by greater regularity and fecundity in reproduction. It is on the lime-rich, unleached, semi-humid soils that animals reproduce well. It is there that the concentrations of disease are lower and some diseases are rare. There beef cattle are multiplied and grown to be shipped to the humid soils where they are fattened. Similar cattle shipments from one fertility level to another are common in Argentina.

In going from midwestern United States eastward to the less fertile soil, we find that animal troubles increase and become a serious handicap to meat and milk production. The condition is no less serious as one goes south or south-eastward. The distribution patterns of milk fever, of acetonemia, and of other reproductive troubles, that so greatly damage the domestic animal industry, suggest themselves as closely connected with the soil fertility pattern that locates the proteinaceous, mineral-rich forages of higher feeding value in the prairie areas but leaves the more carbonaceous and more deficient foods for the East and Southeast with their forest areas. Troubles in the milksheds of eastern and southern cities are more of a challenge for the agronomists and soil scientists than for veterinarians.

Experiments using soil treatments have demonstrated the important roles that calcium and phosphorus can play in the animal physiology and reproduction by way of the forages and grains from treated soils. Applied on adjoining plots of the same area, their effects were registered in sheep as differences in animal growth per unit of feed consumed, and as differences in the quality of the wool. Rabbits also grew more rapidly and more efficiently on hay grown where limestone and superphosphate had been used together than where phosphate alone had been supplied.

The influence of added fertilizers registers itself pronouncedly in the entire physiology of the animal. This fact was indicated not only by differences in the weight and quality of the wool, but in the bones and more pronouncedly in the semen production and reproduction in general. Rabbit bones varied widely in breaking strength, density, thickness, hardness and other qualities beside mass and volume. Male rabbits used for artificial insemination became sterile after a few weeks on lespedeza hay grown without soil treatment, while those eating hay from limed rock remained fertile. That the physiology of the animal, seemingly so far removed from the slight change in chemical condition in the soil, registered the soil treatment, is shown by the resulting interchange of the sterility and fertility of the lots with the interchange of the hays during the second feeding period. This factor of animal fertility alone is an economic liability on less fertile soil, but is a great economic asset on the soils that are more fertile either naturally or made so by soil treatments.

Animal Instincts Are Helpful in Meeting Their Nutritional Needs

Instincts for wise choice of food are still retained by the animals in spite of our attempts to convert the cow into a chemical engineering establishment wherein her ration is as simple as urea and phosphoric acid mixed with carbohydrates and proteins, however crude. Milk, which is the universal food with high efficiency because of its role in reproduction, cannot as yet be reduced to the simplicity of chemical engineering when calves become affected with rickets in spite of ample sunshine and plenty of milk, on certain soil types of distinctly low fertility. Rickets as a malnutrition "disease" according to the soil type, need not be a new concept, so far as this trouble affects calves.

Even if we try to push the cow into the lower levels in the biotic pyramid, or even down to that of plants and microbes that alone can live on chemical ions, not requisite as compounds, she still clings to her instincts of selecting particular grasses in mixed pasture herbages. Fortunately, in her physiology she strikes up partnership with the microbes in her paunch where they synthesize some seven essential vitamins for her. We are about to forget, however, that these paunch-dwellers cannot be refused in their demands for soil fertility by which they can meet this expectation. England's allegiance in war time to cows as ruminants that carry on these symbiotic vitamin synthesis, and her reduction of the population of pigs and poultry that cannot do so, bring the matter of soils more directly into efficient service for national nutrition than we have been prone to believe.

The instincts of animals are compelling us to recognize soil differences. Not only do dumb beasts select herbages according as they are more carbonaceous or proteinaceous, but they select from the same kind of grain the offerings according to the different fertilizers with which the soil was treated. Animal troubles engendered by the use of feeds in mixtures only stand out in decided contrast. Hogs select different corn grains from separate feeder compartments with disregard of different hybrids but with particular and consistent choice of soil treatments. Rats have indicated discrimination by cutting into the bags of corn that were chosen by the hogs and left uncut those bags not taken by the hogs. Surely the animal appetite, that calls the soil fertility so correctly, can be of service in guiding animal production more wisely by means of soil treatments.

Dr. Curt Richer of the Johns Hopkins Hospital has pointed to a physiological basis for such fine distinction by rats, as an example. Deprived of insulin delivery within their system, they ceased to take sugar. But dosed with insulin they increased consumption of sugar in proportion to the insulin given. Fat was refused in the diet similarly in accordance with the incapacity of the body to digest it. Animal instincts are inviting our attention back to the soil just as differences in animal physiology are giving a national pattern of differences in crop production, animal production, and nutritional troubles too easily labeled as "disease" and thus accepted as inevitable when they ought to have remedy by attention to the soil. The soils determine how well we fill the bread basket and the meat basket.

Patterns of Population Distribution Are Related to the Soil

The soil takes on national significance when it prompts the Mayor of the eastern metropolis to visit the "Gateway to the West" to meet the farmers dealing with their production problems. More experience in rationing should make the simple and homely subject of soils and their productive capacity household words amongst urban as well as rural peoples. Patterns of the distribution of human beings and their diseases, that can be evaluated nationally on a statistical basis as readily as crops of wheat or livestock, are not yet seen in terms of the soil fertility that determines one about as much as the other. Man's nomadic nature has made him too cosmopolitan for his physique, health, facial features, and mental attitudes to label him as of the particular soil that nourished him. His collection of foods from far-flung sources also handicaps our ready correlation of his level of nutrition with the fertility of the soil. We have finally come to the belief that food processing and refinement are denying us some essentials. We have not yet, however, come to appreciate the role that soil fertility plays in determining the nutritive quality of foods, and thereby our bodies and minds. Quantity rather than quality is still the measure.

Now that we are thinking about putting blanket plans as an order over states, countries and possibly the world as a whole, there is need to consider whether such can blot out the economics, customs and institutions that have established themselves in relation to the particular soil's fertility. Since any civilization rests or is premised on its resources rather than on its institutions, changes in the institution cannot be made in disregard of so basic a resource as the soil.

National Optimism Arises Through Attention to Soil Fertility

Researches in soil science, plant physiology, ecology, human nutrition and other sciences have given but a few years of their efforts to human welfare. These contributions have looked to hastened consumption surpluses from unhindered production for limited territorial use. Researchers are now to be applied to production, and a production that calls for use of nature's synthesizing forces for food production more than to simple nonfood conversions. When our expanded chemical industry is permitted to turn from war-time to peace-time pursuits, it is to be hoped that a national consciousness of declining soil can enlist our sciences and industry into rebuilding and conserving our soils as the surest guarantee of the future health and strength of the nation.

Chapter 24

FLUORINE IN PLANT AND ANIMAL GROWTH

T HE RECENT interest in the use of Fluorine as an aid in the control of dental caries, has emphasized the need for recording some related data.

The presence of Fluorine in the igneous rocks of the earth's surface, in an amount about equal to that of phosphorus, namely, one part per one thousand, has made it quite universally available for plant and animal growth. Its extreme toxicity, even in great dilution, has been prevented from doing harm by its very low solubility in water, namely, thirty-seven parts per million, for CaF^2. Even a small fraction of this concentration, when present in the drinking water, greatly disturbs normal tooth and bone development, producing the unsightly disfigurement of brown stain and mottled enamel. This curses the people living in the districts having an affected water supply. It may ruin the teeth of grazing animals, by making them so brittle that they break off. Camels, sheep, cows, goats, donkeys and horses are seriously affected in a North Africa district, thus making them unable to pasture.

This increase in Fluorine concentration occurs in water-pools by evaporation and in some artesian water supplies, where the drainage is from distant table lands. These dental defects are caused systemically when the teeth are being formed. Fluorine slightly increases the density or hardness of developed teeth, even in a test-tube. This includes slight resistance to acids, including those due to carbohydrate fermentation. This is the basis for the hope in its reducing the effects of bacterial acids, produced in tooth decay.

Bibby, *The Journal of the American Dental Association*, March 1, 1944. Subject, "Fluorine in Prevention of Caries," reports regarding the experimental efficiency of Fluorine treatment as follows:

> Summary: Experiments on eighty children over a period of two years showed that six topical applications of a one to one thousand sodium fluoride solution, reduced dental caries by somewhat more than one third as compared with results in the corresponding untreated quadrants in the same mouth.

Regarding the theory of acid resistance and methods of treatment, Atkins states, in *The Journal of the American Dental Association*, March 1, 1944: "For lack of a more descriptive word it is explained that the teeth are given an invisible coating of Fluorine in a similar manner as silver nitrate is deposited."

He emphasizes the great care that is needed in applying it because of its extreme toxicity as follows: Because it is one of the violently poisonous elements, Fluorine requires careful handling. In the preparation of solutions one must keep well within the bounds of safety. The highest suggested content here is similar to that of several water supplies, furnished for general consumption. Neither the drug itself, nor the formula, has been given to others than those qualified to handle it. Adding it to the food or water for general use is beyond the practice of dentistry.

In my studies of primitive races in many parts of the world and in many stages of loss of immunity to dental caries, many groups had not changed their location or made changes in their local environment. The water supply, whether from a mountain stream or a well, had remained the same. Ships had made contact with the island, often to carry away local products, chiefly copra, dried cocoanut meat. The payment was made chiefly in three articles of commerce, refined flour, concentrated sweetened fruit jams and highly colored calicos, but no currency. I asked the manager of one of these inter island navigation companies, regarding the proportions. He said ninety percent must be in flour and jams and not over ten percent in cotton goods. The reduction of fluorine intake, if any, was limited to the lowered use of sea foods and land plants. As I have shown in previous chapters, the increase in dental caries averaged about thirty fold.

The great mass of research data, developed during the past fifty years with the mechanisms involved in dental caries, has emphasized the solubility action of acids produced by the breakdown of carbohydrates by bacteria, chiefly those of the acidophilus group. Two controlling factors have been recognized, the type and quantity of carbohydrate present and the presence or absence of depressants to bacterial growth. The emphasis is placed on control of these two factors. Programs involving the use of Fluorine, because of its depressing action on carbohydrate acidity development, should include control of the carbohydrate factor.

It is very important that in the consideration of the dental caries problem it shall be kept in mind continually, that it is only one of a large group of symptoms of modern physical degeneration and when teeth are decaying other things are going wrong in the body. Fluorine treatment, like dental extractions, cannot be a panacea for dental caries.

Evidence of a Need for Fluorine in Optimum Amounts for Plant and Animal Growth and Bone and Tooth Development, with Thresholds for Injury

One of the major problems of dental research for the past three decades has involved phases of hypoplasia of different types. In 1913 the author published an illustrated report presenting an extended series of structural tooth defects, which seemed traceable directly to particular types of baby food. Black and McKay, in 1916, presented data relating to an endemic deformity of tooth structure chiefly expressed as "mottling" and "stain" which has come to be known as the "brown-stain mottled-enamel lesion." McKay's work through the succeeding years has emphasized the relation of this lesion to the water supply. Paleopathology, and medical and dental annals have been recording the exis tence of this disease. The recent studies of Churchill, Smith, and others have emphasized the probable relationship of this lesion to excess of F in the water. The widespread distribution of this lesion throughout large areas of many countries has emphasized the seriousness of the defect and the probability that the causative factors will be found in soil conditions. The present studies have been carried forward to ascertain the method by which F acts when injurious effects are produced. The author's studies of blood chemical changes, as associated with disturbances in mineral metabolism, have emphasized the sensitiveness of the human mechanism not only to shortage of essential minerals and vitamins, but also to toxic quantities of certain metallic and nonmetallic substances. These have suggested the need for more information concerning their effect on mineral metabolism, and on growth for both plants and animals.

Much of the F of the earth's crust occurs in apatite and other Ca-P compounds, being frequently associated with Ca and P. Since approximately one part in a thousand of the earth's crust is P and approximately an equal amount is F, there is no scarcity of either element in the igneous rocks from which soils were developed. There is about thirty times as much Ca as either F or P in the earth's crust. The problem of the chemical form and solubility of F, as compared with other elements, has much to do with its concentration and availability for serious effects. The various phosphate rocks that are used as fertilizers—primarily calcium phosphate—contain from 0.69 to 4.23 percent of F, which is about one tenth the P content. The ratio of F to P^2O^5, as reported by Marshall Jacob, and Reynolds in an extended series of determinations, ranged from 0.06 to 1.32 for continental rocks; from 0.0178 to 0.085 for island deposits. The solubility of F is accordingly an important factor in determining the amount available in various waters and soils. Since igneous rocks are about equally rich in P and F, our problem clearly is not one of limited distribution of F. CaF^2, or fluorite, a common mineral, occurs in abundance in many districts, and is soluble to 37 parts per million of water. Other F salts, such as NaF, and sodium silico-fluoride (Na^2SiF^6) are also soluble— the former, 400 parts per ten thousand; the latter, 65 parts per ten thousand. F presumably has constantly been a factor in the environment of plant and animal life. Since living forms are the product of their environment, F has presumably had a part in vital phenomena. Its low solubility in the forms in which it occurs in igneous rocks suggests that it has not been present in high concentration in surface waters. These studies have accordingly been made to determine the effect of F on plant and animal growth; and on the levels at which it becomes toxic in the water bathing the plant roots, and when ingested by animals in water and food. Various types of plants have been grown in different nutrient fluids in which the concentration of F was varied up to 25 mg.

per liter. F as NaF, added in progressive amounts to sprouting corn—when the plant is utilizing only the stored minerals of the kernel, while growing in distilled water—had a progressive stimulating effect up to 10 parts per million of the water; 20 parts, or more, were very toxic and produced only stunted growth with a bronzed appearance. When, however, Ca and P were added to the fluid, the toxic effect was very greatly reduced. The maximum concentration (37 parts per million) of CaF^2 (the common mineral fluorite) would, if present, prevent this cereal from sprouting; and if it occurred in irrigation waters, would markedly depress plant growth. Surface drainage cannot readily become saturated. Water stored in soil and rocks as artesian water can more nearly do so, and has frequently been found to blight plant growth.

Studies have also been made of the effect on mineral metabolism when F is ingested by rats. In general several chemicals were depressed. The total iron of the blood of a control rat was at 50 mg. per 100cc. (The succeeding numerical data for rat blood indicate mg. per 100cc., when not given as percent.) When F was added as NaF (1 percent of the food), the iron content of the blood was 42.5 mg. The cell-Ca of the blood was reduced from 41.7 to 35. The inorganic P of the serum was reduced from 6.67 to 5.26; of the serum of 100 cc. of whole blood, from 3.89 to 3.42; in 100 cc. of blood cells, from 0.67 to 0.22; in the cells from 100 cc. of whole blood, from 0.88 to 0.28. The cell inorganic-P percent of the total-blood inorganic-P was reduced from 6.7 to 2.3. The inorganic P of whole blood, was reduced from 4.17 to 3.50; the Ca of whole blood, from 9.35 to 7.80. The Mg of blood rose from 2.63 to 3.50. The K of whole blood was reduced from 322 to 267. These data indicate that 1 percent of NaF (diet) caused general disturbance of mineral metabolism. They also suggest that ingestion of F, in amounts above the threshold of tolerance of the tissues, may be very depressing, and may materially influence mineral deposition in bones and teeth. Since, however, the teeth differ from the bones, in that a complete rebuilding process is not possible for the teeth through subsequent months and years, growth defects of the enamel would be permanent.

Field studies gave important data on waters and soils from many districts, including one in Northern Africa where the teeth of humans, and also those of camels, sheep, cows, goats, donkeys, and horses, are seriously affected. The waters from this district contain from 23 to 31 parts of F per million, determined by the Jacob and Reynolds method. The rocks from this district contained 5.38 percent of F, or 53,800 parts per million. This is the highest figure in our series, and higher than any found in the literature. Another series is related to the skeletal breakdown of a group of cattle on a western farm in eastern New Mexico, where both the water and soil contain excessive amounts of F. The blood of afflicted animals showed very marked depression of mineral constituents.

Chapter 25

HOW MOTHER NATURE MADE US

M Y STUDIES of fourteen primitive races in various stages of being modernized, together with our newer knowledge of the role of nutrition in human and animal behavior, help us to visualize what is taking place in our modern society.

It is most significant that where many primitive racial stocks have succeeded superbly, our modernized civilizations are failing dismally. The primitives have retained excellent bodies through many generations, while many moderns wreck theirs early with degenerative diseases.

The explanation as disclosed by the primitives is chiefly in our defeating some fundamental processes of life. We disregard our own physical needs as they are disclosed by our developmental origins. We have used our scientific knowledge largely to change nature's foods and thereby have defeated nature's laws of growth and health. The primitives cooperate with nature where we do not.

To assist in visualizing this I will briefly indicate some steps involved and describe them later.

PHYSICAL BASIS FOR BEHAVIOUR

PHYSICAL FORM	VITAL EXPRESSIONS
1. Prehuman stage of development.	Controlled by two forces, hunger and sex urge.
2. Development of human forebrain.	Reason, mental inhibitions for sex urge and appetite, honesty and unselfishness.
3. Parental nutritional injuries of fetus, with defects of forebrain.	Loss or lowering of inhibitions with character change, delinquency patterns and mentally retarded.
4. Nutritionally produced forebrain growth with increased functions.	Super-mentality, exalted personality, noble music, arts, social reforms and altruism.

Human nature's controlling forces are entirely automatic through a reflex nervous system until the control is divided through higher forebrain development. It is exceedingly important that if we are to stem the tide of modernized self–destruction, that we come to know the nature of and origin of both our physical being and our personalities, in order to ascertain what we have lost and how the loss may be prevented.

As an approach to this it is important that we review and visualize our origin. The current teachings of the three R's and simpler sciences and most of our religious and social philosophies have failed to relate us correctly to our past which so largely controls our physical behaviour and mental attitudes.

Avoiding technical language and using photographs, we can quickly learn much about our physical structure and zoological past. In Figure 142 we see a group of vertebrate embryos as classified by Haeckel and Needham.[1] Figure 142 demonstrates, reading from above downward, the appearance and development of these eight animal forms through three stages. Note particularly that in the early developmental stages of the embryo of these eight vertebrates, there is very close similarity between the Man, Rabbit, Calf, Hog, Chick, Tortoise, Salamander and Fish.

In the second stage shown in line 2 the similarity is retained in all except the Salamander and Fish. It is only in line 3 that the differentiation is complete in all eight groups. All of these forms of life have a similar origin, though clearly this does not demonstrate that man has sprung directly from some ancestral ape, but that both have developed from a common progenitor that lacked their several peculiarities.

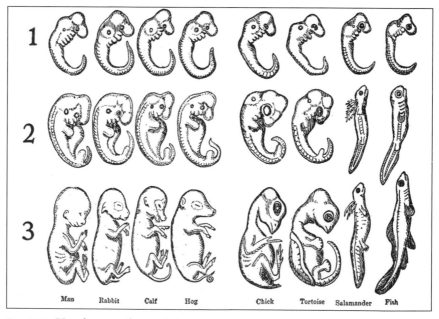

Fig. 142. Vertebrate embryos: 1, 2, 3, successive stages in their development.

Much of modern thinking and teaching has failed to recognize as common the origin of man with many animal forms and its significance for understanding his form and behaviour. Since much of man's expressions, physically and mentally, are related to his automatic behaviour, growing out of his heredity, we see at once the urgent need for a better understanding of him in this aspect, since these controls are the origin of his instincts or inherited behaviour. For all the simpler forms of life, behaviour is automatically controlled by the individual's reactions to the environment. Needham reminds us that many of the lower animals are born educated almost to the full extent of their capacity, the possible lines of action of their whole lives being provided for or being predetermined in their organization. The acts most fundamental to the preservation of races, feeding and reproduction, are thus cared for in the main in all animals and in ourselves. This is very important in connection with our modern tendencies, including human behaviour.

We are familiar with the normal behaviour of domestic animals and birds. For example, a kitten's first response to a dog is to arch its back and spit while bushing its tail and extending its claws. The dog's first response is to halt and back up. We call this instinct. It is wisdom at birth without being taught. Chickens run for shelter, young ones go to the mother at the cry of a hawk, which the mother hen recognizes and responds with her cry of danger. Needham defines instinct as inherited behaviour. He says it is that part of behaviour with respect to which animals are born fully educated. It is automatic and instantaneous in action. It is common to all members of a species. In matters of vital importance all tend to act alike. It is by instinct the animals, birds and insects build their homes, often of great complexity, without having been taught by example. They are instinctive acts, unconsciously performed, being automatic yet made with the full knowledge of the individual.

Pavlov describes instinct as a complex of reflexes. Instinct is knowledge at birth or as soon after as needed. By instinct the kitten knows the dog is its enemy; it is on guard and active even when the individual is not conscious, as in sleep, in which state some animals have violent reactions from odors; for example, sex urge. Humans all start and finish life dominated by these unconscious reactions.

Unlike the simpler forms of life man and the higher forms superimpose willful behaviour in accordance with the dominance of the will and its store of intelligence, which is variable, together with his release from the domination of his impulsive instructor or rather his instructive impulses.

Instructive impulses change radically with internal development and environment. This is strikingly illustrated in many of the simpler animals and insect forms, as shown in Figure 143, of the tent caterpillar.

It has four distinct life stages, viz., as an egg, larva, pupa and moth. Its behavior for all these stages is controlled at the time of the fertilization of the original ovum to produce the egg. The delicacy and power of the mechanism not only persists through these physical transitions, but go forward to motivate similarly all future generations.

The eggs are laid on a tiny twig in July by a small moth, but do not hatch until the following April or May. They must withstand freezing, blizzards of winter and dehydrating sun and wind. The eggs are attached to end tips of live cherry limbs, and for some varieties only cherry will do. Two views of an egg cluster are shown at a and b, Fig. 143. The hatching time of the eggs is adapted to the appearance of green leaves on which the minute caterpillars feed in warm sunshine, and at evening proceed down the twig to the first crotch, laying a web as they go to build their ingenious tent home; see d, Figure 143. The brood from this one group of eggs includes many hundreds. They are laid in pyramid shape, and have a color that matches the cherry branch. When the caterpillars are fully grown, see c, Figure 143, they crawl down the trunk of the tree and find a shelter in which they live alone and spin about themselves a silken cocoon; see e Figure 143. This silken coat is covered by a white creamy fluid secreted to fill the meshes of the cocoon. Within this cocoon the caterpillar changes its form to a pupa (chrysalis) with wings, long legs, antennas and various structures of the moth, male and female; see f and g, Figure 143. This takes about two weeks time. It now can fly, which it does at night after hiding during the day; it no longer has hunger or a digestive system. The controlling impulse is now only sex urge, and it goes forth at night to find a mate that is out on this same mission, which is its only mission in life and for which alone its former stages were provided. The male, too, now cannot eat; after mating he is through with life. His contribution, the spermatozoa, however, lives on through continuing generations as a well-nigh eternal force; they are potentially immortal. The female moth proceeds forthwith to find another cherry tree and plants her fertilized eggs on a twig in systematic order all on end, closely packed and protected by a waterproof covering about the color of the twig. Then her mission in life is fulfilled, her sex-cell caterpillar history and the specifications for future generations are, like the male's, practically immortal.

What is the source of all this energy and can it carry on through countless generations? The only renewal source of energy is the food selected and utilized in only one of its four forms of organized protoplasm, viz., when a caterpillar. That food was required to make it grow to maturity. This involved many score of chemical substances, adequate to build, each, a nervous system, eyes, silk factory and spinning tools, embryonic sex cells, male and female antennas, wings, cocoon parts, moths, etc. These chemicals were all synthesized from the minerals, acids, bases, hormones and vitamins furnished by the rapidly growing green cherry leaves, plus sunshine and atmosphere. These include several minerals from the soil. Clearly this could only occur where Mother

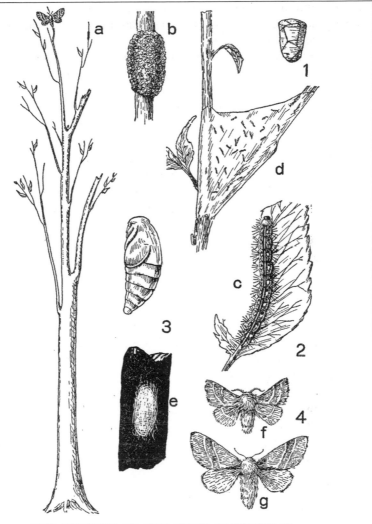

NO. 242 LIFE HISTORY OF THE TENT CATERPILLAR

1. Egg from clusters at *a* and *b*: laid in July, hatch in April.
2. Larva, on leaf at *c*, with others in tent at *d*; active by day: feeds on leaves
   through May.
3. Pupa, removed from the cocoon shown at *e*: inactive until transformation.
4. Adult moths male at *f*, female at *g*: active at night.

FIG. 143

Nature's laws were obeyed at every step. Suppose the caterpillar had learned to rob the plant juice of its carotene, then the vitamin A could not form and no eyes could be made or many of the other structures; or if only starches and sugars were eaten, no body could be built or capacity to reproduce and continue the race. Its safety is provided in both its ignorance and the rigidity of Mother Nature's laws.

While many other cycles may seem more simple than that of this animal they are all controlled by vital forces that we do not yet understand. We are in fact quite as helpless in our dependence on nature's sources and essentials for life as are the insects, animals and birds. All are dependent on land and sea foods, since we cannot create the elements and we can only get them by way of our foods. Ultimately they must come from the sources of all foods, the soil and the sea.

We humans have the same rigid restrictions regarding food selection as the simpler forms of life when foods are evaluated from their chemical basis. Our greater complicity however, introduces new behavior patterns due to injuries to the structure and therefore the functions of the forebrain. All primitive races that have lived on for long periods have done so by obeying Nature's rigid laws.

The insects, birds and animals are provided with a key to direct them to the foods most helpful, namely their instinct; modern man has largely lost this guide, though while young he retains a large measure of it.

It is important to note regarding instincts that they develop and disappear with different stages of development and growth. Children and adults are afraid of snakes but infants are not. With the change in a boy's voice his manners with girls change. In adolescence there is a radical change in the sex urge in which action is automatic in balance with the inhibitions, which in most animals are physiological but in man are primarily mental being provided by education.

The animal or human body is an incubator, nothing can take the place of the germ cells, or change their functions, there is no other starting material for a new generation. Needham's *About Ourselves* explains this clearly as follows:

> Early in the development of the body from the egg there occurs a differentiation of the growing cell mass into two parts that Weismann properly emphasized as "germ plasm" and "body plasm." The germ plasm is a group of cells that will remain unspecialized, that will be segregated within the developing body, and that on the approach of the maturity of that body will produce new germ cells for another generation. They take not part in the labors of the body. They serve no other function than that of reproduction; but they alone leave descendants in future generations. They are thus potentially immortal.
>
> Many of the lower animals are born educated almost to the full extent of their capacity, the possible lines of action of their whole lives being provided for or predetermined in their organization. The acts most fundamental to the preservation of the races, feeding and reproduction are thus cared

for in the main in all animals and in ourselves. So also are avoidance reactions that protect from deadly perils. A chicken flees at the first cry of a hawk although it may be quite unresponsive to the (to us) similar cry of a cat bird. Nature has developed this nice discrimination by the elimination of those individuals that do not act properly and with effective promptness. Racial experience has thus been incorporated into the organism in such manner that vitally important stimuli dominate all the activities of the body and enable it to meet the chief exigencies of life.

There is however, especially in the higher animals, a field of activity in which the reactions are less fixed, and here lies the opportunity for learning by individual experience. This is so large a part of our own life that we have difficulty in realizing how limited it is in many of the lower animals.

These data throw important light on our modern world problems, notwithstanding our declining food resources through loss of fertility, which Needham emphasizes.

Since the units of populations are persons, it is obvious that the basic need is for soundness in body and mind in those persons. There are two sets of factors entering into the making of each person; inherent tendencies and environmental influences; and there are likewise two schools of opinion as to means of social betterment. The programs that they offer bear high-sounding Greek names:

1. Eugenics, looking to nature, to better breeding heredity.
2. Euthenics, looking to nurture, to better environment.

Behind all this crowding is the nature of man, with the irresistible sex urge. Abetting this urge is the demand of war-lords for larger families—more men to man the guns—more men for fodder. There also remains the primitive feeling that the nation is strongest that has the largest population. Obviously this is no longer true.

Nature's inexorable limit is set by the food supply. Mankind must eat to live. Every advance in food production is quickly overtaken by increase in population. Generally the optimum is soon overpassed with men as with caterpillars, and starvation sets in to reduce the excess.

Modern man's mental inhibitions are not strong enough to protect him, as Needham shows.

Studies in widely scattered areas in the United States show that the birthrate among families who have been on relief (Sustained by public funds: 1936) for more than a year is about 60% higher than among families of similar social status who are not on relief.

—James S. K. Bossard, in *Birth Control and Continuing the Depression.*

The normal and proper exercise of the primal altruistic racial instincts is the chief basis of human happiness. The consuming joy that lovers find in each other's company, the captivation of a baby's smile—of one's own baby's smile, the sense of belonging within the family circle; these are far older than church or state or any other artificial products of the social order. They are the product of a natural evolution. They are the greatest of God's gifts to human kind.

It was at this point that several of the primitive racial stocks have displayed superior wisdom, which has enabled them to live on through many centuries even in difficult physical environments. For example the Australian Aborigines controlled the population by limiting the size of families, while permitting each woman to have one or two children but only the restricted number that the territory of that clan could support.

The evidence provided by these studies among the primitives throws an important new light on the confusion regarding which is responsible for modern character disturbances and various mental variations. The general assumption is that it is faulty environment that provides abnormal personalities, since only two causes are considered possible, namely, heredity or environment. In other words, is it the result of nature or nurture? It has not been considered that a third cause may be responsible, namely, intercepted heredity. In the light of these new data our mentally backward and delinquent individuals may be injured and are really abnormal because of this type of injury resulting from parental nutritional germ cell defect. The opposite phase of this, namely, exalted mentality may represent normality. For example, a much larger proportion of Rhodes' scholars than normal are the oldest boy in the family and in general come from districts providing good nutrition. Similarly, data now available illustrate this regarding the leading men of science. Dr. Richard Ashman of Louisiana State University reports in the April 1945 issue of *The Journal of Heredity* a study of the state of birth of American men of science. The map showing this is reproduced as Figure 144.

He closes his interpretation of these finds as follows:

> Since many dysgenic factors are operating in the United States today, it is pertinent to inquire whether our civilization can long endure. For its perpetuation many things are, of course, necessary, including education. But how long shall we have a sufficient supply of educable material? No amount of social and economic reform, however desirable and necessary these may be, can prevail against a downward genetic trend, even though moderate. Civilization in the region or nation which reverses this trend may soon surpass that of the rest of the world.

While his interpretation seems to place the emphasis on genetics it is significant that the states showing the highest population of scientists are those covering the areas that my studies indicate have produced a very high level of body-building foods. It is also significant that Dr. Albrecht has presented data indicating that this district was the one selected by the buffalo herds because of superb pasture, in his discussion of the relation of soils to food qualities.

The relation of brain function to soil fertility is demonstrated in many sources of information. These include a percentage of grade school pupils in classes

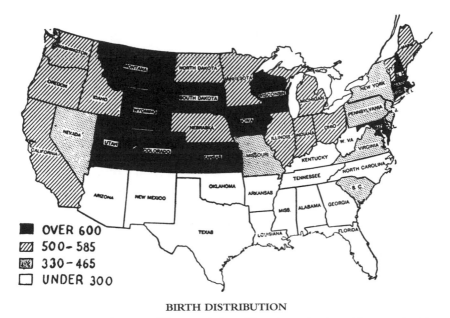

BIRTH DISTRIBUTION

FIG. 144. Concentration per million population of American scientists with respect to state of birth. Climate, education and economic opportunities differ so greatly throughout the country that these differences cannot be attributed mainly to genetic differences.

for mentally retarded and backward children. I have found the proportion in several districts to be above thirty percent, and progressively increasing in several states. In the group of southern states using the same examination, passing from grade schools to high schools, the data show a marked superiority in the proportion of children for the Panhandle area. That area is underlain with caliche subsoil which consists of calcium pebbles cemented together with calcium carbonate.

In Chapter 22 I have shown that the milk and cream produced from wheat pasture in that area are very high in vitamin A and activator X. Many of the children are excellent. The average well above normal. The roots of the wheat plants in this district have been shown to penetrate down six feet, well into the subsoil. The district includes Hereford which has been highly publicized for its low incidence of dental caries. The cattle raised in that area are very superior, both for beef and for reproduction. The people can be also if they are as wise as the buffalo and cattle in the selection of their food.

REFERENCES

[1] NEEDHAM, J. G. *About Ourselves: A survey of human nature from the zoological viewpoint.* Lancaster, PA: Jacques Cattell Press, 1941.

Chapter 26

STEPS IN OUR MODERN DEGENERATION

OUR degenerations like our growths being an unconscious process will be recognized and evaluated best by making comparative measurements. Accordingly, studies of changes occurring in our modern civilization require a set of standards in order to make these comparisons. For evidence of a need for making such studies it will be helpful to note the comments of competent observers in various fields.

Ernest Thompson Seton has been a critical student of the early American civilization that preceded modern European invasion and conquest. In his analysis of the relative virtues of the American Indian as recorded in his book *The Gospel of the Red Man*[1] he makes this observation:

> The civilization of the white man is a failure; it is visibly crumbling around us. It has failed at every crucial test. No one who measures things by results can question this fundamental statement.

Referring to the comparative physical qualities of our modern whites he says:

> All historians, hostile and friendly, admit the Indian to have been the finest type of physical manhood the world has ever known. None but the best, the picked, chosen and trained of the Whites, had any chance with him.

In his discussion of the comparable cultural qualities of the modem whites and the Indians he states:

> The culture and civilization of the White man are essentially material; his measure of success is "How much property have I acquired for myself?" The culture of the Red man is fundamentally spiritual; his measure of success is, "How much service have I rendered to my people?"

The severe expressions of modern degeneration as they affect various organs and tissues constitute the every day experience of surgeons. This group of specialists has developed because of the imperative need that diseased parts of organs and tissues should be removed in order to prolong the function and comfort of other structures. Sir Arbuthnot Lane, a world renowned authority on the disturbances of the intestinal tract of the modernized whites as compared with the more normal functioning of primitive races, has expressed his deep impressions in his Preface to *Maori Symbolism*[2] as follows:

Long surgical experience has proved to me conclusively that there is some-
thing radically and fundamentally wrong with the civilized mode of life, and
I believe that unless the present dietetic and health customs of the White
Nations are reorganized, social decay and race deterioration are inevitable.

Sociologists emphasize strongly the evidences of an alarming increase in
the percentage of individuals in our modernized cultures who cannot manage their own lives successfully, and hence require some supervision by those
who are more competent. Laird in discussing this problem under the title *The
Tail That Wags the Nation*[3] states:

The country's average level of general ability sinks lower with each generation. Should the ballot be restricted to citizens able to take care of themselves? One out of four cannot....The tail is wagging Washington, and Wall
Street and LaSalle Street.

The seriousness of the decline in modern physical fitness has been emphasized by many individuals and organizations. An expression of the deep interest and concern is seen in the large contributions amounting to many millions
of dollars yearly for scientific research to find the contributing factors. This
generous response by philanthropists has made possible the engaging of the services of many prominent research workers in various fields of investigation.
Among these, the contributions of Dr. Alexis Carrel have been outstanding.
In his profound studies of the problem under the title *Man, the Unknown* he
has made a most forceful review of the present dilemma and places great importance on modern man's increased susceptibility to degenerative diseases.
In relating this phase to modern medicine he states:

Medicine is far from having decreased human suffering as much as it en-
deavors to make us believe. Indeed, the number of deaths from infectious
diseases has greatly diminished. But we still must die in a much larger proportion from degenerative diseases.... All diseases of bacterial origin have
decreased in a striking manner.... Nevertheless, in spite of the triumphs of
medical science, the problem of disease is far from solved. Modern man is
delicate. Eleven hundred thousand persons have to attend the medical needs
of 120,000,000 other persons. Every year, among this population of the
United States, there are about 100,000,000 illnesses, serious or slight. In the
hospitals, 700,000 beds are occupied every day of the year.... Medical care,
under all its forms, costs about $3,500,000,000 yearly.... The organism seems
to have become more susceptible to degenerative diseases.

While it has been a matter of general knowledge that progressive deterioration was in operation, the search for contributing factors has not adequately revealed the causes. The forces at work have been largely assigned
to either heredity or environment. The exponents of these two views have
marshalled impressive evidence in support of their interpretations. It is of

particular importance that practically all of the efforts at correction have been built around either the prevention of reproduction by defective individuals or the modifying of the environment of defectives in order to prevent or correct the development of the disturbance. A widely accepted interpretation of the controlling factors in heredity has been the acceptance of the principle that the carriers of individual qualities, as involved in the function of the sex cells and the entire processes of reproduction and development, are practically immutable and as such cannot readily be modified by the environment into which the individual is born. These principles have been supported by impressive evidence from both animal and plant life illustrating the laws of transmission of Mendelian qualities. The very principle on which racial and tribal characteristics are evaluated and classified implies a faithful transmission from generation to generation. This view requires that these dominating forces prevail over disturbances in prenatal environment and provide normal offspring from normal ancestry.

That the journey of the fetus resulting from the fertilized ovum encounters grave experiences in the prenatal environment is indicated by the report of the American Association of Obstetricians and Gynecologists[4] as follows: "Out of every one hundred pregnancies in the United States, 25 are lost before birth."

An evaluation of the controlling forces requires that light be thrown on the role of each heredity and environment and on the forces at work—each— prior to fertilization, during gestation and after birth. As an approach to this phase it is important that we have in mind the nature of the defects, for which we must find the causes.

The ills of modern man have required the services of large groups of specialists trained for rendering service in the various fields. The dental profession is organized to serve civilization and treat and care for the ills of the oral cavity including dental caries, dental arch deformities and diseased supporting tissues of the teeth. Similarly, each organ of the body has its corps of specialists equipped to furnish first aid and make repairs and adjustments where possible. Their greatest effort, and in the dental profession nearly the entire effort, is expended in repair and replacement of defective or removed organs. Available data indicate that from 90 to 100 percent of the individuals in our modernized groups have suffered from dental caries.

A comprehensive study of modern degeneration will require the use of controls in order that standards of excellence may be established. Not finding adequate controls in our affected groups it became necessary to look elsewhere in Nature's great biological laboratory which has been in operation throughout the history of life. For this the primitive racial stocks that have persisted through centuries have been selected. These have been located both where still protected by the isolation, and where they were in the process of being modernized by contact with the culture and commerce of the white man. For this fourteen primitive racial stocks have been studied by comparing the individuals of the more isolated groups with groups of the same stock in various stages of modernization, also with modernized Europeans and Americans. The following primitive racial stocks have been studied: Swiss, Gaelics, Eskimos, North American Indians, Polynesians, Melanesians, Africans, Australian Aborigines, New Zealand Maori, Malay Micronesians, Ancient Peruvians, Isolated Peruvian Indians, High Andes Indians and Amazon Jungle Indians. The data obtained from these comparative studies together with the results of animal experimentation are the basis for this report.

It is clearly impossible in the limited space available for this text to include extended supporting data. The data presented here will be classed under two heads; injuries that result from forces at work after the individual is born, and those that are produced prior to birth. For brevity and to avoid confusion arising out of extended details only general results are provided in this text.

Were it not for the greater importance of the larger problems involved in modern degeneration, it would be appropriate to use the available space for this chapter in the discussion of new light on the dental caries problem since the detailed data are so illuminating. Under the circumstances the dental problem will be discussed here only briefly. Clearly the personality and behaviour problems are most important.

However the comparative incidence of dental caries in the various isolated groups and the same groups when modernized, expressed in terms of affected teeth, ranged from an average of about one percent for the isolated to thirty percent of all teeth studied for the modernized. In several groups the effect of contact with modern white culture and its commerce involved an increase in the incidence of dental caries of several hundred fold. The one factor in the contact with modern civilization that was universally found to be present and always associated with loss of immunity to dental caries and in proportion to its use, was a change from the native foods as selected by the isolated groups to the commercial foods of commerce. In many groups the loss of immunity occurred promptly after the change in nutrition was established and existed only during the period of the change, immunity being reestablished with the return to the original nutrition of the tribe.

This is illustrated by the calling of ships to isolated islands in the Pacific to purchase copra (dried coconut meat) when the price suddenly rose from forty dollars to four hundred dollars a ton. This lasted for only a short time and in two years the price dropped to about four dollars per ton, which changed factor that could be found in the environment was the displacement of the native diets with the foods of commerce that were used to make the exchange. I was informed personally by the administrator in charge of the out-fitting of trading vessels that 90 percent of the exchange was required to be taken in white flour and sugar and only 10 percent could be taken in cloth-ing and other products. In ports of regular call on ship routes the displacing diet included also canned foods, polished rice, vegetable fats, etc.

My studies on isolated Pacific Islands were made a few years after the tem-porary calling of copra ships. They revealed that teeth that had recently erupted, particularly first or second molars, at the time there was a change in the nutri-tion, had evidence of past active caries related directly to the period of changed nutrition. The cavities were open but immunity had been reestablished by a return to the native foods.

The data obtained from these various studies strongly indicated that the presence or absence of immunity of the teeth to dental caries was not depend-ent upon a change of structure in the formative period. The problem of im-munity to dental caries has seemed clearly to be related to nutrition of the affected individual at the time the dental caries is active. Similarly other effects such as rickets, avitaminosis diseases, were found to relate to changes in the structure of the organs and tissues rather than being transmitted qualities from the ancestry. A large group of affections were found to be directly related to forces that were operative before birth. These contribute the principal discussion of this chapter.

A glimpse of the dental tragedy which ushers in the disappearance of many of these primitive racial stocks is easily shown.

The girl (Figure 38) is an Hawaiian. She is not only suffering from abscess-ing teeth but is coughing with tuberculosis, from which her mother and a brother recently died. The boy (Figure 32) upper right is a Fijian, typical of many suffering from abscessing teeth. The woman to the right below is a typ-ical illustration of the Australian Aborigines confined in reservations in Aus-tralia being fed by the government. The woman at the lower right (Figure 26) is a typical modernized Florida Indian.

A bird's-eye view of factors found associated with mental and moral expressions of physical deficiency shows common biologic contributing agents.

The end result has been the same in all the primitive racial stocks studied when they changed from their native dietary as selected in accordance with the accumulated wisdom of their race to the foods of modern commerce. These have been largely the same for the different groups. It is a matter of great importance in connection with the world problem of dental caries that these several racial groups that established immunity for themselves by using a proper selection of available food did so on very different dietaries when judged on the basis of type and name of the foods. Their efficient diets, how-ever, were very similar when reduced to mineral and vitamin content. The outstanding difference from the chemical standpoint is the comparative level of body-building and body-repairing materials in proportion to heat and energy factors or calories. In general all the efficient dietaries were found to contain two to six times as high a factor of safety in the matter of body-building material, as the displacing foods.

The people in the isolated valleys of Switzerland provided a high immunity by the use of exceptionally high-vitamin dairy products and entire rye bread, with meat about once a week and vegetables as available, chiefly in the summer.

The people of the Outer Hebrides accomplished high immunity with the use of sea foods, oat cake and oat porridge with limited vegetables in season. Marine plants also were used.

The Eskimos and Indians of Alaska and the Far North accomplished a high immunity with sea and land animal tissues used as foods but limited vegetables and very limited seeds. Green foods were used in season and in some districts were stored. The organs of animals were used liberally.

The people of the South Sea Islands whether Polynesian, Melanesian or Micronesian provided a high immunity with a liberal use of sea animal foods, marine and land plants, limited seeds and lily roots or taro.

The cattle tribes of Africa established their high immunity by the use of milk, blood and meat supplemented by plant foods. The agricultural tribes of Africa used domestic animals, utilizing their organs, fresh water animal life, insects and a variety of plants.

The Australian Aborigines established their high immunity by the use of large and small wild animal life, wild plants, and where available, fresh water or marine sea life, large and small.

The New Zealand Maori had a high immunity to dental caries by a liberal use of sea animal life, marine plants, marine birds and their eggs, land birds, seeds of trees and plants and vegetables, particularly fern root.

The Indians of the plains of North and South America provided a high immunity by a liberal use of the organs and tissues of wild animal life, a large variety of plant foods and fresh and salt water animal life, as available.

The coastal Indian tribes of North and South America provided a high immunity by a liberal use of sea animal life together with plant life of the coastal region.

The Amazon Jungle Indians provided a high immunity with a liberal use of fresh water animal life, small land animals and birds, and wild plants and seeds.

In all of these groups the displacing diets that consisted of the foods of commerce were more or less highly refined sugars, refined flours, canned goods, vegetable fats and polished rice.

My investigations have included, when visiting these tribes, the gathering of samples of foods utilized by them. These were carried or sent to my laboratory for chemical analysis. Clinical investigations also were made in which individuals who had lost their immunity to dental caries in our modern highly susceptible groups were provided special dietaries which were modified to make them as nearly as possible equivalent in minerals and vitamins to the efficient primitive dietaries. The result of doing so not only has prevented the development of dental caries (when caries is the problem involved) in practically all cooperating individuals but has controlled it where active in over ninety percent of the individuals so studied.

Departure from Racial Types

An important new light has been thrown by these studies among primitive races on modern departure from racial types. Whereas it has been assumed that gross changes in physical form could only result from influences operative through a vast number of generations, these studies have revealed that gross changes can occur in a single new generation.

I have referred to the view in physical anthropology that has provided for the classification of skeletal material and its assignment to races on the basis of uniformity of structure and design. This has also enabled individuals to be classified into racial groups while living. It is based on recognition of similarity of facial and body form in various individuals in a given racial stock and recognizes a constancy regardless of location. This constitutes a fundamental expression of the laws of heredity.

This is illustrated in Figure 98 in which four Melanesian boys are shown who were photographed on different islands where the stock was still isolated. While they probably have never seen each other the family resemblance is purely a racial resemblance and demonstrates that under an adequate environment the racial characteristics were perfected in these various locations some of them hundreds of miles apart.

Similarly in Figure 99 will be seen Polynesian girls. They look like sisters but only so because they look like Polynesians. They have been born and lived in locations many hundreds of miles apart. In these groups the accumulated wisdom regarding nutrition was similar.

We are concerned to know how quickly gross changes like these can occur. An important part of these studies included an examination of parents and their offspring, both where still isolated and where recently modernized. In Figure 101 above is shown an African father and son of the Wakamba tribe. The father was born before the advent of imported foods. He works for the railroad which furnishes the family nutrition and his son has a marked change in facial form as may be seen. In Figure 101 below will be seen a Fiji father and son. The father was born before the influence of foods of commerce had reached that group. He and his wife have excellently developed faces and normal dental arches. Their son was born after the change in nutrition. The father works for a sugar plantation which provided the commercial foods. The son has a narrowed upper dental arch, and modified facial form.

In Figure 100 (page 276) above is seen a father and his son of a coastal Indian tribe in Peru. Note the father's excellent facial and dental arch development. He was born when his parents lived largely on sea foods. He is now working for the International Oil Company at Talara which furnishes the food for the family. The boy has badly deformed dental arches. In Figure 100 is shown an Indian father and son living in the High Andes in Peru. The father is the product of the primitive nutrition as used by his parents, and the son is the product of the use by his parents of modern foods of commerce.

These marked changes in facial form are characteristic of many individuals in our modern civilization and in the modernized groups of the primitive racial stocks represented in this study.

If space for illustrations permitted we would use many obtained in various parts of the world indicating the superior physical structure including facial and dental arch design as found among primitive races in many countries. People do not require to be specialists to recognize a large percentage of individuals in modern European and American life with deformities of the face and dental arches. My studies in many parts of the United States and Europe have disclosed that from 25 to 75 percent of the population carry injuries of these types. In some communities the percentage is even higher.

In contrast with this, in a study of twenty-seven native tribes in eastern and central Africa, I found thirteen tribes in which I did not record a single instance of even moderate deformity of facial and dental arch form. Similarly, in studies in Peru of the ancient burials along the coast, an examination of 1,276 skulls in succession did not reveal one with deformity of the facial design and dental arch form. The modernized natives in these as in all modernized groups showed a considerable percentage of the population with gross deformities. The change that occurs in even the next generation after the parents have adopted the modern foods of commerce is so marked that one would expect that some other force like mixture of bloods would be involved. This is typically illustrated in figures. While a considerable variety of pattern changes occur in each racial group with modernization, I have selected as an example a very common type of deformity consisting of a dropping inward of the upper laterals with a narrowing of the upper arch and consequent prominence of the cuspids. This will be recognized as a very frequently occurring deformity in our modern civilization. In many figures this has developed in (a) a modernized Eskimo; (b) an Indian of northern Canada; (c) a Polynesian of the South Sea Islands; (d) an East Indian of Mombasa; (e) a Negro of Belgian Congo and (f) an Arab of Khartoum. Similar illustrations are abundant in each of the primitive racial stocks examined wherever they are in the process of modernization, occurring even in the first generation after the adoption by the parents of foods of modern commerce.

The gross physical changes occurring promptly after modernization were not limited to structures of the head. The narrowing and lengthening of the face was usually only a small part of the change in body form. The hips and chest were usually narrowed with a tendency for narrowing throughout the length of the body. As we will see later, the bones of the head, particularly the maxillary bones, seem to suffer most severely.

An important development occurs in a large percentage of our modern families which, so far as I know, has been entirely overlooked by even the members of the dental profession. This is expressed as changes within the family group in individual facial and body form, which disturbances tend to occur more severely in late members of a family than in the first or early born. Orthodontists will have an opportunity to study this phase by noting the birth rank of the children of a family who have greatest need for orthodontia. Where the child needing this service is the oldest, it is very often the only child in the family. Another factor operates of course, namely, that an only child will often receive professional service because the expense can be afforded while it cannot always be afforded for the children of large families. The fact that among both the modernized primitives and our modern whites there is a tendency for a greater injury to occur in the late children in the family is of great significance, because of its indication that a lowering of capacity for reproduction has occurred in the parents.

REFERENCES

[1] SETON, ERNEST THOMPSON. *The Gospel of the Red Man*. Garden City, 1936.

[2] LANE, A. Preface to *Maori Symbolism* by Ettie A Rout. London, Paul Trench Trubner, 1926.

[3] LAIRD, D. The tail that wags the nation. *Rev. of Revs.*, 92:44, 1935.

[4] The report of the American Assn. of Obstetricians and Gynecologists at their meeting September, 1939, indicated that out of every 100 pregnancies in the United States 25 are lost before birth.

Chapter 27

NUTRITIONAL PROGRAMS FOR
RACE REGENERATION

OUR MODERN civilizations are doubly indebted to the primitive races for they have both demonstrated what we might be like in physical form and health and have indicated the nutritional requirements for doing so.

We will consider these expressions of modern degeneration under two main headings, namely, (see group 1) those caused chiefly by the faulty nutrition of the affected individual, and, (group 2) those caused in large part, by parental deficiencies which affect function.

Typical expressions of the former are: dental caries, peridontal inflammations, so-called pyorrhea alveolaris, types of eye inflammations, failing vision, scurvy, un-united fractures, recurring spasmodic fractures, skeletal affections, joint pains, berri berri, pellagra and sterility. Over ninety have been reported by McCarrison.[1]

The second group of affections are associated with prenatal injuries, caused by parental vitamin and mineral deficiencies, before and at the time of fertilization. These affect the germ cells, thereby producing a defective fertilized ovum and defective fetus.

In this group (2) are hare-lip, cleft palate, narrow hips, narrow face, constricted nostrils, mental backwardness, juvenile delinquency, skull defects of the face and the floor of the brain, brain defects, mongoloidism, idiocy, etc. These two groups will be discussed and illustrated separately in this chapter.

At the point of contact of modern commerce with large areas in which the primitive racial stocks have been protected by their isolation, we find degeneration of the human stock in its worst phase.

In order to reach the Pelly Mountain Indian tribes in the interior of the far north of Canada, just inside the continental divide, the only method of approach that seemed justified or practical was to travel up the Stikine River, which flows into the Pacific in the vicinity of Wrangell. A high-powered, Diesel-engined, shallow-draft boat has been constructed for this purpose. The river winds through snow-capped mountains, which progressively rise to higher heights as one approaches the continental divide. The river finally becomes so narrow and the gorge so deep that for forty miles beyond the last landing stage the banks are so steep that, we were advised, moose could not leave the water and scale the banks. In order to cross the divide a truck is used over an old moose trail.

The engineering problems involved in making that journey call for the finest craftsmen. For example, the experiences crossing the divide were so harrowing that a young man, who was being sent to a Hudson's Bay post, the one farthest north in the interior to relieve the man who had been in charge, made the comment that if he had to go over that road again in order to get out to civilization, he would rather die there than endure the frights he had on that trip. At places on the road, we were shown where two trucks and their loads had slipped down the river wall and all were lost.

The chief industry that has used the Stikine River navigation has probably been the Hudson's Bay Co. in order to obtain the furs collected by the Indian tribes. These are carried across the divide from one to several hundred miles. The commodity of exchange, as in most parts, is not money but goods. In this district, this means blankets, for which the Hudson's Bay Co. is so famous, and other apparel, together with foods such as are used by the modern whites outside. This latter consists chiefly of white flour, refined sugar, jams.

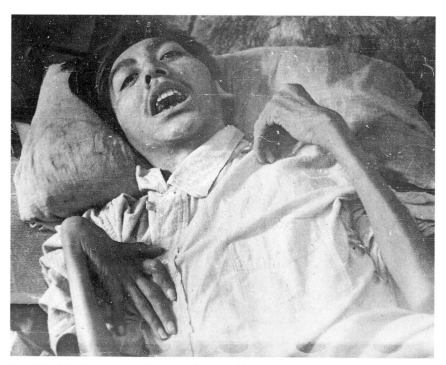

FIG. 145. This Indian boy's dilemma is heartbreaking. He is physically helpless, is in terrible pain, and cannot eat and was kept alive by an old Indian mother who fed and cared for him.

At the terminus of navigation, Telegraph Creek, in addition to the important Hudson's Bay post, the government Indian Agent is located. It was through his highly esteemed assistance that we were able to arrange in advance, both for the permission to enter the north country and for transportation. At this point is also located a group of missionaries who are teaching the people modernized methods for living.

Several score of Indian families and half-breeds, a few families of whites, have congregated around this business center.

We visited a number of their homes and found many bed-ridden cripples, including boys and girls in their late teens. A striking illustration is shown in Figure 145. This young man's jaw is locked in the open position and note that his right hand has been distorted by the pull of the muscles so that the hand is folded back on the forearm. The extremity of his suffering cannot readily be imagined.

In Figure 146 are seen three children suffering with tuberculosis. The two boys have tubercular infection of the glands of the neck. The girl, above, pulmonary tuberculosis in the late stages. The fence in front of her tent, we were told, was to keep the dogs away.

These children were in the vicinity of the interior post over the divide and had been and were living on the imported foods whereas their parents and untold generations before had lived on the native foods of moose meat, moose livers, caribou, bear, ground nuts, dried berries and dried buds of trees.

A picture of a typical native Indian family in the far north, who were and had been living on their native foods, is shown in Figure 147. The meat on the drying racks, shown in the picture, consists of moose liver and slabs of moose meat. The hardihood of the native Indian men is splendidly illustrated by an incident that happened on the last trip of the truck across the divide, prior to our crossing. The truck broke down about half way over the two or three day return trip and the driver had to leave his two passengers and walk the sixty-five miles back to Telegraph Creek for another truck. This he did without stopping to rest or eat, a journey which took eighteen hours.

The lesson we should learn is that these primitive Indians living in that very inclement climate were able, before the advent of the modern foods, to build superb bodies and that, in even the first generation after the arrival of modern foods, their children broke down with typical nutritional deficiency diseases.

Under the second group of infections, namely those due to prenatal defects, caused by deficient nutrition of one or both parents prior to fertilization, we will emphasize the wisdom of the primitives in providing sources of food that will be adequate for preventing this type of injury.

I have presented evidence in Chapter 17 "One Origin of Physical Deformities" using illustrations from several of the primitive groups which indicate the nature of these defects.

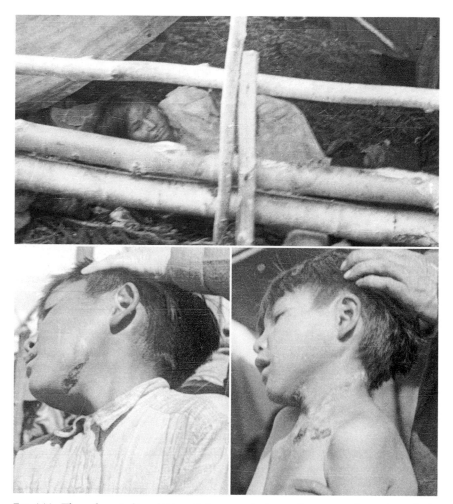

FIG. 146. These three Indian children, living near the last exchange store have tuberculosis. Pus is running from the infected glands of the neck of the two boys; one boy wore only a sweater because the flow of pus was so great. The girl has tuberculosis of the lungs.

On pages 274, 275, 276 and 277, I presented data indicating the normal facial structure of several primitive groups and then have shown members of the next generation with marked changes in physical form, particularly of the face. I have emphasized that this appears in severe form in even the first generation.

On pages 278, 279, 280 and 282, I presented data demonstrating that the injury is more severe in later children born in the family as compared with the first. This seems clearly to show a lowering of reproductive capacity of one or both parents and usually of the mother.

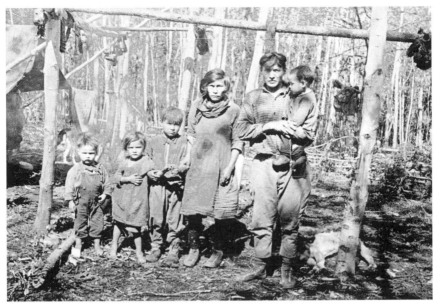

FIG. 147. This happy healthy Indian family live in the deep woods of the far north on Nature's natural foods.

On pages 284, 285 and 287, I presented evidence showing that the injury is progressive through three successive births. The data strongly emphasize that many structures of the body may be involved. Among them, the deformity of club feet is very frequent. This is illustrated on pages 287, 289, 290 and 291.

Chapter 18 covers data emphasizing the frequent association of lowered defense against infection. On pages 297, 298, 299 and 301, I have shown cases of individuals with low capacity of resisting tubercular infection, all of whom show physical evidence of prenatal injury by deformities of the dental arches.

Fortunately, experimental animals can be used to demonstrate the types of deficiencies that produce typical physical deformities. I have emphasized this phase by giving the history of several animals used in the study of the problem. On pages 307 and 308 are shown pigs, presenting a large group of defects, all born to the same mother. In that group, six mother pigs were purposely deprived of vitamin A by Prof. Fred Hale. Fifty-nine little pigs were born of these six sows, not one of which had an eyeball. Other lesions produced were defective ears, club feet, cleft palate, hare-lip and spinal bifidae. Later litters were produced by these same sows, while on an adequate nutrition, without the production of any defectives and still more important, when these blind pigs were mated they produced litters with normal eyeballs. This is contrary to the tenets of the hereditary transfer of these defects.

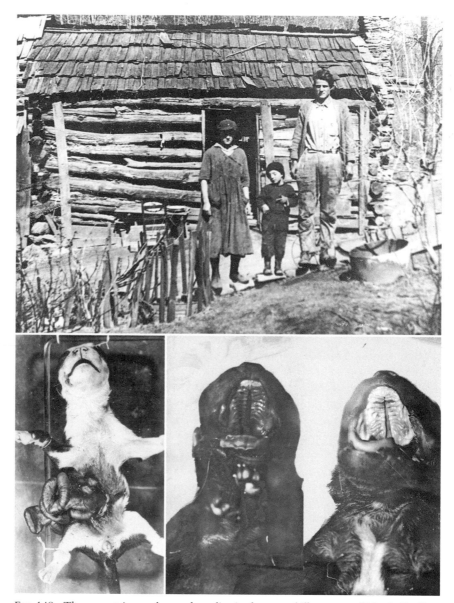

FIG. 148. The mountaineers shown above live in the waste hill country of North Carolina. Their only child is an idiot. The three defective pups shown below were produced by inadequate food of the parents.

I also presented data illustrating the serious loss amongst dairy cattle and sheep herds during drought periods. In Figure 148 are shown, in the lower group, three pups. In the first from the left, the pup was born with the intestines outside the abdomen. The next two have an unique history, they both show cleft palates. The mother of these pups has had five litters the first four all by the same sire. In the first three litters, when both were on an adequate nutrition, all pups were perfect. In the fourth litter ten pups were born of which eight had cleft palates and only two were normal. Both parents were on an inadequate nutrition prior to and at the time of this fertilization. In the fifth litter this mother dog was mated to her own son and if this factor had been of hereditary origin, this defect would have to appear according to Mendel's law. Three pups were born, all of which were perfect.

In my correspondence with an observing teacher in the hill country of western Pennsylvania, she reported that in her school a condition was frequent in the families, namely, that the children could not carry prescribed textbook work because of low mentality. This is often spoken of, though incorrectly, as delayed mentality. In one family of eight children only the first child was normal. The mental and physical injuries were progressively more severe. The eighth child had both hare-lip and double cleft palate. The seventh child had cleft palate and the sixth was a near idiot. The second to the fifth, inclusive, presented increasing degrees of disturbed mentality.

In my cabin-to-cabin studies of families living in the hill country of North Carolina, I found many cases of physical and mental injury. Among these cases arthritis and heart disease were very frequent, many individuals being bedridden. A typical case is shown in the upper part of Figure 148 of a father and mother and their one child. The child is so badly injured that he is mentally an imbecile. They are living on very poor land where even the vegetable growth is scant and of poor quality. Their food consisted very largely of corn bread, corn syrup, some fat pork and strong coffee.

In my studies amongst the primitive races, I was continually impressed with the increase of population where foods were most efficient. This is strikingly demonstrated by the physical evidence of dense populations which lived through several centuries along the west coast of Peru.

The Chimu tribe make their burials in the dry sand. The scantiness of rain in that area is demonstrated by the fact that their clay walled cabins, built hundreds of years ago, are still standing in large numbers. There has not been sufficient rainfall to wash down these walls. That they obtained ample water is shown by the many aqueducts, one of which extended for many hundreds of miles into the Andes mountain wall, which rises to twenty and twenty-two thousand feet, some of the passes being sixteen thousand feet above sea level.

An important part of nutrition was provided in the sea food. This is supplied by abundant food for sea animal life, from the vicinity of the South Pole ice caps. In many parts of the world the primitives made their habitation by those seas where an abundance of fish eating birds were in evidence and where seals and sea lions lived in large numbers. This is splendidly illustrated, for the Peru coast, in Figure 149, in the upper part of which is shown a flock of fish-eating birds, that range in size comparable to ducks and geese. They fly over the sea and dive into it to catch the fish. The splashes show where they have just dived to make their daily catch. In the lower part of the picture is a herd of sea lions, which I was advised included over a million. Each sea lion was said to eat an average of seventy-five pounds a day.

That the earlier members of the Chimu tribe were good fishermen is readily shown by the extensive fishing nets removed in large numbers from the burials. I personally examined many hundreds of the skeletons and in not one did I find a dental arch which was constricted or the teeth out of line. Tooth decay was apparently practically unknown to this cultural group.

Our war department records reveal that in both world wars, one and two, from thirty to seventy percent of the young men of the draft age were found to be unfit for field service. It is urgent that we learn why.

Modern civilization is in a dilemma. The biggest problem in the world today is not war, but means for race betterment. Epidemics, plagues and infectious diseases are largely under control. Today, the members of the healing professions are engaged in alleviating suffering from degenerative diseases by means of remedial surgery and makeshift repairs.

A prime requisite is a new orientation; first, for recognizing our dilemmas, and second for establishing educational programs and leadership for human conservation through race betterment. As an aid to this new orientation, let us review the observations of some of our leaders in social sciences.

1. Modern man is delicate.... The organism seems to have become more susceptible to degenerative diseases. (Carrel)
2. Nearly one-third of the whole population (of two dozen states) is of a type to require some supervision. (Laird)
3. Of 2,000,000 babies to be born in 1941, 738,386 will be wholly or partially wasted, 37%. (Nat'l Committee for Planned Parenthood)
4. Measurable brain can be correlated with testable mind. (Waverly Researches)
5. Thinking is as biologic as digestion. (Thorndike)
6. Of all the psychological causes of crime, the commonest and gravest is usually alleged to be a defective mind.... (Burt)
7. ... Gross human congenital malformations arise solely from influences which affect the germ cells prior to fertilization.... (Murphy)

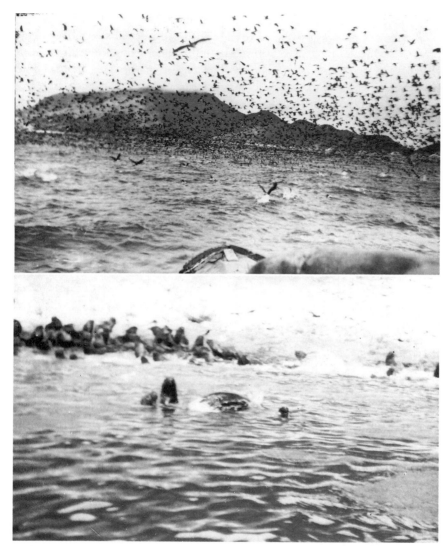

FIG. 149. Above: This vast flock of fishing birds is enjoying meal time in a fish-laden polar icecap current off the coast of Peru. Below: A herd of sea lions, part of a million feeding in this current.

8. Eggs (fertilized ova) are not all of equal quality, 25% are not good enough to be born as living individuals. (Streeter)
9. It is store food which has given us store teeth. (Houton)
10. There is a nutritional basis for modern physical, mental and moral degeneration. (Price)

Evidence of our modern degeneration is developing at an increasing rate and has now reached a point where the continued existence of modern civilization is threatened. This is well illustrated in the alarming death rate from several modern degenerative diseases. The report of the Metropolitan Life Insurance Company under date of August 1941 reveals that death rates per hundred thousand policy holders had reached, for the month of July 1941, 714 for all causes. Of these, 185 were from heart disease and arterial conditions and 100 from cancer, death rates from all other causes combined being 429. Whereas, formerly infectious diseases accounted for the large proportion of deaths, these are now well under control, but the degenerative diseases have increased to such an alarming extent that in this total of 714 deaths for the month of July for each hundred thousand policyholders, the degenerative diseases now constitute 420, or 60 percent, of the total. Of the degenerative diseases, conditions of the heart and arteries and cancer took 285, or 40 percent; while all of the other causes took only 293, or 40 percent. The latter number included automobile accident. Even this wastage of human life is not adequately expressed by a consideration of the principal causes of death after birth; since of every hundred pregnancies in the United States, twenty five are reported to end before term.

In order that we may get a bird's-eye view of simply one factor in progressive modern degeneration, let us consider the problem of depletion of soils. In Figure 150, we see expressed diagrammatically the ratio of the various minerals that make up the soil of the earth from which all our plant foods must develop. It is of interest that calcium and phosphorus are limited to the small section at the left of the circle. Calcium and phosphorus, in the group of minerals classed as apatite, constitute only a minute percentage of the earth's surface. These two minerals, forming as they do the principal constituents of bone, are in greatest demand in the growth of animal life.

It will aid us in visualizing the difficulties involved in obtaining these minerals by plants and animals to observe with regard to phosphorus that it constitutes only about one part in 1,000 of the earth's crust. Plants, dry weight, require about 30 parts per thousand; while animals with skeletons, dry weight, require it in the ratio of 100 parts in 1,000. The only source of phosphorus is the soil on which the plants grow, and we must realize that the top 7 inches of an acre of ground contains only about 1,000 pounds of phosphorus in a chemical form in which plants can use it. Now when we realize that a 60-bushel crop per acre of wheat or corn will remove from the soil about 25 pounds of phosphorus per acre, or one-fortieth of the total content of the top 7 inches, we are immediately confronted with the fundamental, controlling problem that we have, accordingly, only enough phosphorus in the average soil for forty excellent crops. This is why we see so many farms that have been abandoned because they have been exhausted of their minerals, particularly phosphorus. It is also the reason that the annual death rates are so rapidly increasing in certain parts of the country, particularly those districts that have been longest settled or where the soil is shallowest.

While it is true that only about one-thousandth of the original earth's surface consists of available phosphorus, Nature's system of management of plant and animal life provides for an accumulation of the minerals most used by increasing the concentration of these minerals on the surface of the soil. In Nature's program, plants and animals return to the earth what they borrow. The roots of plants, large and small, particularly forests, bring up the required minerals from the various depths to which the roots penetrate and deposit them as fallen leaves and trunks, to decay on the surface. By this method, Nature builds an enriched top soil, production of one inch of which requires

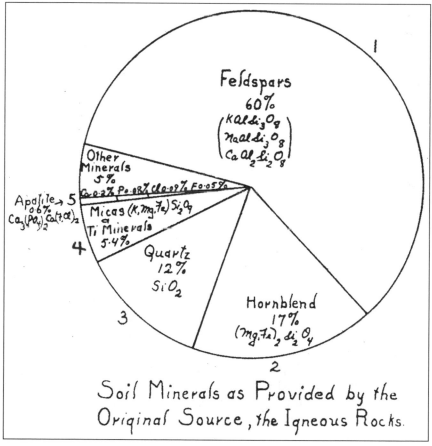

FIG. 150. All our calcium and phosphorus came originally from apatite, which constitutes only six-hundredths percent of the earth's surface.

400 years. Our prairies have from 4,000 to 10,000 years of accumulated top soil, which greatly reinforces the capacity of the surface for plant growth. The top soil is normally held by the roots of grasses and shrubs. When the roots are all removed, the wind and water rapidly carry away top soil, chiefly to the ocean, where it is lost for human use.

The death rate from heart disease in 1925 as reported by the American Heart Association has for many areas increased 50 percent or more, in the last fifteen years. The states of New England and those bordering the Great Lakes, together with the Pacific coast states, constitute the areas where the death rates are the highest, and these are the areas that have been occupied for the longest time. Large areas of these states now have a greatly reduced capacity for human maintenance, requiring that food be shipped in from other areas.

My studies of this problem of reduced capacity of soils for maintaining animal life have included correspondence with the agricultural departments of all of the states of the union with regard to maintaining cattle. The reduction in capacity ranges from 20 to 90 percent, and large areas are reported to carry successfully now only 50 percent as many head of cattle as formerly. I am advised that it would cost $50 an acre to replace the phosphorus alone that has been shipped off the land in large areas.

There is an important fact that we should consider; namely, the role that has been played by glaciers in grinding up and distributing rock formations. One glacier, the movement of which affected the surface soil of Ohio, covered only about half the state; namely, that area west of a line starting east of Cleveland and extending diagonally across the state to Cincinnati. It is important for us to note that, in the areas south and east of this line, several expressions of degeneration are higher than in the areas north and west of this line. The infant mortality per thousand live births in 1939 is very informative. In the counties north and west of that line, the death rate was from 40 to 49 per thousand live births; whereas, in the area south and east of that Line, the death rate was from 50 to 87.

It is of particular interest to us as dentists that studies show the percentage of teeth with caries to be much higher southeast of this line than northwest of it.

The effect of depletion of soils on animal life is striking. In a district in which I was studying this phase of the problem, I examined ranch cattle that were pasturing on a badly depleted soil where there was adequate water. These cattle had been shipped into the area to provide food for human beings. In one district, in traveling about 5 miles, I counted ten head of cattle that had starved to death for lack of certain minerals that had been depleted from the soil. A typical example is shown in Figure 151.

Another excellent illustration of the effect of change of pasturage on cattle is shown in Figure 152. A number of well-fed long horn cattle were trans-

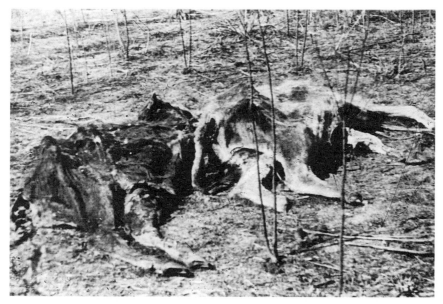

FIG. 151. These two cows died for want of essential foods. I found ten in about five miles. They were shipped in as a reserve supply of beef for the declining population in Florida.

ferred from a good district to a poor one. Figure 152 shows two views of the same steer, at the left while pasturing on a good soil and at the right after being transferred to pasture on a depleted soil, indicating the results of depletion of the soil of minerals. Because the long rangy horns have been demineralized at their base, they have dropped down so that their tips extend far below the nose and mouth. This condition constituted a barrier to eating grass because the horns prevented the animal from reaching its food. In the picture to the right, the steer is badly emaciated.

Another approach to this important problem is directly related to the quantity of animal life, large and small, that can be maintained on grain food such as flour. This is of special concern because of the effect of depletion of our cereal foods of natural minerals and vitamins by processing. Modern white flour has had approximately four-fifths of the phosphorus and nearly all of the vitamins removed by processing, in order to produce a flour that can be shipped without becoming infested with insect life. I have been advised by millers that they could not ship flour if the minerals and vitamins were not removed. At once, we have an important measure of the value of a food; namely, the quality of insect life that it can support. The more valuable the product for human food, the more insect life it will support. Whereas highly refined white flour

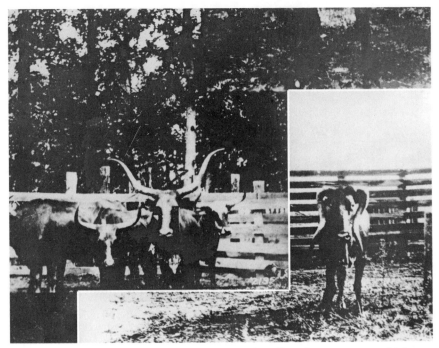

FIG. 152. These two views of the same steer show the effect of poor pasture on his horns; his wasting body is being kept alive by borrowing from his skeleton.

will support almost no insect life, a good product will support a relatively large amount of insect life in proportion to the volume of flour.

When I was studying this problem in the high Alps of Switzerland, I found an excellent state of physical development and health in adults and children living in all the high valleys. While the summers were short, the rate of plant growth was rapid, and rye was the only cereal that developed well for human food. Herds of cattle pastured near the glaciers. Mountaineer cabins were located near the foot of the glaciers. The children living in these cabins were exceptionally healthy. On the side of the valleys, rye was grown for bread. I obtained a piece of the bread that was made in one of these homes and put it in a bottle and carried it with other foods to my laboratory for chemical analysis. It was rich in minerals and vitamins.

In Figure 153, the dish to the right contains all of the residue of that bread after it had been eaten by the bugs which later developed in it. The one at the left shows the quantity of skeletons of bugs that had developed in and lived upon this one small piece of bread. This explained why the human life living upon it was so exceptionally fine. Bugs and children require the same minerals and vitamins. Our modern white bread cannot support much insect life.

This is one of the evils that has accompanied our progress in modernization. We do not realize how much modern human beings are handicapped and injured since they learned how to modify Nature's foods.

The wild animal uses Nature's foods as Nature makes them. This was true of the earlier races of mankind. In proportion as man has learned to modify Nature's foods, he has degenerated.

The physical qualities of the Neanderthal man as he inhabited southern Europe are attested by the perfection of his skeleton. Prof. Sergio Sergi, of Rome University shows what is called the most perfect Neanderthal skull. I visited him in Rome and studied his wonderful collection in 1935. Whereas only four skulls out of 4,000 belonging to the pre-Christian era and gathered from Italy and surrounding islands showed serious malformations, approximately 40 percent of the skulls in the collection of people who died in the last fifty years showed gross imperfections and abnormal formations. These people had all died in mental institutions.

I have been impressed many times in my studies with the superior physical development and acuteness of the senses of primitive races. This is strikingly illustrated in the visual acuity of the Maori of New Zealand, the Aborigines of Australia and some African tribes. Figure 154 shows a caveman. He did not need a telescope to correctly draw the position of the stars constituting the constellation of Pleiades.

I was advised that the Australian Aborigine could see a mile away animals which the white man could not see.

It has been my privilege to study the skeletal remains of primitive groups in many parts of the world. I have been continually impressed with the superior qualities exhibited, particularly skull development and design of dental arches. Among the skulls of the Maoris of New Zealand, of individuals who

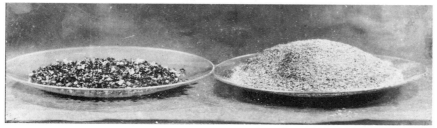

FIG. 153. The half slice of whole rye bread, grown up near the glaciers in Switzerland, fed all the bugs in the left hand dish; the refuse is shown at the right. They cannot live on our highly refined white flour bread.

lived before the coming of the white man, only one tooth per thousand teeth had been attacked by decay. This is in striking contrast with the condition of the teeth of this same people today since it has become largely modernized by contact with the white population. In my studies of modernized Maori groups, I found from 300 to 600 per thousand teeth attacked by dental caries. This is a typical and striking illustration of modern degeneration. The whites of New Zealand, according to their own dentists have the poorest teeth in the world today. A typical primitive Maori skull shows excellent dental arches.

I have recently made a study of pre-Columbian Indian burials in seven of the southeastern states. It has been impressive to see that those groups that lived near the coast and used sea-animal life abundantly, as evidenced from the material found in the burials, had excellent skeletal development, usually with complete freedom from dental caries. This was also true of skeletal material in the interior districts where they used fresh-water clams liberally. In contrast with this, in those areas where they were largely dependent on plant foods and small animals, the skeletal material was fragile and tooth decay often had been extensive. A striking difference in skeletal quality was found. Whereas the skeletons of both men and women were in a state of complete preservation and physical perfection, with little or no caries where sea foods

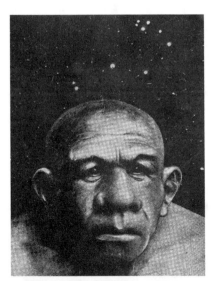

He Saw Stars . . .
you need a telescope to see.

FIG. 154. The primitives did not need glasses, their eyes were so good. Like the animals they knew what foods to select.

STARS IN A CAVE

Delighted were archeologists to discover a prehistoric cave-wall painting of the Pleiades star group, "Seven Sisters." But surprised were they that the ancient artist painted ten stars, four of which we need telescopes to see. Natural guess: stars were brighter then. Astronomers said "No.". . . the artist had seen all ten stars with his naked eye. Correct assumption: cave men had better eyesight than modern men.

were eaten, those in the interior districts showed a marked difference in quality of the skeletons of adult women and adult men. This was illustrated by skeletons which show what is presumed to be a husband and wife buried together. While his skeleton is well preserved and its structure excellent, most of her teeth had been lost and her bones were of much poorer structure. This may have been due to the overload of pregnancies. This condition did not occur where sea foods were used liberally.

There is a marked tendency in modern civilization to substitute synthetic products for Nature's foods. This has been particularly true of vitamins. While these tendencies are fortunate so far as Nature's requirements can be duplicated, the limited knowledge regarding the number and kind of activators and their individual roles in conjunction with other necessary activating substances and body-building minerals has resulted in serious injuries and some unfortunate misapprehensions. For example, it has been assumed that so-called vitamin D as viosterol included much that is required for the control of mineral utilization, particularly calcium and phosphorus.

Since the reduction in skeletal growth constituted the most easily observed deficiency in nutritional interference in infancy as expressed in rickets, the growth process was assumed to adequately express Nature's requirements for mineral utilization. It was early found that exposure of affected infants to ultraviolet light, either from sunlight or from an artificial source, and the use of materials that had been exposed to suitable radiant energy were comparable procedures, since both were effective in preventing rickets. Thus, the activation by irradiation of ergosterol marketed as viosterol or calciferol was supposed to accomplish all that was needed for reinforcing the body enough to maintain normal mineral utilization. A patent was granted covering the entire process of activating drugs and food substances by irradiation. Notwithstanding the fact that I was one of the first, by some considered the first, to report this process, I have never interpreted my data as indicating that irradiation of ergosterol satisfies Nature's requirements. In the first volume of my work on *Dental Infections, Oral and Systemic*, published in 1923, page 342, I presented a preliminary report, in a chapter on irradiation. Later, in a paper read before the National Academy of Sciences at Washington, I included the activation of cholesterol by this means.

For nearly two decades, the product activated ergosterol has been accepted as meeting Nature's requirements for mineralization as expressed by a need for vitamin D. Recent studies, however, have shown that Nature's product is not activated ergosterol, now known as vitamin D^2, but activated cholesterol, now known as vitamin D^3. During the years in which activated ergosterol has been used extensively to aid in mineral utilization, many clinical reports have indicated marked inadequacy as expressed by clinical results. Dr. Brehm,[2] for example, has reported that a very large percentage of infants born to mothers that had received activated ergosterol and minerals in tablet form during the gestation period were abnormal at birth, showing such conditions as stone in the kidney and abnormal closure of the sutures of the skull and the fontanel at birth. Calcified islands were also found in the placentae. Several reports have appeared of infants dying soon after birth with gross calcification, including involvement of the coronary artery and myocardium and arteries of other parts of the body.

With the newer knowledge of the determining role of nutrition in the development of degenerative diseases, which, according to the data previously quoted, now cause 60 percent of deaths, it is evident that, in many cases, conditions which do not cause death are primarily vitamin deficiency, including dental caries. The new role of nutritional control for disease prevention challenges the attention of the various groups engaged in public health service. Almost weekly, reports appear of additional findings throwing light on the contributing factors in heretofore obscure nutritional diseases.

An important illustration is a report in *Science News Letter* for August 2, 1941, presented under "Medicine" with the following headline: "Cancer Growth Prevented in Mice by Yeast and Vitamins; Vitamins Alone Had Little Effect, but Riboflavin and Pantothenic Acid with Yeast Succeeded with 62%."

These advances in knowledge emphasize the necessity that a change be made from relief of the symptoms of these degenerative diseases by surgery and repair to measures that are adequately conceived and applied for their prevention. While I am not suggesting that a cure for malignancy has been found, data available from several sources indicate that this and other serious disturbances of the digestive tract and associated organs are directly related to nutritional deficiency. In my contacts with government hospitals and medical missions that had been established among primitive races, these diseases were reported to be rarely found among the strictly primitive groups, but to be found in the same stock after they were modernized. Two things are strongly emphasized: the imperative need for substituting prevention for repair, and the need for programs for teaching the public regarding means for prevention.

This at once raises an important question: By what means will the public be informed and who will be their teachers? A report of the survey of the American Dietetic Association made of schools teaching nutrition indicates that of seventy-six medical schools reporting, only twenty had separate courses on nutrition, and of thirty-nine dental schools reporting, only fifteen had separate courses on nutrition. This survey was made in 1939. On the basis, it would seem that we have an explanation for much of the confusion in the minds of the members of the dental and medical professions in this matter of preventive medicine, including dentistry, through nutritional means.

One of the most serious of the present confusions is failure to appreciate that an adequate, well-balanced diet is capable of building people strong and well in all respects and adequate from maintaining health and strength. This is the right of all mankind and their sacred birthright. The primitive races have demonstrated a score of different nutritional formulas, any and all of which will accomplish this. These, when reduced to their bases, are chemically equivalent. The primitives' methods of living give them excellent appetites, enabling them to provide a good factor of safety for the essential minerals and vitamins. While they do not understand the chemical nature of the needed foods, they know and teach the use of the special foods that are needed for providing normal development and continuous health of the various organs and tissues of the body. The Chinese, for example, in a treatise written 1,600 years ago, listed more than sixty foods that were good for the eyes, more than twenty of which we now know to be very high in vitamin A, an essential for the development and the function of the eyes.

My investigations have included, when visiting these tribes, the gathering of samples of foods utilized by them. These were carried or sent to my laboratory for chemical analysis. Clinical investigations also were made in which individuals who had lost their immunity to dental caries in our modern highly susceptible groups were provided special dietaries which were modified to make them as nearly as possible equivalent in minerals and vitamins to the efficient primitive dietaries. The result of doing so not only has prevented the development of dental caries, when caries is the problem involved, in practically all cooperating individuals but has controlled it where active in over ninety percent of the individuals so studied.

REFERENCES

[1] WRENCH, G.T. *The Wheel of Health: The Sources of Long Life and Health Among the Hunza.* London, The C. W. Daniel Company Ltd., 1938.

[2] BREHM, W. Potential dangers of viosterol during pregnancy with observations of calcification of placentae. *Ohio S.M.J.*, 33:990,1937.

Chapter 28

SOCIAL REFORMS BY EDUCATION

PREVENTION can be our salvation. Our greatest need, therefore, is to teach the masses by every means possible. This will save millions both in lives and money. We can prevent but we cannot cure. Whom and what will we teach? Fortunately, our experience is enlightening. It has been found that grade and high school pupils get the prevention idea clearly and naturally.

The masses must be taught that "LIFE IN ALL ITS FULLNESS IS MOTHER NATURE OBEYED."

These lessons from Primitive Races are already being used in many places. Miss Alfreda Rooke has given me a note with her experiences. She says, *Nutrition and Physical Degeneration* by Dr. Weston A. Price has been used as a textbook on three different teaching levels: elementary, adult education and teacher training. Each program covered three phases of nutrition:

1. Nutrition and physical degeneration
2. Inadequate diets due to deficient foods
3. Adequate nutrition from present day foods.

The dramatic evidence presented by Dr. Price of the effect of diet on growth and development, captivates the interest of students of every age level. His description and picturization of the change in primitive man who has lived on the vital foods of his country, after he adopts the food habits of the civilized world, proves both startling and thought provoking; a stimulating introduction to the teaching of nutrition.

On the elementary level, a program in nutrition, based on this book was developed in the Chula Vista Union School District, San Diego County, California, by the supervisor of Physical and Health Education. (Chula Vista Union Elementary School District, San Diego County, California, J. C. Lauderbeck, District Superintendent. Alfreda F. Rooke, Supervisor of Physical and Health Education.)

The foundation for the work in the elementary schools was laid in teachers' meetings and conferences. The Supervisor provided recent books on nutrition, pertinent medical and dental reprints, government bulletins, and other available material for teaching fundamentals of nutrition.

Every other week, in each fifth and sixth grade class, the Supervisor presented nutrition material, throughout the district. This brought the newer

456

nutritional knowledge to both teachers and pupils. On alternate weeks, the classroom teachers correlated the subject with social science and other studies. Stories, maps, pictures from such periodicals as the *National Geographic*, as well as interesting objects from various countries, served to add color and interest.

To the children, the Supervisor introduced Dr. Price as the dentist who locked his door, and set out with his wife, to discover why many people in primitive countries had healthy mouths. After they had completed their study of the travel pictures from Dr. Price's book, which were shown on class room walls by means of a large projector, they made a summary of the things they had learned. From notes, voluntarily taken, they drew a comparison between the diet and health of primitive peoples and that of civilized peoples. They demonstrated quite plainly they had learned, that there is a difference between animal and plant proteins in building blocks for the body; that protein is a "grow" food, whereas carbohydrate is a "go" food; that animal proteins differ in nutritional quality depending on the fertility of the soil where the animals graze; that processing of foods destroys heat labile factors that are necessary to maintaining normal health.

At the University of Missouri, the same material and procedure was again used in teaching a nutrition unit in Health Education for secondary teachers. This was an inter-departmental project, including the Department of Physical Education, in which the course in Health Education was given, and the Department of Soils, of the College of Agriculture. (Department of Physical Education, Miss Mary McKee, Director, Miss Ethel Mitchell, instructor in Health Education. Department of Soils, Dr. Wm. A. Albrecht, Chairman; Miss Alfreda F. Rooke, Graduate Student in Soils and Nutrition.)

Miss Rooke is devoted to helping the next generations of children by teaching the new generations of parents-to-be.

My contacts have included all ages and people of many colors. Children are always more receptive than adults. Note the two essays below.

A grade school boy, aged 9, writes:

> From the pictures I see that the sugar rationing in the United States is O.K. because people here will start using more honey and maple syrup as well as other natural sweets. This will do much to improve their health and teeth. I have seen that there are 30 insects in the brown flour and none in the white flour so now I know that the insects and bugs are smarter than we are and go for the whole wheat which is nourishing and do not touch the white flour which is not nourishing because the minerals and vitamins are not in it. I learned from the pictures that if we want healthy children when we grow up and are married, we better learn to eat right now. When we eat right it makes our bodies right, it makes our bodies healthy and when we're married and have children they'll be good and healthy too.

This next is a high school girl of sixteen, who heard my thirty-five minute talk a week previously.

> Good bodies are essential to good minds. Healthy bodies are made by proper food. That means enough vitamins and minerals. If one's parents are healthy, you will have a good chance to be happy and healthy. If the egg and sperm cells are the best one can produce, good bodies will follow. Children should be spaced for several reasons. A mother gives so much of her vitamins and essential needs to her child that it requires several years to rebuild her body. The youngest child is likely to be the one most lacking. The mother gives her best to her first child and if she has many children her body elements slowly decline. Yes, the parents should have a good diet before fertilization. A healthy egg does not come from sickly or deficient parents. A healthy egg results in a healthy child. A good diet would insure good health. The source of the criminal person Dr. Price thinks is the parents. A criminal is born of dietary deficient parents or parents deficient in other ways. Educate the parents and the criminals will disappear. His information applies to everyone who will heed it. We, as the future parents should realize and take into consideration his information. We know he is right because good common sense will tell us the same thing.

Similarly the modernized primitives respond readily. The Maori in New Zealand are materially benefited and I quote from a previous report as follows:

> An excellent illustration of the application of this principle is provided by the history of the Maori stock in New Zealand. The skulls of the native New Zealanders before the coming of the white race and at the time of its arrival showed that only one tooth per thousand teeth had been attacked by dental caries. My studies of the modernized Maori revealed that from 30 to 60 percent of the teeth had been attacked by dental caries, or from 400 to 600 per thousand teeth. The present Maori dietary is very similar to that of the white of New Zealand. In contrast with the original high immunity of the natives to caries, the modern whites of New Zealand are credited by their own dentists with having the poorest teeth of all groups in the world.
>
> The Hukerara Girls' School in Napier for native Maori girls had, as I have reported, a high incidence of dental caries in the student body when I visited the school in 1936. Dr. Tocker has undertaken to improve the conditions there by modifying the food selection for this group in accordance with a program that I have outlined for him. This included a liberal increase of sea foods and seeds as used by the original Maori. His report recently made in the *New Zealand Dental Journal*, indicates a reduction in dental caries of 75 percent since the establishment of the program. Another item of importance that he reports relates to a flu epidemic in which not one of the girls in this group under the nutritional program contracted the flu, whereas, in the Maori boys' school in the same vicinity, approximately half of the boys developed influenza. Similarly, diphtheria, which was epidemic, failed to attack any of the girls on this special dietary program.

The available data reveal that our greatest need is for better nutrition for parents-to-be, particularly mothers. The public must know of the relation of prenatal injury to the vast group of physical, mental and moral defectives. For example, Burt of London reports: "Of all the psychological causes of crime, the commonest and the gravest is usually alleged to be a defective mind."

Hickson of Chicago reports, regarding the origin of young delinquents: "85.8% of our female cases are distinctly feeble-minded, and 84.5% of boys under arrest are morons."

The general idea assumes that delinquent boys can be trained to be normal. The United States Department of Labor, bulletin 203, states: "Out of 621 paroled from five of the best known correctional institutions 66% were later arrested and 59% convicted."

The economic problem associated with defectives includes both support and expense of teaching. From *Time*, June 17th, 1940, we learn: "Detroit spends $287 a year to educate a subnormal child, $58 for a smart one."

The economic problems involved for education of mentally retarded individuals is increasing rapidly in most of the country because of the general lowering of nutritional level. Nutritional education is the only foundation for individual, national and world peace and must be fostered by state and national organizations.

Since the greatest asset of a nation is the quality of its citizenship, the responsibility of the government includes the prevention of nutritional degeneration by making adequate foods available to the masses. For large areas of the earth the supply of adequate foods from the land has been reduced below the population level. Fortunately, there is a vast store house of excellent food still available in the oceans. The polar currents which flow from the icecaps are teeming with fish, the waters near the icecaps are loaded with high protein food which accumulates there by subocean currents. The temperature of the water adjoining the polar icecaps is four degrees below freezing, at which temperature bacterial breakdown does not occur. This provides a huge storage of nutrition for animal life by way of algae. These feed the myriad crops of first small, then larger and larger animal forms until we come to the billions of seals, whales, sea cows, walrus and sea lions. These together consume more fish, the world's best food, than the entire human population could consume. Some civilizations in the past, like the cultures along the coast of Peru, tapped this great reservoir. Today's cultures there disregard it.

Technicalities have been avoided in this book to make it useful to any teacher. Practically every community today has this problem and its teaching literature should increase rapidly.

Great care must be taken to guard against commercial encroachment for gain.

For additional information, write to Price-Pottenger.

Chapter 29

ADDITIONAL PHOTOGRAPHS FROM
DR. WESTON A. PRICE'S TEACHINGS

THESE additional photographs from the archives of the Price-Pottenger
Nutrition Foundation were used by Dr. Weston A Price during his
teaching presentations. All associated text is in Dr. Price's original words.

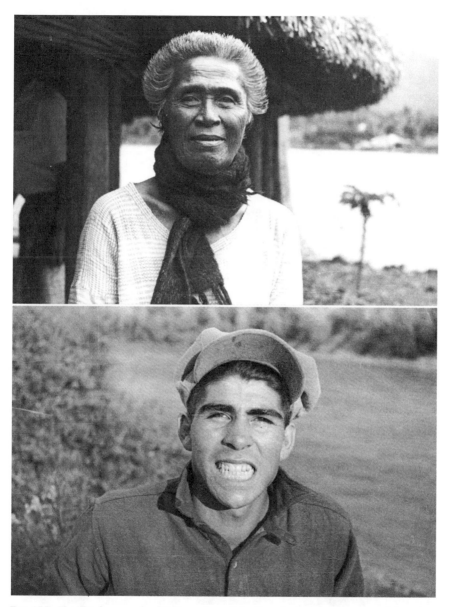

FIG. 155. Top: We have a splendid illustration of the fine physical development of the primitive Polynesians. This woman is nearly 90 years of age. She has splendid teeth and excellent facial and body build. She represents typically what Nature can do and will, when adequate nutrition is provided. Bottom: This photograph shows an Indian boy twenty-two years of age with magnificent facial and body build. He too, is the product of native environment.

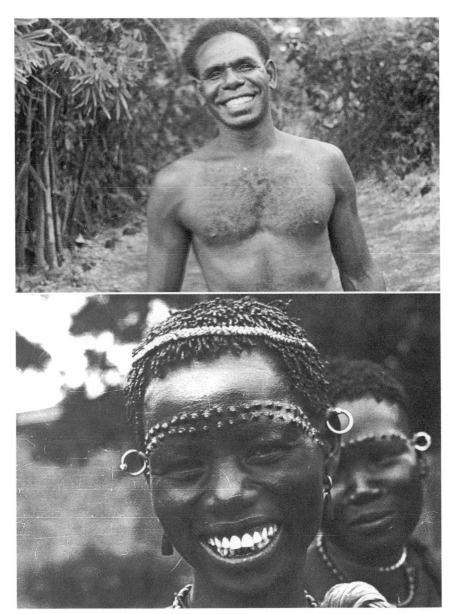

FIG. 156. Top: This photograph illustrates the fine physical development of this Malaysian racial stock. They are wonderful divers, as required in the pearling industry. They build fine native boats and are skilled navigators. They live on the plant food of the islands and the shell-fish and scale fish of the equatorial seas. Bottom: This photograph shows an African belle with broad dental arches and facial design like her tribe.

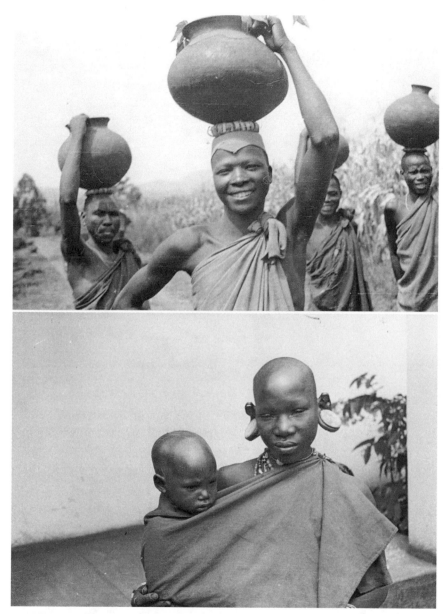

FIG. 157. Africans. Top: Splendidly illustrated here is the strength of their necks for carrying loads. Below: Here we see a young mother and her child of the Kikuyu tribe. In this agricultural tribe, girls are required to eat special foods for six months before marriage, during which time they must not be required to do hard work.

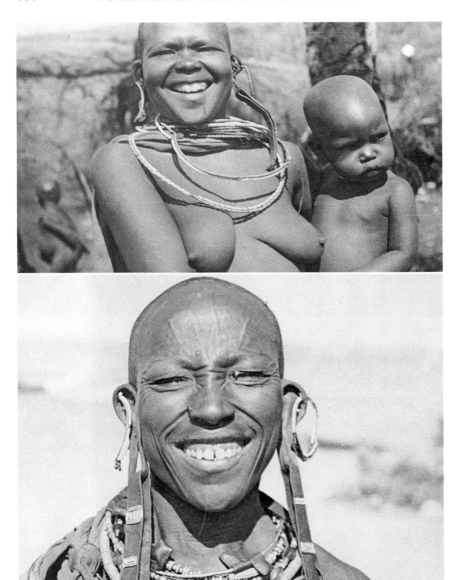

FIG. 158. Top: Here we see another splendid illustration of the wisdom of the primitives in the matter of preparation for motherhood by use of special foods. This young mother belongs to the Masai tribe in Central Africa. Their foods are dairy products, milk, meat and blood. In their more primitive condition girls are required to delay marriage until after the drought period in order that she may use the milk products produced after the cows are on the rapidly growing young grass following the rains. It is their belief and practice that by the use of fresh grass milk for three moons, they will prepare their bodies for marriage and reproduction. Bottom: We see a typical Masai belle with her glistening teeth. This particular primitive tribe, wherever I studied them, used the organs of animals. During the drought periods there is very little vegetation, during which time they get their special vitamins from the blood of steers which they bleed once a month. They milk the cows daily.

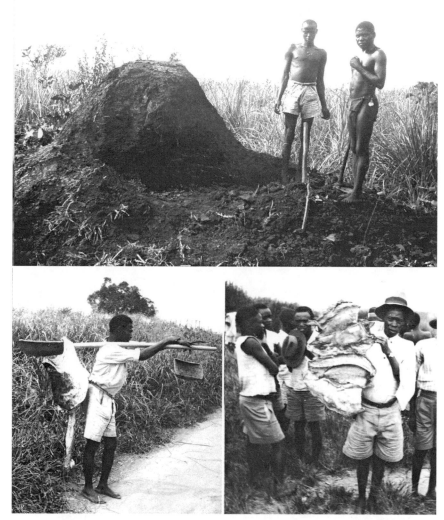

FIG. 159. Africans. Top: Robbing an ant hill for food. The eggs are distributed on galleries for hatching. Bottom Left: Shows the head of a monstrous fish caught in one of the lakes of the headwaters of the Nile. Bottom Right: Among the special foods used, fresh water fish play an important part. Here we see fish being carried off to great distances from the lakes and streams as special food.

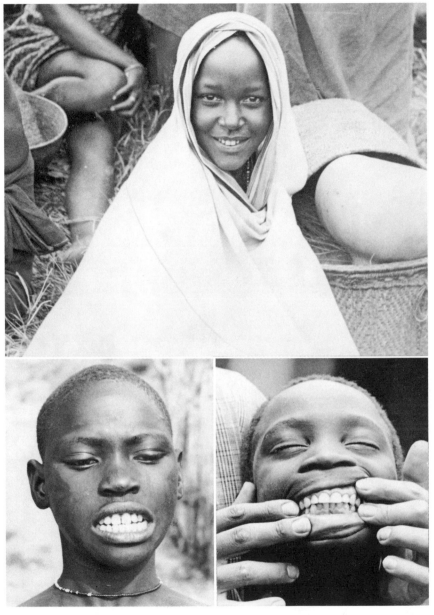

FIG. 160. Top: We see an African girl who is the product of the accumulated wisdom of her tribe in the selection of the native foods. Bottom: These African primitives were well built and handsome. Their tribal wisdom was highly efficient.

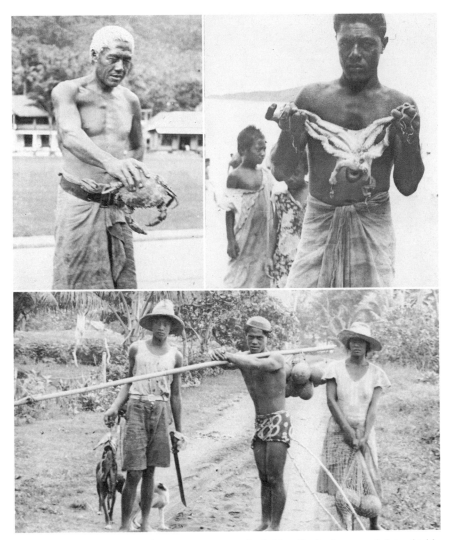

FIG. 161. Polynesians. Top: The Samoans use sea foods liberally. At the upper left is a highly prized crab; At the upper right is an octopus. Bottom: Here is a splendid illustration of the management of the food problem in a Polynesian family. The father, mother and son are out gathering the day's food supply. The mother is carrying breadfruit. The father is carrying coconuts and the son is carrying a string of fish. They will probably have from their garden, taro, a species of lily of which they use the root like we use potato. The young taro tops are also used. This makes splendidly balanced nutrition competent to prevent tooth decay and many other evidences of degeneration.

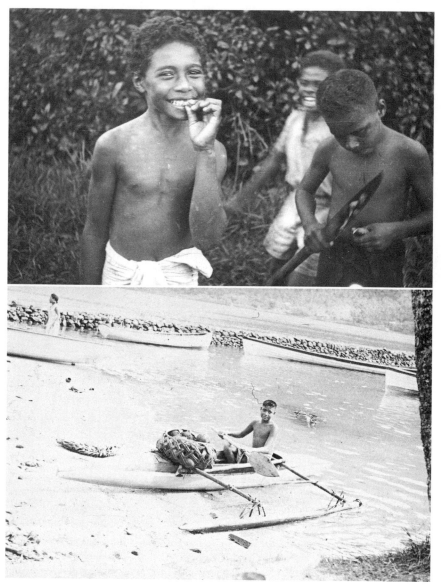

FIG. 162. Polynesians. Top: The boy is eating a delicious and highly prized sea worm. Bottom: Gathering and trading coconuts.

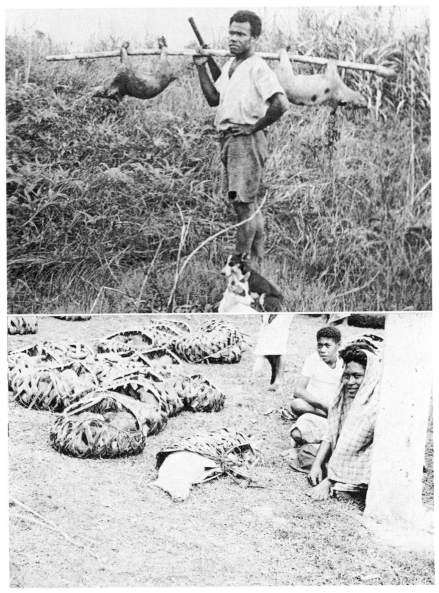

FIG. 163. Top: Typical foods used by the Melanesians. Bottom: Taro roots and a wild pig used by the Polynesians.

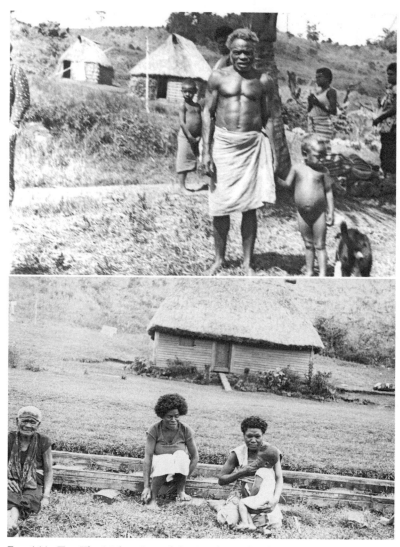

FIG. 164. Top: The Melanesians of the South Pacific islands are a very strong and sturdy race, as illustrated in the splendid development of this man. The warm climate in which they live makes very little clothing and shelter necessary. Bottom: Melanesian women. Note the size of child still nursing.

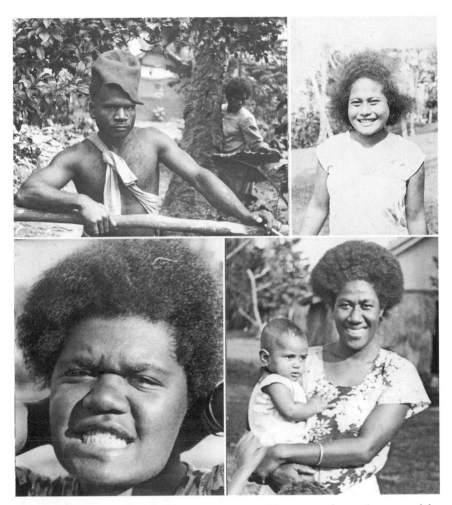

FIG. 165. Melanesians. Top left: Here we see the rugged keen type of man who mastered the southern sea. He lives on the Island of Caledonia. Top right: We see a typical young lady of the Melanesian race of the South Sea islands. Note her splendid facial development and beautiful teeth. Bottom: The typical primitive mothers have broad faces and regular dental arches with no tooth decay. They live on islands of the western pacific. They are very happy in disposition and are very conscious of the need for great care in the selection of their foods which are largely from the sea.

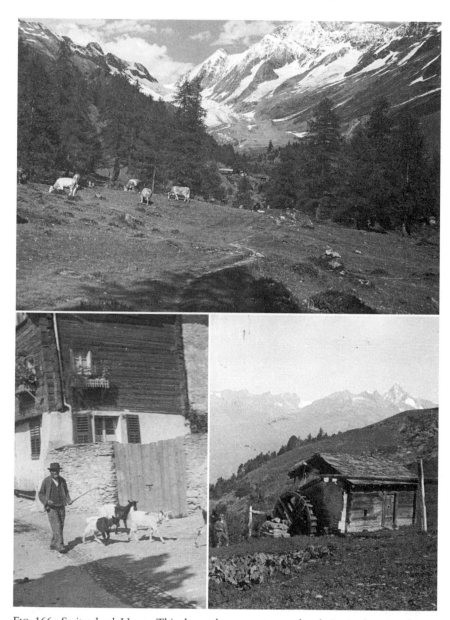

FIG. 166. Switzerland. Upper: This shows the cows up near the glacier in the Löetschental Valley, Switzerland. (Editor's Comment: The grinding action of the massive glaciers provided the minerals in the water as the glacier melted providing rich liquid fertilized for the soil below.) Lower left: Goats also were used for furnishing milk of very high nutrient value. Lower Right: For food the Swiss are largely dependent on dairy products from cattle and goats, and on rye bread. The rye was either ground in hand mills or water-driven stone mills, as shown.

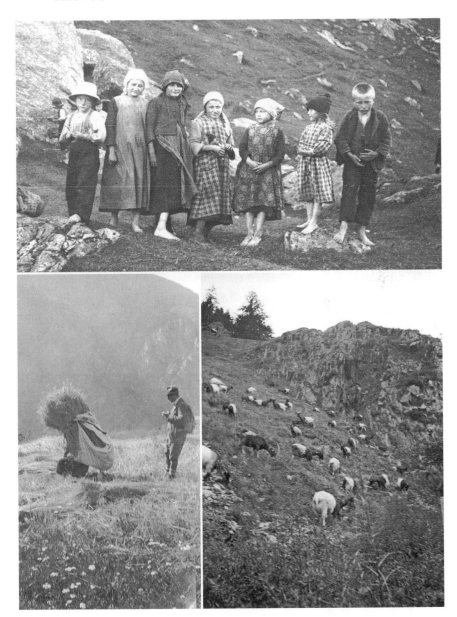

Fig. 167. Swiss. Top: Typical Swiss children living near the snow line. Bottom Left: A grand-mother of 65 harvests the rye, altitude over a mile. Bottom Right: A typical herd shown here. Rye proved to be the only grain that would develop and ripen in the short summer of the high mountainsides.

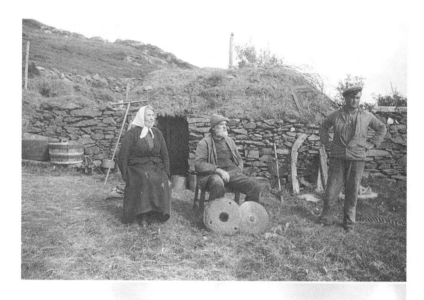

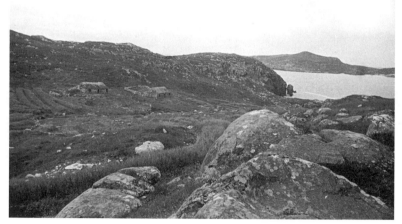

FIG. 168. Gaelics. Top: Typical primitive Gaelics. Note ancient mill stones. Bottom: There is scarcely a tree on these islands.

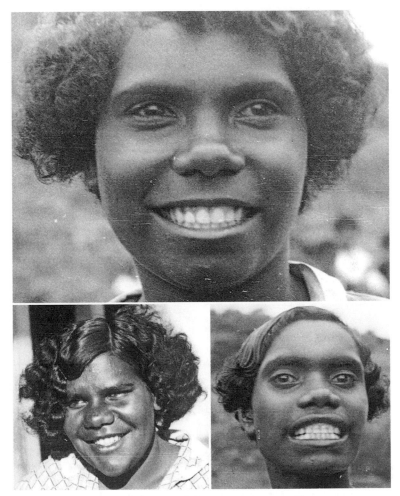

FIG. 169. Some of the Aborigine girls have a unique type of beauty.

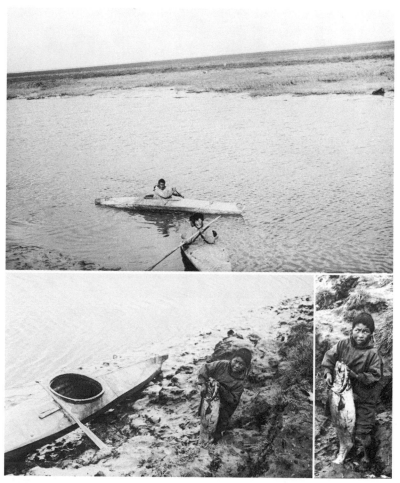

Fig. 170. Top: Here we see two of their small kayaks used for fishing. These Eskimos have lived almost entirely on a meat diet for most of the year. They have been required in many places to build their shelters of snow and ice and depend upon burning the fat of the large animals of the sea for fuel. They are living in their isolation just as their ancestors did ten thousand years ago. They have mastered the cruel forces of Nature of the Arctic. Bottom: Eskimo child holding onto a fish that he caught. Eskimo boys are taught the balancing of kayak by being tied in and put adrift with only a short paddle. They become very expert and catch large salmon with line or spear.

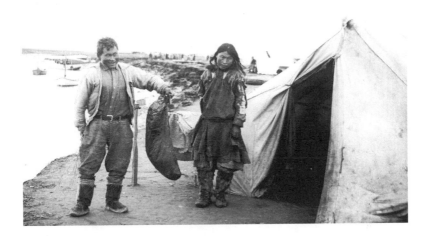

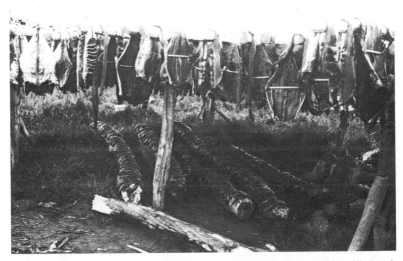

FIG. 171. Here we see an Eskimo and his wife. He is holding up a sealskin filled with seal oil. A sample of this oil brought to my laboratories for testing revealed it to be the richest source of vitamin A of any single food I have analyzed. Each piece of food, which consists largely of fish and large animals of the sea, is dipped in seal oil before being eaten. Bottom: This photograph shows the Eskimos method of drying the fish in the wind. The fish are often laden with sand which clings to their wet surfaces. On the logs below the hanging fish are the fish eggs being dried for food for the babies, young children, and mothers when raising families.

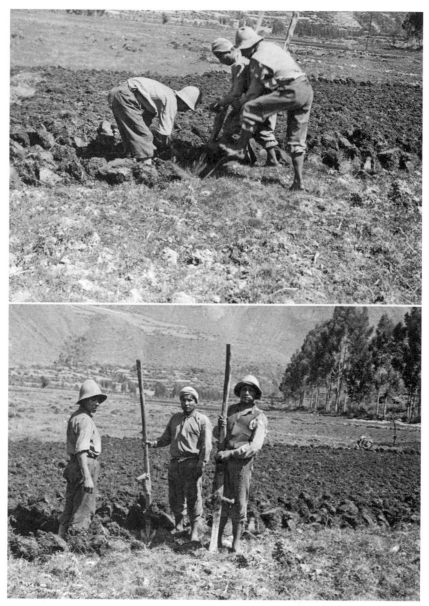

FIG. 172. The Andean Indians have long been expert agriculturists. We see typical Indian agricultural equipment, similar to the devices used by them for centuries. The ground is turned by hand.

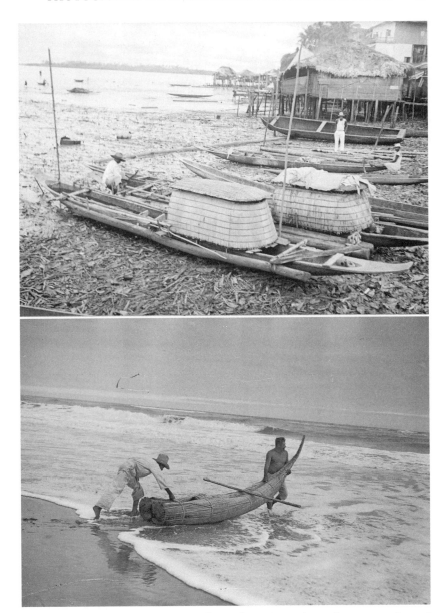

FIG. 173. Peruvians. Top: The river craft are of very interesting native construction and many of them house the family. Bottom: Here we see a type of canoe with which they ride the waves as they come crashing in on the coast. They go out to their fishing nets which provide a large and important part of their daily nutrition.

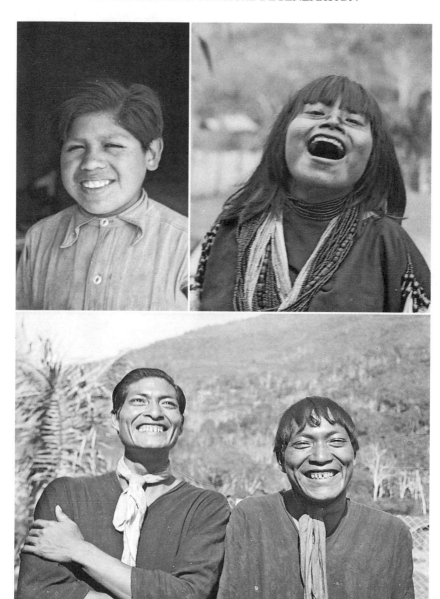

FIG. 174. Peruvians. Top Left: Here we see a thirteen-year-old Indian boy who is one of the brightest chaps of his age that one could find anywhere in the world. Note his beautiful face, broad nostrils and fine dental arches. Top Right: We see a beautiful Amazon girl showing her splendidly developed dental arches. Bottom: We see two young men demonstrating their magnificently developed dental arches and faces.

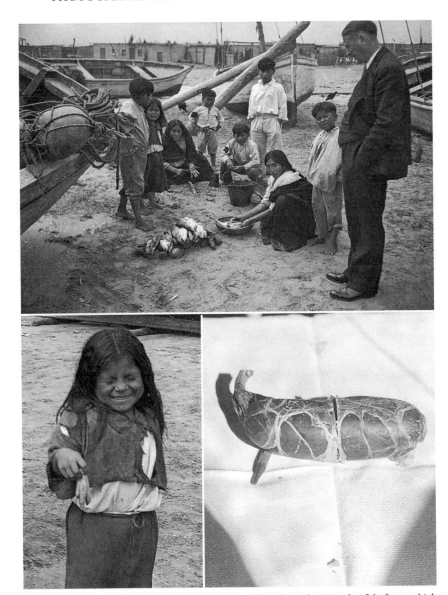

Fig. 175. Peruvians. Top: Here we see a group of mothers cleaning the fish from which they select special parts for special purposes. Bottom Left: During the period of growth of the children the girls are taught to eat fish eggs liberally in order to complete the building of excellent bodies for highly efficient reproduction. This little girl has been down to the beach where the women were cleaning the fish, to get her ration of fish eggs which she is holding in her hand. She was on her way back to her cabin to have them cooked for her breakfast. Bottom Right: Here we see a special fish product that is used by the men who are to become fathers, in order to prepare their bodies for efficient reproduction. This is an organ of the angelote, a species of fish between the skate and the shark.

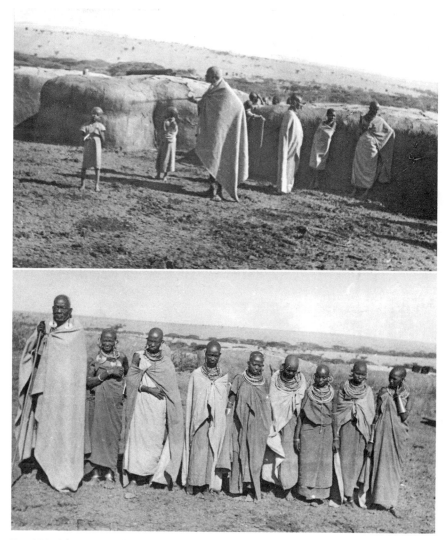

FIG. 176. This Masai African chief is past 80 years of age and is 6'6" tall. He has eight wives and many young children, two are shown. Masai men eat sex glands of male animals.

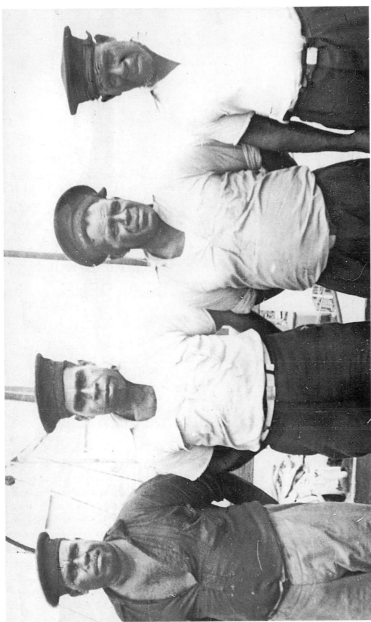

FIG. 177. These natives of the Torres Strait are men of the sea and are very dependable sailors.

Chapter 30

ACID-BASE BALANCE OF DIETS

(Read before the New York Dental Centennial Meeting, New York. N.Y., December 4, 1934; reprinted from the Dental Cosmos for September 1935.)

ACID-BASE BALANCE OF DIETS WHICH PRODUCE IMMUNITY TO DENTAL CARIES AMONG THE SOUTH SEA ISLANDERS AND OTHER PRIMITIVE RACES

By Weston A. Price, D.D.S., M.S., F.A.C.D.
CLEVELAND OHIO

★　★　★　★　★　★　★

AMONG the many theories regarding the controlling factors for immunity to dental caries, "potential alkalinity" has been stressed by many as playing the controlling role. This has been strongly emphasized in the paper by Dr. Martha Jones entitled "Our Changing Concept of an Adequate Diet in Relation to Dental Disease." She and her associates have emphasized this factor in several previous communications. I do not find in her reports, however, the type of quantitative data which seem to be needed for evaluating this problem. The fact that a given potentially basic diet has been found associated with immunity may have little significance regarding the role of acid-base balance in establishing that immunity.

It is very clear that a satisfactory approach to this problem will require the consideration of many diets which have been competent to establish and maintain a very high immunity. No modern civilization provides such a control group, since dental caries is active and in certain groups rampant among the individuals of all of our modernized peoples. It is for this reason I have been making expeditions during several years to reach the remnants of primitive racial stocks who, like their ancestors, are characterized by a very high immunity to dental caries and who by their isolation make possible a critical study of the variables at the point of contact with modern civilization where the high immunity changes to a high susceptibility to tooth decay.

I have previously reported on my studies among the Swiss in the high Alps[1] in isolated valleys. The people of the Outer Hebrides[2], the Eskimos of Alaska[3] and the Indians of northern and central Canada[4] have also been reported. In addition to these we now have very extended data obtained during the past summer from studies among the Melanesians and Polynesians on eight archipelagos of the Pacific.

In this report we shall include a consideration of the acid-base balance of the foods for both these racial stocks and for groups with high immunity to dental caries and for those who have lost that high immunity.

In order to make these data more readily understood when a comparison is made of the potential acidity of the various diets that have been found capable of producing and maintaining high immunity, it is important that we visualize, first, the levels of incidence of tooth decay in these groups while they are isolated and also the levels of those of the same racial stocks who had lost their immunity at the point of contact with civilization. These are shown for the different groups in Fig. 1. There are five groups. We are using all of the people of the South Sea Islands in one group for convenience in this study. It will be noted that the isolated Swiss of the high Alpine valleys had forty-six teeth attacked by tooth decay out of each 1000 teeth examined. The modernized Swiss who were eating our modern foods had 298 teeth involved with caries for each 1000 teeth examined. For the primitive Gaelics in the Outer Hebrides these figures were eleven teeth of each 1000 teeth examined which had been attacked by dental caries and for the modernized groups 300 teeth. For the isolated Eskimos less than one tooth, 0.9, was attacked by caries in each 1000 teeth examined and for those at the point of contact with our modern foods 130 teeth were involved. For the Indians of the far north and interior of Canada living on their primitive native foods, 1.6 teeth were attacked with dental caries, while for the modernized Indians 215 teeth. For all of the groups in the South Sea Islands living on their primitive native foods 3.4 teeth per 1000 teeth examined had been attacked by dental caries, whereas among those eating foods of modern civilization this was increased to 308 teeth. It is important that we keep these figures in mind as we observe the total acidity and total base provided in the average daily diets of these various groups.

FIG. 178

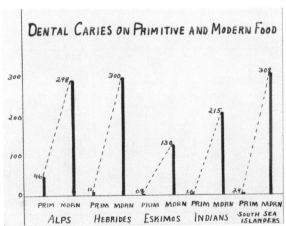

The figures for acidity and base content are shown in Fig. 2. We have in this chart the same groups in the same relationship as in Fig. 1. The method of determining the acid and base content of a given food involved determining the quantity of each of the basic elements—calcium, magnesium, sodium and potassium—and the acid elements—phosphorus, chlorine and sulphur. These determinations have been made by using Sherman's tables with special determinations of special foods. These are expressed in terms of cc. of normal acid and normal base, using the method suggested by Salter, Fulton and Angier in the *Journal of Nutrition* for May 1931. The excess of acid over base or base over acid is expressed as potential acidity or potential alkalinity. It is important to note that in four of these five groups of primitive racial stocks, living on entirely different native foods and in widely divergent climates and entirely different living habits, the immunity-producing diets were found to be higher in acid factors than in base factors. In some the divergence is quite small and in others, quite large. It is also important that, in changing from high immunity to high susceptibility diets, there was no increase in potential acidity with increased susceptibility to tooth decay. This

graph shows the quantity of acid and base in each of the diets associated with immunity and also with susceptibility to tooth decay, and it is of interest to note the very great difference in total acid and total base contained in the nutritions of the various groups.

The clinical work that has been done by Dr. Jones and her associates in the Hawaiian Islands has been on a diet that is potentially alkaline, consisting, as we have learned from her, of poi and milk. The poi is made from powdered cooked taro to which water has been added and fermentation allowed to take place for a definite period. We are primarily concerned with the inorganic acids in evaluating the role of potential acidity, since the organic acids are largely, if not completely, oxidized in the body. Fermenting the poi does not therefore materially change the acid-base balance. The following are the figures for both acid and base factors for each of the primitive and modernized diets for the five groups: for the primitive peoples in the Alps we have as cc.N. acid 369 and base 355; for the modernized groups we have acid 165 and base 171. For the Gaelics of the Outer Hebrides in the primitive groups we have acid 248 and base 152; for the modernized groups, acid 171 and base 152. In

FIG. 179

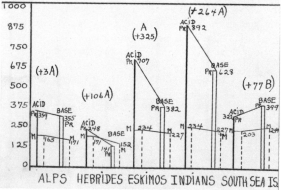

the primitive Eskimos' diet the acid is 707 cc.N. and the base 382; for the modernized Eskimos the acid is 234 cc.N. and the base 227. In the primitive groups of Indians the acid content is 892 cc.N. and the base 628; for the modernized groups the acid is 234 cc.N. and the base is 227. For the primitive South Sea Islanders' diet the acid is 322 and the base 399, and for the modernized groups the acid content is 203 and the base 244. My data, accordingly, do not support the theory advocated by Dr. Jones.

It is of particular interest that in my studies of the South Sea Island groups, taro was found to be one of the most universally and extensively used articles of food. When used with adequate primitive diets of all the Island groups studied, except the Hawaiian Islands, which would include the Marquesas, Society, Cook, Tonga, New Caledonia, Fiji and Samoan Islands, the taro, which was cooked by baking in ovens consisting of heated stones covered with leaves and dirt, produced a very high level of immunity to dental caries in every instance where the groups were isolated from contact with foods of modern civilization and where they were using only their native vegetables and fruits and animal life of the sea. The nutrition of these people will be discussed from a chemical and activator basis in another communication, since space does not permit including it here.

It is very important that dependable data be accumulated as rapidly as possible which bear upon this problem of acid-base balance of foods, since many enthusiasts are advocating strongly the elimination or reduction of potentially acid foods such as cereals, meats and fish. Indeed, a great deal of propaganda is reaching the profession and laity which places great stress upon the importance of keeping the diet potentially alkaline.

It is my personal belief, based on the extensive data that I am accumulating from a study of these various primitive groups and their breakdown at the point of contact with civilization and its foods, that several constitutional factors may be involved besides

tooth decay, and which are very important. My investigations are showing that primitive groups have practically complete freedom from deformity of the dental arches and irregularities of the teeth in the arches and that various phases of these disturbances develop at the point of contact with foods of modern civilization. It is not my belief that this is related to potential acidity or potential alkalinity of the food but to the mineral and activator content of the nutrition during the developmental periods, namely, prenatal, postnatal and childhood growth. It is important that the very foods that are potentially acid have as an important part of the source of that acidity the phosphoric acid content, and an effort to eliminate acidity often means seriously reducing the available phosphorus, an indispensable soft and hard tissue component.

It is my belief that much harm has been done through the misconception that acidity and alkalinity were something apart from minerals and other elements. Many food faddists have undertaken to list foods on the basis of their acidity and alkalinity without the apparent understanding of the disturbances that are produced by, for example, condemning a food because it contains phosphoric acid, not appreciating that phosphorus can only be acid until it is neutralized by combining with a base.

An illustration of this is the following case: A girl was brought for assistance and study who still had her childhood face at sixteen years of age. There had been marked delay in physical development and function other than this growth factor. I was advised that the nutrition of this child had been very largely guided by the literature of the Defensive Diet League which, as one of its principal premises, has urged the keeping down of the acid producing foods. This girl was so conscious of her underdevelopment that she disliked to go to social events with those of her age. When brought to me for assistance and correction of her facial deformity I did not deem it wise or feasible to undertake to change the position of the facial bones by use of orthodontic appliances. I depended entirely on a reinforced nutrition. We supplied mineral and activator carrying foods, with the hope that the growth factors might be in part latent and still be capable of stimulation. There was a very marked improvement in the facial development. In one year she largely developed her adult face. She is very conscious of this improvement and, instead of being reticent and reserved, she has become the leader in her group.

It is very unfortunate that medical and dental science has not looked to the primitive people earlier for standards of not only physical perfection but also of nutrition.

Indeed, while I am dictating this text I have been interrupted by a nurse who has come to inquire whether the teachings so strongly heralded by certain groups should be followed, namely, that proteins and carbohydrates should never be eaten together.

I have seldom found anywhere in the world such a high percentage of physical excellence with high immunity to our modern degenerative diseases as among these people of the South Sea Islands. Their diet practically every day consisted of eating the proteins from the animal life of the sea with the carbohydrates of their land vegetables, many of which were very rich in starch. This was equally true of the Gaelics in the Outer Hebrides, living almost entirely on oats and sea foods.

By studying primitive people who have exceedingly high immunity to dental caries and those people at the point where they lost that high immunity, we were able to reduce the total number of variables to a minimum. It was then possible to study critically those factors of the nutrition which are found to be changed and the varying amounts which can be directly related to the changed incidence of dental caries. This provides still another approach to the problem since, by adding those factors to a deficient diet which are found to constitute the difference between that diet and one that has been demonstrated by those primitive peoples to be efficient, we have a means for checking and determining whether these factors when added will change susceptibility to immunity. It is by this procedure that we can now control dental caries when active, or completely prevent it from developing.

It is of particular significance that when all of the foods of these various primitive groups are reduced to their chemical and activator content they are found to be relatively equivalent. This strongly indicates the direction in which the dental profession can profitably move in this matter of the prevention of tooth decay. Since many other degenerative processes are found to develop simultaneously, or nearly so, with the loss of immunity to dental caries, we have strong evidence that these physical afflictions are, like dental caries, symptoms rather than unit diseases. This clearly is the direction that modern preventive medicine will take in order to establish high immunity to the degenerative diseases.

In every instance in my studies of these primitive racial stocks where I found that they had made contact with our modern civilization, with the result that they had lost their immunity to dental caries, that contact included displacing part of their native diet with imported white flour and sugar and sweetened goods. These foods are exceedingly low in Nature's building material for growth and repair. Refined sugar has practically no minerals or activators, and white flour has had removed about four-fifths of the minerals and nearly all of the germ with its contained activators. Molasses, or sorghum, carries very little phosphorus, though it does carry calcium, which is usually provided easily in safer foods like milk and vegetables. It also carries potassium liberally. Concentrated sweets of all kinds are too high in caloric value to be safe in liberal quantity. Our daily limit of two or three thousand calories, together with our requirement of about two grams of phosphorus in the foods (in order to obtain two-thirds of that amount for body building), means that to obtain this amount we would have to eat enough molasses to supply about 13,300 calories, or about ten pounds. This, if possible, would probably do much harm. To get sufficient phosphorus from white flour products usually requires eating about four and one-half pounds of white bread daily, which would provide about 10,000 calories.

In my clinical practice, in which I am endeavoring to put into practice the lessons I am learning from the primitive people, I do not require that the foods of the primitive races be adopted but that our modern foods be reinforced in body-building materials to make them equivalent in mineral and activator content to the efficient foods of the primitive people. This usually is accomplished by displacing white-flour products with whole-wheat products, together with eliminating or reducing the high caloric foods such as sugars and other sweets, and adding foods that are good providers of the fat-soluble activators, such as the butter of milk as produced by cows that are eating liberally of fresh or cured rapidly growing green wheat or rye, together with the organs of animals and the use of sea foods such as these primitive people have used so successfully in providing not only high immunity to dental caries but excellent bodies, with high defense for the degenerative diseases. We are learning Nature's methods and undertaking to utilize them. The chemical content of all of these primitive foods is comparably high in minerals and activators, especially the fat-soluble activators, while being relatively low in calories. In no instance have I found the change from a high immunity to dental caries to a high susceptibility among these primitive racial stocks to be associated with a change from a diet with a high potential alkalinity to a high potential acidity, as would seem to have been the case had the high alkalinity balance theory been the correct explanation. If the requisite is so simple as a potential alkalinity, why has not the addition of sodium bicarbonate to a deficient diet controlled dental caries?

BIBLIOGRAPHY

[1]PRICE, WESTON A.: "Why Dental Caries with Modern Civilization?" *Dental Digest*, 39:94, 147, March and April 1933.
[2]*Idem: Dental Digest*, 39:225, June 1933.
[3]*Idem: Dental Digest*, 40:210, June 1934.
[4]*Idem: Dental Digest*, 40:130, April 1934.

Chapter 31

PERSONAL CORRESPONDENCE
TO AND FROM WESTON A. PRICE

[Transcript of a letter believed to have been, written about 1934 - Donald Delmage Fawcett (grand-nephew of Weston A. Price)]

Weston A. Price, D.D.S., M.S.
Dental Research Laboratories
8926 Euclid Avenue
Cleveland, Ohio

My Dear Nieces and Nephews:

I am deeply interested not only in your health individually but in the efficiency and welfare of your families. It is particularly important in these times of industrial and financial stress, that children shall not suffer defeats which may mark and handicap them for their entire life. Fortunately, an adequately defensive nutritional program can be provided without much expense and indeed often more cheaply than the currently selected foods. There will be no necessity for any child of yours to develop dental caries or tooth decay if the simple procedures that I am outlining, shall be adequately carried out. Your cousin, Alice, desired to send some suggestions to Olive and Julia and I suggested to her that I would outline something that would be helpful to all of you. I think Alice will be glad to assist in making copies to supplement those that I am sending her.

There are two ways in which I could make suggestions relative to the mineral and vitamin problem in the selection of food, the one on the basis of detailing a special menu for each day, which is very unsatisfactory, and the other would be in the form of general principles which should control and guide you in selecting the foods which will meet the body's daily needs. I would suggest the latter and the following is an outline of the principles involved.

If you will think of an automobile into which you would have the choice of putting two kinds of gasoline, one that would furnish only power, corresponding with ordinary gasoline, and the other capable of making new tires grow as fast as the old ones are worn out, continually putting on a new coat of paint and even making an Austin grow into a Pierce-Arrow, there is no doubt as to which gasoline you would use, even though there would be a great deal of difference in the price. This very closely represents the condition that is found in our bodies.

490

Letter on Nutrition by Weston A. Price - Page 2

We have a sense of hunger which expresses itself as appetite and we eat until this is satisfied, but this only applies to that part of our food which produces power and heat. We have almost no sense of hunger for the minerals and other chemicals and vitamins that are needed for building and repairing old tissues. Modern civilization is making a tragic mistake in getting away from the natural foods that are low in energy and high in minerals, and teasing the intake of the heat and energy producing foods. This energy can be quantitatively expressed by the amount of oxygen that may be utilized when modern foods are burning either by the wet process within our bodies or by the dry process in special apparatus. We speak of this in terms of calories.

Most people need from 2000 to 3000 calories a day, according to the nature of their physical activities. Similarly, we need two grams of phosphorus and one and one-half grams of calcium a day in our food in order to keep up the body's daily requirements. Our problem then is to get enough of the minerals and vitamins without exceeding our limit in calories. Our bodies call a halt usually when they have taken in enough calories to satisfy the appetite but at the same time they probably have not obtained enough of the minerals and vitamins sufficient for the daily requirement. Cereals, milk and sea foods are the foods that Nature has provided us with in natural form, which will satisfy our hunger and will at the same time take care of our body's requirements. Modern civilization has modified this by providing us with menus that tend to be too high in calories and too low in mineral content.

Our next great problem is to keep the battery of our car charged sufficiently so that we will utilize the fuel efficiently. The vitamins provide the battery charge for animals including humans. One of our greatest struggles is to get sufficient amounts of the vitamins, particularly the fat-soluble vitamins. There is a great tendency toward trying to supply these with synthetic products which are not a substitute. The amount of minerals that are in the food that we eat, that will be utilized by the body, will be largely determined by these activating substances. We may apply these principles to the daily diet.

It is not wise to fill the limited space with foods that are not doing our bodies any particular good. You would be interested to know that while you would have to eat 7 1/2 pounds of potatoes or 11 pounds of beets or 9 1/2 pounds of carrots to get the daily phosphorus requirement, all of which would provide too high a number of calories, you would obtain as much phosphorus from 1 pound of lentils. This would also provide the calcium. You would also supply the entire day's requirement of minerals from 0.8 pounds of fish or 0.6 pounds of cheese. Milk is one of the best, if not the best single food, since you obtain the minerals rapidly in proportion to the calories. The main thing is to get the daily phosphorus and calcium requirement and sufficient of the vitamins, particularly the fat-soluble vitamins.

Letter on Nutrition by Weston A. Price - Page 3

There is a misapprehension regarding the value of fruits as food. Of course fruits are desirable as an adjunct, but most of them are very low in minerals. You would for example, have to eat 37 pounds of apples a day or 26 pounds of oranges to get your two grams of phosphorus and when these fruits are sweetened into jams or jellies, you would have to eat 32 pounds of orange marmalade a day, which would provide 33,000 calories; few of us could take care of more than 3000 calories. You would also have to take over 30,000 calories of honey to get your two grams of phosphorus, for which you would need to eat 28 pounds per day. Similarly, you would have to eat 34 pounds a day of maple syrup which would provide 85,000 calories. Among the poorest foods we could feed children would be white bread and jam or pancakes with maple syrup or similar combinations, and these are no better for adults than they are for children, for we all have the same problems except that the stress is greater during periods of rapid growth.

The basic foods should be the entire grains such as whole wheat, rye or oats, whole wheat and rye breads, wheat and oat cereals, oat-cake, dairy products, including milk and cheese, which should be used liberally, and marine foods. All marine or sea foods, both fresh and salt water, are high in minerals and constitute one of the very best foods you could eat. Canned fish such as sardines, tuna, or salmon are all excellent; also the fresh fish such as oysters, halibut, haddock, etc. The protein requirement can be provided each day in one egg or a piece of meat equivalent to the bulk of one egg a day. The meals can be amply modified and varied with vegetables, raw and cooked, the best of the cooked vegetables being lentils used as a soup. The cooked vegetables are better since raw vegetables are usually too bulky to allow very much mineral to be obtained from them. Some of the best of the cooked vegetables are cauliflower, brussels sprouts, asparagus tips and celery. Lettuce is the best of the raw vegetables.

Cut down on starches and sugars. Sweet things satisfy the hunger and provide calories and thus not only displace foods higher in minerals, but reduce the total amount of food eaten by satisfying the appetite. Reduce all white flour products and pastries to a minimum. One of the best sources of minerals is provided in cheese. Use freshly cracked wheat for cereal, muffins or bread. Much of the value of the wheat germ is lost by oxidation if the product is not fresh.

There are only a few foods that would give you your fat-soluble vitamins. These are the fish products, including practically all fresh water and salt water foods, milk, cheese and butter made from cows that have been on a rapidly growing green young wheat, either fresh or stored grass, particularly butter made in June. This is much richer than butter made during other seasons of the year. Eat butter chiefly for its vitamin content.

One of your greatest difficulties will be to provide the children and yourselves with sufficient of the fat-soluble activators and vitamins. We being mammals, have bodies prepared to get these

Letter on Nutrition by Weston A. Price - Page 4

from milk and its butterfat, which is not in Skimmed milk. There
is not much left for the children when the cream has been taken
from the milk for the parents' coffee. Where possible, have June
butter stored for winter use. Cod liver oil can be given in moderate doses without injury and to great advantage. Seldom however,
should the child be given more than a teaspoonful a day for
extended periods, because of toxic effects that often develop.
It is better to take the cod liver oil with the meal rather than
before or after, as it aids in the utilization of the minerals
in the food.

We are now able to determine from a chemical analysis of an
individual's saliva whether or not tooth decay would be likely to
be present in that particular mouth. Remember, it is the defensive chemicals that must be present in the saliva to prevent
tooth decay and these are provided to the saliva by having the
food amply high in minerals and fat-soluble vitamins. The saliva
furnishes the greatly needed minerals which aid in the digestive
process; hence the great advantage in having the food in a physical form to require chewing, which makes the saliva flow. Do not
let the children wash their food down with their drink. They
should drink about a quart of milk a day, preferably after each
meal or part of it between meals.

An excellent program then will be to use a cooked cereal made
from freshly cracked wheat or oats, this to be eaten with cream
or milk and a limited amount of sugar sufficient to flavor the
cereal. Have them follow this with one or two glasses of milk.
Recently baked whole wheat muffins made from freshly cracked wheat
and spread liberally with a high-vitamin butter are excellent in
both their mineral and vitamin content. These can be eaten to
advantage with cooked applesauce or other cooked fruits not too
highly sweetened. The highly sweetened marmalades and jams check
the appetite and make a disproportion of the calories to the minerals and vitamins. There is no objection to having the children
fill up on bulky foods such as potatoes and vegetables, if the
daily mineral and vitamin requirements have been satisfied first.
If June butter cannot be obtained, which is usually the case for
most of the year, and unless arrangements can be made for having
some put in storage for winter use, it will be well to reinforce
the diet with a little cod liver oil during the winter months.

In my studies of growing children in other countries as well
as in this country, in every instance where they were eating
foods that were found to be high in minerals and vitamins, there
was no tooth decay and in every instance where modern foods high
in calories and low in minerals were used, rampant tooth decay
was prevalent. Remember that it would take three large loaves of
white bread a day to provide our requirements for phosphorus, but
this would give us 10,000 calories, an amount which it would be
physically impossible to utilize. Eating this with skimmed milk
would be one of the surest ways to produce dental caries and in
some cases might even produce convulsions. The safety of the
primitive people has been the impossibility of their getting hold
of any foods that were high in calories and low in minerals, but

Letter on Nutrition by Weston A. Price - Page 5

my studies have indicated that they break down and develop dental caries as readily as any other people when they go on modern diets.

Practical demonstrations of the way this program works out will shortly be available in a series of articles which I have provided for one of our journals, The Dental Digest. These articles will emphasize that tooth decay is a symptom and not a disease. It is evidence of a faulty nutrition and not as so many have thought, entirely the result of the lack of mouth care. Mouth care is, of course, desirable. Preventive diets usually cost less, besides preventing the expense of repair of the teeth.

These are times when these practical problems should be and must be considered carefully.

I hope I have not seemed to be lecturing to you. I love you all dearly and am deeply concerned for your best welfare.

Lovingly,

Uncle Weston

MEMORANDUM FROM

H. H. TOCKER
DENTIST
MASSON HOUSE,
DALTON STREET, NAPIER
New Zealand

SURGERY PHONE - 318
RESIDENCE PHONE 1022

4th August 1939.

Dr. Weston A. Price
Dental Research Laboratories
8926 Euclid Avenue
Cleveland, Ohio
U.S.A.

Dear Dr. Price,

Your letter of June 21st, and autographed copy of your book
NUTRITION AND PHYSICAL DEGENERATION, were received with the very
greatest interest and pleasure. I am immensely grateful. Your
data supplies just the knowledge I lacked and needed so much to
arm me with power in my work to improve the health of the Maori
people in particular. Immediately on reading, I sent the chemical
analysis of the old time Maori foods to the Maori Bishop of New
Zealand, contrasting the former abundance with the existing deficiencies, and anticipate collaborating with him to disseminate
this invaluable information among his people. The 180 scholars of
two Maori schools will also carry this information, and its lesson, throughout New Zealand, to Rarotonga and the Cook Island
group, thanks to your work.

Our Branch of the N.Z.D.A. recently gave a dinner to a member
who was retiring on account of age and ill health. This member
said that on looking back over a life of fillings and extractions, he could see nothing that he had done to improve the condition either of his profession or his patients; that for all the
good he had done, he might just as well not have lived at all.
He represented 99% of dentists. You have accomplished a magnum
opus by sustained effort that lifts dentistry to a higher plane
and patients to better health. It is a great work that justifies
pride while memory lasts.

You have interpreted natural law for us all, and once interpreted, the obscure becomes obvious. Human life can exist without
air 5 minutes; without water about one week; without an adequate
intake of essential chemical elements somewhat longer, say three
generations, in which the signs and symptoms of degeneration give
warning. As I read your book, my pre-conceived ideas of the hori-
zons of the nutrition problem, ever receded, and new and wider
vistas appeared; dental health, public health, the contrasting
birth rates of the Pacific border peoples and sequelae, economic
and military aspects; influence of ocean currents; soil depletion
and renewal.

I am located in a sparsely populated country, without access
to technical libraries, and my appreciation is profound.

2.

At my home, I have followed your suggestion of installing a motor driven grain mill, and am spreading the gospel. The Hukarere test, on diet amended according to your suggestions, completes its 1939 6 months in Sept. 1939, when results will be sent to you. Arrested decay has been established in some mouths, with deposition of secondary dentine. Control is incomplete, school holidays interrupt diet. Data will be sent to N.Z. Dental Journal,and to Dental Branch of Government Medical Research Committee.

I should be grateful if you would be able to supply me with information I have failed to get in New Zealand. Even the Wheat Research Institute refers me to the Rowett Institute, in Abderdeen, Scotland.

My problem refers to the length of time taken for the loss of vitamins after milling wheat.

In supplying freshly milled wheat for Hukarere bread, a crude local mill was first used, which was without cleaning apparatus. Repeatedly, sand present with the wheat caused complaints, and ultimately the abandonment of this mill. Wholemeal from a Christchurch, South Island of New Zealand mill was then used. I have since been dependent on the millers' assurance that the meal is freshly ground immediately before shipping to the local baker, the minimum time being 5 days, and the average at least a week between milling and baking, possibly more. I am concerned to know whether the interval of 7 to 10 days between milling and consumption is sufficient to cause the loss of vitamins by oxidation. It is possible that there is such deterioration of the volume and strength of vitamin action, due to this interval, that mineral absorption is so retarded as to defeat the object of the test.

In view of the fact that local bakers estimate that it takes 8 weeks for "green" or freshly milled white flour to age, (i.e. to lose its vitamins by oxidation) I am calculating on a slight, not a major, loss.

While a recent influenza epidemic infected 50% of Te Aute Maori boys, Hukarere girls were protected by their diet and contracted no influenza. The girls were jubilant, crowing over the boys "Who are the tough guys now?" The whole school is convinced of the efficacy of the diet, and take their convictions into their homes.

With sincere thanks,
Yours faithfully

H.H. Tocker

September 1, 1939

Dr. H. H. Tocker,
Nasson House,
Dalton Street,
Napier, New Zealand.

Dear Dr. Tocker,

Your interesting and very informative letter of August fourth is received. I am hastening to reply so it will catch the return boat.

I am, of course, greatly interested in the scholars in the two Maori schools and the comparative studies you are making. Your observations regarding the flu correspond with many other reports here to the same effect.

The comment made by the retiring dentist in New Zealand is in substance the experience of dentists throughout the world who are concerned that their life shall contribute to our civilization rather than only receive benefits and those because of the misfortunes of others.

Your question with regard to wheat and the length of time the germ will be useable is important. In your winter climate the flour should contain most of its vitamin E for a week. In hot weather, however, the oxidation takes place rapidly. I asked an old Indian whom I saw grinding corn between two stones why he did not use larger stones and grind a lot at a time. His reply to all of my questions was "no good". When I reduced the time down for the flour to be used in three days he still said "no." When I asked him why, he said "something gone". His magnificent physical condition at a very advanced age strongly testified to the wisdom of his program. His tribe lived largely on sheep and goats, the milk and flesh, and on corn and some green foods. One of the greatest difficulties in making bread from whole wheat flour is the dryness and the ease with which it crumbles. This is largely overcome by an increase in the amount of yeast used which should be doubled for that required for white flour.

I hope the cooperation of your girls will be adequate to permit you to demonstrate a hundred percent control of tooth decay. I am anxious to cooperate in every way that I can.

I am greatly interested in the comments of your Bishop. I am enclosing herewith a personal letter to him addressed in your care. I am sorry I did not meet him personally. I greatly enjoyed my contact with Bishop Williams when in Napier and my correspondence before and after going to New Zealand. Because of the great importance of the Bishop's work and his opportunities I am sending him, in your care, a complimentary copy of my book so he will have one to take with him to show the officials in the Cook Islands. I had a very interesting and pleasant contact with the officials at Rarotonga while there in 1934 and also by correspondence with them before and after my visit there. I am enclosing a copy of my letter to the Bishop for your files.

2-HHT-9-1-39

I look forward to a very important contribution to world betterment that will come through the demonstration that Bishop Williams and his associates will make at Cook Island and which will be applicable to bettering conditions of all of the primitive groups in the Pacific archipelagos.

I will appreciate highly your cooperation and advice in my efforts to help the Bishop in his work among the splendid native tribes in his large parish.

You will be pleased to know that the interest in my book wherever it has been reviewed has been enthusiastic and considered promising for the betterment of humanity.

I am looking forward with keen interest to our report of the second six months' studies with your group. You will please extend my personal greeting to the young ladies in the Hukarere school. I will send them a little token as an expression of my appreciation of their cooperation.

                              Yours very sincerely,

                              Weston A. Price

WAP:RWM
Encl.

September 1, 1939

Presiding Bishop,
New Zealand and Cook Island Dioceses,
c/o Dr. H. H. Tocker,
Dalton Street, Napier, New Zealand.

My dear Bishop,

Dr. Tocker has told me of your kind interest and cooperation in behalf of the natives of your diocese. I had the great pleasure of meeting your predecessor, Bishop Williams, and having correspondence with him before and after going to New Zealand. He gave me very important assistance in the study of the nutrition of the primitive Maori. I am especially happy to know that the Cook Islands are in your diocese. I consider the natives there among the finest studied in the eight archipelagos of the Pacific, though I only met those on Rarotonga Island. From the information I was able to obtain I have the impression that some of the finest primitive groups still remaining are on the most isolated of the Cook Islands due to their absence of contact with modern civilization.

It would be most fortunate if someone could make studies in those isolated islands on the accumulated wisdom of the natives. If special foods are used for special purposes forward those data to me or to someone who will utilize them for the betterment of humanity.

I am having special foods sent from several parts of the world for chemical analysis. I will write you further regarding this and as to the method of preparation of the samples so that they will be acceptable for entry into the United States. In general plants that are sent in preservative are not subject to quarantine. Certain plants and roots are subject to quarantine unless specially preserved.

In order to assist you in your important work, I have pleasure in sending you a copy of my book NUTRITION AND PHYSICAL DEGENERATION so you may have it for reference in your various contacts with officials. The book is going to you in care of Dr. Tocker. I have advised him that it is being sent.

I have dreamed that someday I might be able to go back to the Cook Islands and learn more of their splendid accumulated wisdom. They and their cousins who migrated to New Zealand are among the finest examples of primitive culture.

2-Bishop-9-1-39

　　I am sure you will have great happiness and satisfaction in
your work among these primitive people who had learned so well
Nature's laws regarding life and for whom contact with the white
civilization and its foods of commerce have brought so much mis-
ery and harm. I deem it a great privilege to have a small part
in cooperating with you in your work. I shall look forward with
pleasure in being of any assistance that I can at any time in
your important work.

　　　　　　　　　　　　　　　　　Yours very sincerely,

　　　　　　　　　　　　　　　　　Weston A. Price

WAP:RWM

Rodale Press

Publishers of:
FACT DIGEST
EVERYBODY'S DIGEST
YOU CAN'T EAT THAT
SCIENCE AND DISCOVERY
YOU'RE WRONG ABOUT THAT

EMMAUS, PA.

July 26, 1939

Dr. Weston A. Price
8926 Euclid Ave.
Cleveland, Ohio

Dear Dr. Price,

We are reading your book called "NUTRITION AND PHYSI-CAL DEGENERATION" and are very much interested in it because of the fact that we have been so much interested also in the findings of Drs. L. J. and P. H. Belding. If you are not familiar with their work, perhaps you could write to DENTAL ITEMS OF INTEREST and get a copy of the paper that was read by the Beldings at the dental meeting in New York.

They seemed to show that the eating of wheat products, and to a much more limited extent rye and corn, gave rise to a condition in the mouth which not only causes caries but also might possibly lead to some of the degenerative diseases that you mentioned. Bread seems to be a very acid food.

As a result of the Beldings findings, the writer and his family have been away from bread now for about eight months. It is only recently that I started to eat the pure rye bread. It has done very much for me in connection with colds. A friend of mine who had a case of constipation for twelve years standing has been cured most beautifully by means of a breadless diet.

I am writing to Dr. Belding, as I believe that you folks should get together, as you have a community of interest.

Sincerely yours,
RODALE PRESS

J. I. Rodale, Pres.

JIR:VR
CC to Dr. Belding

August 8, 1939

J. I. Rodale, President,
Rodale Press,
Emmaus, Penna.

My dear Sir:

Your letter of July twenty-sixth is before me. I am glad you
are finding my book NUTRITION AND PHYSICAL DEGENERATION helpful
as well as of interest.

I am quite familiar with the work of Drs. L. J. and P. H.
Belding. I know them both personally and esteem highly their
earnestness and sincerity.

We who are engaged in research in Nature's laboratory are
ourselves on trial and when our findings do not agree with
Nature's established standards it is important that we recheck
using Nature's standards. This is the criterion that I try to
use in interpreting my own findings.

The matter of the role of cereals when used as modified and
refined products may be very different from that which Nature has
provided. A striking illustration of data from Nature's laboratory that does not check with the findings of the Beldings is the
magnificent physiques of the Gaelics of the Outer Hebrides whose
diet has consisted so largely of oats in the form of oat meal
porridge and oat cake used in connection with a sea food diet.
Similarly the magnificent tribes that I have studied in the
high Andes of South America living so largely on corn and beans,
the superb physical development of the Swiss in the isolated
valleys of Switzerland were living on rye and dairy products; the
agricultural tribes in central Africa living on native cereals
together with an assortment of intelligently selected supplement-
ing foods, all emphasize the need for checking with Nature before
making too general an application of data which seem to conflict
with Nature's laws. It is important to note that all of these
primitive groups insisted that the cereal products be used quickly
after the grains were cracked and therefore all of the material
that Nature provided in each grain is utilized.

The problem of acid or alkaline balance in the diet has been
very confusing to many earnest students of nutrition. I found
Indians of the far north presenting whole villages without a
single tooth that had ever been attacked by tooth decay and yet
living for ten months of the year almost entirely on the meat of
wild animals, chiefly moose and caribou, bear and mountain goat.
Similarly the Eskimos were using a food providing a high acid
balance. Physical fitness of the individuals and freedom from
tooth decay was as high in these groups and in fish eating groups
as in those using the plant foods that gave a high alkaline
balance.

2-JIR-8-8-39

It usually seems to be forgotten or not appreciated that chemical reactions required to make skeletal material are based primarily on the unknown equivalent amounts of acid and base. The
facts are that we require more phosphorus than any other single
element for maintaining body function from day to day and phosphorus can only exist as an acid or in stages of combinations
with bases.

The above does not mean that I am an exponent of modern bread.
You will have noted from my book that I have put much of the
responsibility for modern degeneration on the demineralization
and devitalization of foods by modern processing.

I believe that primitive tribes have demonstrated to us that
the use of natural foods when selected with an adequate intelligence can create a very much higher perfection and immunity to
disease including immunity to dental caries than is accomplished
by our modern civilization. I strongly advocate adopting the
means used by the primitives, namely, using an adequate selection
of native natural foods for the control of dental caries and the
development of excellent bodies and for preserving them, rather
than waiting until we understand all the chemical processes
involved in digestion, immunity and metabolism.

Let us suppose that the particular organism responsible for
dental caries is the one the Beldings report finding. How much
better off will we be for the prevention of dental caries than we
are now. Whether the active organism of dental caries belongs to
the lactobacillus group as advocated by Bunting, Jay and associates of the University of Michigan, or an acid producing strep as
suggested by the Beldings is relatively insignificant compared
with the fact that neither can produce dental caries if the
selection of the food is adequate. What humanity needs is practical procedures for the control of dental caries and for building
efficient bodies and maintaining them so.

                              Yours very sincerely,

                              Weston A. Price

WAP:RWM

Conclusion

ARE TWO OF OUR MAJOR DILEMMAS SOLVED?

WHAT produces our so-called bad boys and girls, and why? This concerns every thoughtful citizen and all parents.

Only two forces have been considered as capable of producing both our juvenile delinquents and the increasing population of so-called mentally retarded individuals who drive both our parents and our teachers to despair, since they are blamed. Heredity and environment have been the only forces understood to be associated with birth and childhood. The mystery of where we came from and how, have been but vaguely understood and for most of us a carefully closed and almost sealed book, through ignorance and prejudice. Our environment is simple and is always presided over, presumably by parents, hence they must be to blame for their children's behavior. Our California law now implies their blame by recording that whenever a juvenile offender, boy or girl, is reported, the parents must be hailed into court to explain why. The present increase is explained by the fact that both parents are now employed in war work, statistical data however easily refute this since in only about 4%, of the cases, are both parents so employed. The origin of this law may have been inspired by conviction that since heredity is a perfect process of divine origin its processes are beyond human knowledge and indeed are not proper and appropriate topics for Christians to consider. This is strongly demonstrated by the opposition to any interference with *unregulated* childbirth.

In this situation both juvenile delinquents and mentally retarded individuals have increased decade after decade all over the country. This increase has been much greater in some districts than in others which incidentally gives us a clue. Another factor has been recorded in which certain physical divergencies from normal, tend to be found present in the delinquent, regardless of where born.

These two sources of influence, inheritance and environment, have been the limit of consideration or knowledge. The fact of similarity, regardless of birth place, has led me to investigate primitive races in various parts of the world, to learn whether humans there have indicated any other wisdom than that which we possess. Since many a long-buried skeleton shows superfine bone formation, they apparently had good physical form. I have accordingly gone to many remnants of old civilizations to find the reasons and fortunately so, for I have found that the more perfect groups physically, are duplicates of our best form and their defectives are duplicates of our imperfect moderns. This latter group however, is their group of modernized individuals who have been touched and changed by contact with our modern commerce. We made them with our demineralized and vitamin-free foods.

Even heredity with all its complicated nature, while in a sense immortal is itself purely physical and composed of units of proteins, minerals and vitamins called genes and in the transfer from one generation to the next must be re-built by the special sex cells of the parents and only by complete rebuilding can perfect hereditary traits, physical and physiological, be expressed as personality and character. These modernized primitives produced typical juvenile delinquents with abnormal personalities and the associated physical defects of our modern defectives. Their undoing is not caused by heredity but is intercepted heredity. Yes, their parents produced them but they are not the product of their external environment. They are cripples produced at the time of conception, their defects can never be cured, but, with proper education and parental nutrition they could have been prevented. Nature has been making normal birds, butterflies and animals for millions of years. If wild animals can do it why cannot we? Is it because they, by their instinct, select the right foods and do not meddle with nature's foods by changing them? A part of the bird and animal at birth is its education or instinct, for it knows how to build a home and how to select its food. They are protected by their ignorance, including a natural absence of a profit motive.

In my recording of these studies of primitive races I have made thousands of photographs which show the constant similarity of given defects in all humans and animals in which many changes in shape of the head and structure of the body are shown. These also demonstrate that it is not normal heredity since the next generation is not affected whenever the defective parent had the proper food. This is the burden of this book *Nutrition and Physical Degeneration* here reprinted and enlarged.

It is very significant as I have shown that the Rockefeller Foundation has, in May of this year, made a grant of $282,000 to the Jackson Memorial Laboratories, at Bar Harbor, Maine, for the study of what goes on in genes in normal and disturbed hereditary processes. The director, Dr. C. C. Little, in announcing the grant, made the following statement:

> . . . It has become evident that neither heredity nor environment could go far without the other.
>
> If for example, the tiny concentrated centers of chemical organization known as genes—the basic unit of heredity, had no living organism provided by food and growth on which and in which to express their directive powers, they would be incapable of description, measurement or identification.

Dr. Little is one of the world's leading students of the problems associated with the complicated structure of the genes, which must carry to the new generation the parental characteristics.

Dr. Ernest A. Hooton, who has written the foreword to this book, has closed with the following statement:

> So I consider that Dr. Price has written what is often called "a profoundly significant book." The principal difference between Dr. Price's work and many others so labeled is that in the present instance the designation appears to be correct. I salute Dr. Price with the sincerest admiration (the kind that is tinged with envy) because he has found out something which I should have liked to have discovered for myself.

We can all see, as in my many illustrations from primitive races and from animals, this problem of physical degeneration expressing itself in the younger members of the family, indicating that the parents were running out of something. Even the personality may show it, if they are more backward than the first born child and if they are more than ten years of age, look for narrow nostrils, crooked teeth or narrow hips. Nature does the best she can with the available material. Twenty-five percent of our modem babies are not perfect enough to have a live birth, and thirty-seven percent of those born alive are either dead or have become a burden on society in fifteen years.

Our immediate need is for means to prevent the building of defectives which is primarily a matter of education of parents to be, long before the problems arise. This is the method used by many of the primitive races that I have studied. It does not involve parading sex problems but simply telling the story of biology to both grade and high school pupils, which now is being done very successfully. An adequate nutritional program will indicate in detail the nature of the defects produced by faulty foods, in both the individuals themselves and in their offspring. The needed better foods for both are indicated. It is significant that the proper foods have been found available in all the countries where primitive races have succeeded: very often however, certain foods, recognized as necessary, were carried long distances.

With adequate teaching we can save millions both in money and in lives besides building a living, instead of, a dying civilization.

WHO WAS MY MOTHER? Was it that sweet soul who conceived me and gave me a physical birth? The land of my birth first claimed me and provided food and shelter; the church where my father was so active, sponsored controlling tenets for guiding my young and wavering feet. Or is there a *force* back of all these that is *parent to them all*? As I go to remnants of ancient cultures I find that, though differing in color and size, they are all true to type and all disclose the same constant relation to variations in physical form and behaviour and share these variations with all the animal forms of their district. They all fit into an endless scheme revealing interrelationships exceeding the most varied assortment of known vital forms. They include all the geologic strata of the epochs through which this earth has passed and hence must be related to its very structure. Living forms have been adapted to the changing physical environments. Earnest students of living cultures find them each sympathetic to some controlling motive. Ernest Thompson Seton, an earnest student of the American Indian, summarizes the Indians' motive as being "fundamentally spiritual, his measure of success is, 'How much service have I rendered to my people?'"

Dr. M. F. Ashley-Montagu, distinguished anatomist and anthropologist, in discussing the motives of the Australian Aborigine and the average Eskimo, states:

> We are very definitely their inferiors. We lisp noble ideals and noble sentiments—the Australians and Eskimos practice them—they neither write books nor lecture about them. Theirs are the only true democracies where every individual finds his happiness in catering to the happiness of the group, and where any one who in any way threatens the welfare of the group is dealt with as an abnormality.

Similarly the many creeds of today have differing points of emphasis, though with many qualities in common. The association of the concept of human beings often carries over to chemicals of which they are made, giving them almost parental relationships. Thus heavy elements break down slowly into slightly lighter elements, but always according to atomic weight of the elements and in doing so, give off radiant energy as in the splitting of uranium and production of radium. It is common practice today in biological laboratories to start the breakdown of a substance, for example phosphorus, by making it radioactive, by exposure to neutrons, negatively charged particles, and thus making it capable of recording its position photographically in its passage through animal tissues. In 1900 I reported in Paris the use of Roentgen rays for making skiagrams of bone specimens, and in 1922 I reported at the Mayo Institute, Rochester, Minn., on the ability of foetal tissues to collect irradiation from the circulating blood. I injected a solution of radioactive salt into the leg of a living guinea pig and made records of the changing location by photographing through black paper. At first the plate was darkened only opposite the leg. An hour later the entire body gave off diffuse radiation and in another hour the radiant energy was accumulated in the unborn foetus. The embryo was removed and covered with black paper and its photograph shows a halo about it in the resulting illustration. Many viruses are now grown in embryonic tissues, for example the viruses of our common colds are grown in unhatched chicken eggs, these viruses are ultra-microscopic, like the building blocks in the parental tissue of genes.

These genes, which carry all the physical characters in heredity, are so small that their entire mass for providing the blueprint for an elephant is so small that only the highest magnification of the best microscopes are able to reveal them. They are the parental transfer of life in all its details. A pollen floating invisibly in the air far above the earth, is a seed, capable of producing a plant, or a chemical reaction in our bodies as hay fever, yet it is invisible. Such invisibly small structures are the carriers of life in all its forms. We are familiar with slow oxidation producing body warmth and with rapid oxidation as in the open fire. Similarly, atomic energy is expended slowly in nature in all living forms and its prodigious energy as heat and light. The carriers of hereditary factors call for force prodigious in small units *comparable to, if not identical with atomic energy.*

We can now visualize our universe, its light, gravity and heat, its seasons, tides and harvest, which prepare a habitation for the universe of vital forms, microscopic and majestic, which fill the oceans and the forests. We have a common denominator for universes within and around each other, our world, our food and our life have potentials so vast that we can only observe directions, not goals. We sense human achievements or ignominious race self-destruction. Every creed today vaguely seeks a utopia; all have visualized a common controlling force or deity as the most potent force in all human affairs. Yes, man's place is most exalted when he obeys *his Mother Nature's laws.*

Neither heredity nor environment alone cause our juvenile delinquents and mental defectives. They are cripples, physically, mentally and morally, which could have and should have been prevented by adequate education and by adequate parental nutrition. Their protoplasm was not normally organized.

This atomic energy which may be liberated in large amounts as light and heat from the sun, or in small amounts from decaying elements in nature at varying rates, builds all the foods by its reactions in living plants. It thus provides the plant and animal protoplasms which gives them life. Needham, from whom I have quoted in Chapter 25, emphasizes protoplasm as the first of the four units of the living world. He says:

> In all living creatures there is one common substance, protoplasm, the physical basis of life, the only known living substance. It is a semi-fluid substance, transparent, well nigh structureless, and apparently inert, yet possessing the unique powers that distinguish living from nonliving things, the powers of *growth and reproduction.*
>
> The living substance throughout is protoplasm; seemingly one substance, alike in all, and yet in the course of its onflow, marvelously dispensing to every individual some mark of his own that no other individual in all the

world possesses. Protoplasm organizes itself in cells, its working units; and behind the cells that build our bodies, that do the work of our bodies and of our minds, is the great mystery of life itself—the driving power of an unexplained control that shapes the course of self development in the individual, and carries on by cell lineage through successive generations.

This driving power must have qualities like this universal but obscure atomic energy.

We now see new and greatly enlarged meaning in each Activator, the various hormones and the vitamins. We learn how they have changed many prospective mothers and their babies as illustrated on page 372.

There has been intelligent purpose in the strange practices of many of the primitive races. Those terraced gardens in the high Andes and Himalaya mountains are evidence of the struggle toward a better radiated atmosphere, by those superbly built Incas and Hunzas who constructed them. They beautifully reveal cause and effect.

All human growth demands this struggle towards these sources of life produced by atomic energy.

"LIFE IN ALL ITS FULLNESS IS THIS MOTHER NATURE OBEYED."

—*Weston A. Price, DDS*

EPILOGUE

D R. Weston Price's legacy to mankind lives on in Price-Pottenger (previously known as the Weston A. Price Memorial Foundation), founded in honor of Dr. Price and Dr. Francis M. Pottenger, Jr., pioneers in teaching the fundamentals of optimum health using natural dietary methods. A principle purpose of Price-Pottenger is to ensure that this volume, *Nutrition and Physical Degeneration*, will always be available to individuals who are searching for superior health, and who are willing to trade the "displacing foods of modern commerce," for foods that build strong bodies and minds.

Dr. Price's extensive scientific documentation from five continents proves that only a diet composed of whole, mineral-rich foods, including sufficient fat-soluble activators found exclusively in animal fats, can provide continuing generations of parents and children with perfect teeth and bone structure and freedom from degenerative diseases, as well as the achievement of the highest spiritual ideals that accompanies absence of mental illness, emotional problems and criminality.

Price-Pottenger provides both health professionals and the public with information on such diverse topics as traditional whole foods and their preparation, soil improvement, natural farming, pure water, nontoxic dentistry and holistic therapies in order to conquer disease and prevent birth defects, thus enabling people to achieve excellent health and long life into future centuries.

Members of Price-Pottenger receive a quarterly health journal containing articles by leading nutritional writers and researchers, as well as information about therapies based on dietary, environmental and ecological principles. Price-Pottenger also provides a healthcare professional members' list and a catalog of well-chosen books.

Membership fees and donations help Price-Pottenger maintain its precious archives and library, which house the extensive files, notes, and photographs of Dr. Price and Dr. Pottenger, along with those of Dr. Royal Lee, vitamin researcher; Dr. Melvin Page, specialist in the relationship of the endocrine system, diet and disease; Dr. Emanuel Cheraskin, renowned nutrition researcher; Dr. William Albrecht, famous soils specialist; and practicing physicians Dr. John Myers and Dr. Henry Beiler, both known for their successes in treating chronic fatigue and degenerative illness, as well as many others.

510

Through access to its archived materials, its quarterly journal, and its booklist of reprints and modern publications, Price-Pottenger serves as a trustworthy source of accurate information on the principles of good nutrition and on the biological cycle of which man is a part.

Nontoxic farming and the nontoxic home are natural adjuncts to obtaining optimum health and happiness. Information on natural therapies for man and soil are among the many topics covered in the collections.

Future generations of healthy robust children and the conquest of infectious and degenerative disease can only be accomplished by a public that is well informed. Price-Pottenger's services are designed to provide practical, accurate and educational information on nutrition, food preparation, nontoxic dentistry, holistic therapies, soil enrichment, natural animal husbandry and environmental enhancement. The future depends on your financial support of Price-Pottenger.

Please write or call Price-Pottenger for membership information and your free catalog.

Price-Pottenger
7890 Broadway
Lemon Grove, CA 91945
www.price-pottenger.org
info@price-pottenger.org

Price-Pottenger is a 501(c)(3) nonprofit, tax-exempt organization. Membership donations and general donations are fully tax deductible.

INDEX

Other Works Available By
Weston A. Price, DDS

Dental Infections, Oral and Systemic & Dental Infections and the Degenerative Diseases,
Volumes 1 & 2
1174 pages, 2 volumes in 4 parts...$150.00
PPNF member price $135.00

Dr. Price's Search for Health
This tape surveys the research of Weston A. Price, DDS, and reveals the effect of diet on
native peoples around the world, showing that dental cavities, misalignment of teeth, increased susceptibility to disease & physical & mental degeneration are largely attributed
to modern processed foods, and that optimal health starts with sound nutrition.
DVD $35.00
PPNF member price $31.50

The Price-Pottenger Story on DVD
Morley Video Productions, Licensed to Price-Pottenger Nutrition Foundation
For the first time in our history, the story of PPNF as well as the story of Drs. Price
and Pottenger's research is available on one DVD
1 hr. 25 min $25.00
PPNF member price $20.00

Dr. Price's Original 7 Teaching Lessons
The lessons include over 350 photos and Dr. Price's original text written for each photo.
7 CD Set on Power Point...$350.00
PPNF member price $300.00

Weston A. Price, DDS Bibliography is available at www.ppnf.org

Based on the Works and Research of Weston A. Price, DDS

Root Canal Cover Up
George E. Meinig, DDS, FACD
Learn how hidden bacteria in teeth cause side effects that can endanger your life.
Discover how germs trapped in teeth and tonsils mutate and metastasize like cancer
cells and how these bacteria migrate to heart, kidneys, eyes, brain, arthritic joints and
countless other body tissues. Learn how Dr. Meinig discovered that a meticulous
25-year research program, conducted by Weston A. Price, DDS, under the auspices of
the American Dental Association's Research Institute, was buried by disbelievers of the
focal infection theory.
227 pages $19.95
PPNF member price $17.95

To Order:
1-800-366-3748 (U.S. only)
619-462-7600
www.ppnf.org

ALL PRICES SUBJECT TO CHANGE WITHOUT NOTICE

Become a Member

Join Price-Pottenger, an educational nonprofit committed to keeping you healthy. Prevent cancer, heart disease, diabetes, and the other degenerative conditions that threaten your well-being.

Visit **price-pottenger.org** to access the many exclusive benefits available to our members and health professionals. Sign up for a *free one-month trial membership* and explore topics such as Nutrition, Recipes and Food Preparation, Natural Medicine, Vitamins and Minerals, Dental Health, Fertility and Prenatal Nutrition, Antiaging, Detoxification, Mental Health, and more.

Become part of the community that has discovered the power of traditional foods and the rewards that come from a truly healthy lifestyle. Reclaim your health and join the organization that, for over 60 years, has been helping people feel better, live better, and live longer. ***Sign up today!***

**www.price-pottenger.org • info@price-pottenger.org •
1-800-366-3748 (U.S. only) • 619-462-7600**

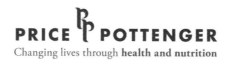

PRICE P POTTENGER
Changing lives through **health and nutrition**

Price-Pottenger is a 501(c)(3) nonprofit. All membership dues are fully tax-deductible.

Dr. Price's Search for Health DVD

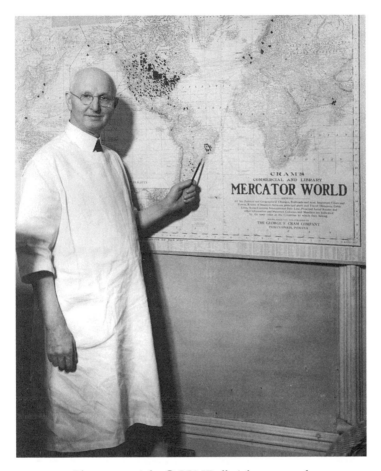

A survey of the research of Dr. Weston A. Price, DDS, revealing the effect of diet on native peoples around the world. Vividly shows that dental cavities, misalignment of teeth, increased susceptibility to disease, and physical and mental degeneration are largely attributed to the use of modern processed foods, and that optimal health starts with sound nutrition from whole foods from both vegetable and animal sources, eaten fresh or prepared with methods that do not remove essential fats, vitamins and minerals.

DVD 25.30 Minutes
$35.00
$31.50 Member Price
Wholesale Discounts Available

ALL PRICES SUBJECT TO CHANGE WITHOUT NOTICE

Dental Infections, Oral and Systemic & Dental Infections and The Degenerative Diseases, Vol 1&2

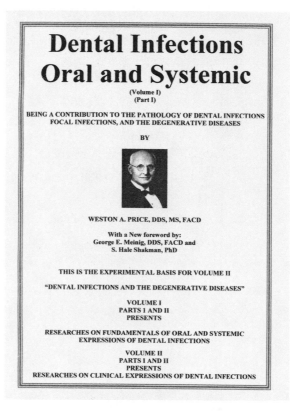

Weston A. Price, DDS, conducted a 25 year project under the auspices of the American Dental Association's Research Institute, on the subject of infected teeth and how they cause disease. This is Dr. Price's complete research report:

Volume 1: A contribution to the pathology of dental infections, focal infections and the degenerative diseases (experimental basis).

Includes 262 illustrations with 8 color illustrations and 261 charts

Volume 2: Researches on clinical expressions of dental infections.

Includes 6 color illustrations

Weston A. Price, DDS
1174 pages, 2 volumes in four parts steel spine bound by PPNF
$150.00
$135.00 Member Price

ALL PRICES SUBJECT TO CHANGE WITHOUT NOTICE

Root Canal Cover-Up

ROOT CANAL
COVER-UP

A Founder of the Association of
Root Canal Specialists
Discovers Evidence That
Root Canals Damage Your Health
Learn What to Do

GEORGE E. MEINIG
D.D.S., F.A.C.D.

Root Canal Cover-Up shows how hidden bacteria in teeth cause side effects that can endanger your life. Discover how germs trapped in teeth and tonsils mutate and metastasize like cancer cells and how these bacteria migrate to heart, kidney, eye, brain, arthritic joints and countless other parts of the body. Learn how Dr. Meinig discovered that a meticulous 25 year research project conducted by Weston A. Price, DDS, under the auspices of the American Dental Association's Research Institute, was buried by disbelievers of the focal infection theory.

George E. Meinig, DDS, FACD
227 Pages, softcover
$19.95
$17.95 Member Price
Wholesale Discounts Available

ALL PRICES SUBJECT TO CHANGE WITHOUT NOTICE

Pottenger's Cats: A Study in Nutrition

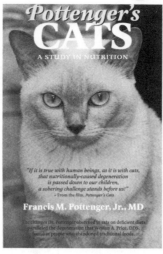

Dr. Francis M. Pottenger, Jr., MD, was an original thinker and keen observer whose imagination, integrity and common sense gave him the courage to question official dogma. Dedicated to the cause of preventing chronic illness, he made significant contributions to the understanding of the role of nutrition in maintaining good health.

In his classical experiments in cat feeding, more than 900 cats were studied over 10 years. Dr. Pottenger found that only diets containing raw milk and raw meat produced optimal health: good bone structure and density, wide palates with plenty of space for teeth, shiny fur, no parasites or disease, reproductive ease and a gentle temperament.

Cooking the meat or substituting heat-processed milk for raw milk resulted in heterogeneous reproduction and physical degeneration, increasing with each generation. Vermin and parasites abounded. Skin diseases and allergies increased from 5% to over 90%. Bones became soft and pliable. Cats suffered from adverse personality changes, hypothyroidism and most of the degenerative diseases encountered in human medicine. They died out completely by the fourth generation.

The changes Pottenger observed in cats on the deficient diets paralleled the human degeneration that Dr. Price found in tribes that had abandoned their traditional diets of whole, unprocessed foods.

Francis M. Pottenger, Jr., MD
123 pages, softcover
$9.95
$8.95 Member Price
Wholesale Discounts Available

ALL PRICES SUBJECT TO CHANGE WITHOUT NOTICE

The Pottenger Cat Studies DVD

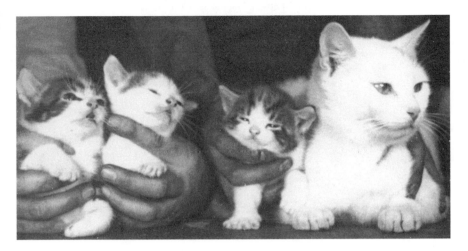

Raw Food Cat and Kittens
Photo copyright © PPNF, all rights reserved

A survey of the famous 10-year nutrition study conducted by Francis M. Pottenger, Jr., MD, on more than 900 cats. The research documents how a diet of cooked meat and pasteurized milk led to progressive degeneration of the animals.

Comparison of healthy cats fed raw foods with those on heated foods is made, with mention of parallel findings among humans in Dr. Weston A. Price's worldwide studies. Behavioral characteristics, arthritis, sterility, skeletal deformities and allergies are some of the problems the cats experienced that were associated with the consumption of a diet consisting entirely of cooked foods.

DVD 28.30 Minutes
$30.00
$27.00 Member Price
Wholesale Discounts Available

ALL PRICES SUBJECT TO CHANGE WITHOUT NOTICE

The Price-Pottenger Story DVD

Morley Video Productions, Licensed to Price-Pottenger Nutrition Foundation

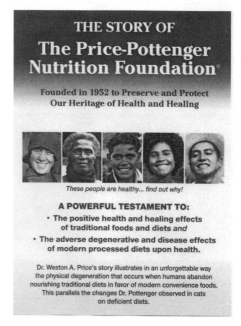

The story of PPNF as well as that of Drs. Price and Pottenger's research is now available on one DVD. In three parts, Janet and Don Morley have created a wonderful gift to Price-Pottenger by presenting this valuable information.

Part 1 - The Price / Pottenger Studies

        This section is a synopsis of the works of Dr. Weston A. Price, DDS and Dr. Francis M. Pottenger, Jr., MD. The stories of Dr. Price's and Dr. Pottenger's studies are intermixed with modern relevance that shows that the findings from their research of many years ago are still relevant today.

Part 2 - The Foundation: The Story of The Price-Pottenger Nutrition Foundation

        The history of the foundation from staff interviews from our beginning to where we are today and where we are going in the future.

Part 3 – Staff Interviews

        The complete interviews that are partially used throughout the entire DVD.

DVD 1 hour and 25 minutes
$25.00
$20.00 Member Price
Wholesale Discounts Available

ALL PRICES SUBJECT TO CHANGE WITHOUT NOTICE

Share the Knowledge and SAVE!

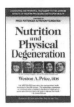 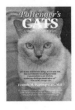 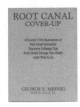

The most important books on health and nutrition ever written!

*"**Dr. Weston Price** was one of the most prominent health researchers of the 20th century.... This extraordinary masterpiece of nutritional science belongs in the library of anyone who is serious about learning how to use foods to improve their health."* — **Dr. Joseph Mercola**

*The changes **Dr. Pottenger** observed in cats on deficient diets paralleled the degeneration that Weston A. Price, DDS, found in people who abandoned traditional foods. "If it is true with human beings, as it is with cats, that nutritionally-caused degeneration is passed down to our children, a sobering challenge stands before us!"* — **From the film,** *Pottenger's Cats*

Root Canal Cover-Up: The Founder of the Association of Root Canal Specialists Discovers Evidence That Root Canals Damage Your Health. Learn What to Do.
- By George E. Meinig, DDS, FACD

The <u>PERFECT GIFT</u> for family or friends.

<u>ESSENTIAL INFORMATION</u> for both patients and healthcare practitioners.

NEW Discount Rates!
When you purchase in quantity to help disseminate this important work.

<u>*Pottenger's Cats: $9.95*</u> (64 books per case)
10-19 books . . . . .35% off
20-39 books . . . . .45% off
One or more cases (40+) . . . . .50% off

<u>*Nutrition and Physical Degeneration: $27.95*</u> (20 per case)
10-19 books . . . . .30% off
One case (20-39). . . . . .40% off
Two or more cases (40+) . . . . .50% off

<u>*Root Canal Cover-Up: $19.95*</u> (18 per case)
10-18 books . . . . .30% off
19-36 books . . . . .40% off
37+ (2 or more cases) . . . . .50% off

All prices subject to change without notice.